T0213331

Immunoepidemiology

Peter J. Krause
Paula B. Kavathas
Nancy H. Ruddle

Editors

Immunoepidemiology

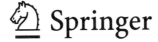 Springer

Editors
Peter J. Krause
Department of Epidemiology of Microbial Diseases
Yale School of Public Health and Departments of Medicine and Pediatrics
Yale School of Medicine
New Haven, CT, USA

Paula B. Kavathas
Departments of Laboratory Medicine and Immunobiology
Yale School of Medicine
New Haven, CT, USA

Nancy H. Ruddle
Department of Epidemiology of Microbial Diseases
Yale School of Public Health
New Haven, CT, USA

ISBN 978-3-030-25555-8   ISBN 978-3-030-25553-4   (eBook)
https://doi.org/10.1007/978-3-030-25553-4

Cover design: © Krause, Kavathas, and Ruddle 2020

This Springer imprint is published by the registered company Springer Nature Switzerland AG
The registered company address is: Gewerbestrasse 11, 6330 Cham, Switzerland

We dedicate this book to our families and students

Preface

This textbook focuses on the nascent field of immunoepidemiology that addresses how differences in immune responses among individuals affect the epidemiology of infectious diseases, cancer, hypersensitivity, and autoimmunity. The idea for the book originated from a course entitled "Immunology for Epidemiologists" at the Yale School of Public Health that was required for MPH students in the Epidemiology of Microbial Diseases Department. While many fine textbooks are available that address the immunological responses of *individuals* to pathogens, these provided very little information regarding how immunological variation among *populations* affects the epidemiology of disease. And yet, it has long been recognized that there is great immunologic diversity among people, which can have a profound effect on the epidemiology of disease. Careful review of the immunologic and epidemiologic literature revealed that there have been relatively few publications concerning immunoepidemiology and that no textbook is available on the subject. This textbook, therefore, aims to fill this void by providing a much-needed tool to comprehensively and efficiently teach immunoepidemiology.

The emphasis of the book, as in the course that inspired it, is on infectious diseases, autoimmunity, and cancer. We recognize that many of the same immune principles can be applied to chronic diseases that are not covered here. The roles of acute and chronic inflammation are becoming ever more recognized in cardiovascular, metabolic, and neurologic diseases.

The book includes a section on the basic principles of immunology and then applies them to particular examples of disease in human populations. The primary target audience for this textbook is Masters of Public Health students. Others who should also find it of interest include PhD students in epidemiology and immunology, medical students, generalists, and specialists in immunology, infectious diseases, cancer, and rheumatology.

New Haven, CT, USA

Peter J. Krause
Paula B. Kavathas
Nancy H. Ruddle

Acknowledgments

We thank the following individuals for their excellent illustrations: Yexin Yang (major illustrator), Trisha P. Gupte, Jennifer Yoon, Francesica Tizard, and Wendolyn Hill. We thank Francesica Tizard for her administrative help. We thank our Yale colleagues for their continual scientific input, particularly Najla Arshad, João Pereria, Peter Cresswell, Marie Landry, Michel Ledizet and Kenneth Kidd. We thank the Gordon and Llura Gund Foundation for their support (PJK).

Contents

Section IV   IMMUNOEPIDEMIOLOGY OF INFECTIOUS DISEASES AND CANCER

Contributors

Marwan M. Azar Department of Medicine (Infectious Diseases), Yale University School of Medicine, New Haven, CT, USA

Amy K. Bei Department of Epidemiology of Microbial Diseases, Yale School of Public Health, New Haven, CT, USA

Richard J. Bucala Departments of Medicine (Rheumatology), Pathology, and Epidemiology, Yale School of Medicine, New Haven, CT, USA

Kara Fikrig Department of Epidemiology of Microbial Diseases, Yale School of Public Health, New Haven, CT, USA

Paula B. Kavathas Departments of Laboratory Medicine and Immunobiology, Yale School of Medicine, New Haven, CT, USA

Peter J. Krause Department of Epidemiology of Microbial Diseases, Yale School of Public Health and Departments of Medicine and Pediatrics, Yale School of Medicine, New Haven, CT, USA

Xiaomei Ma Department of Chronic Disease Epidemiology, Yale School of Public Health, New Haven, CT, USA

Diane McMahon-Pratt Department of Epidemiology of Microbial Diseases, Yale School of Public Health, New Haven, CT, USA

Eric Meffre Departments of Immunobiology and Internal Medicine, Yale University School of Medicine, New Haven, CT, USA

Linda M. Niccolai Department of Epidemiology of Microbial Diseases, Yale School of Public Health, New Haven, CT, USA

Kate Nyhan Harvey Cushing/John Hay Whitney Medical Library, Yale University, New Haven, CT, USA

Jane O'Bryan Department of Epidemiology of Microbial Diseases, Yale School of Public Health, New Haven, CT, USA

Camila D. Odio Department of Internal Medicine, Yale School of Medicine, New Haven, CT, USA

Elijah Paintsil Departments of Pediatrics, Pharmacology, and Epidemiology of Microbial Diseases, Yale School of Medicine and Yale School of Public Health, New Haven, CT, USA

Sunil Parikh Department of Epidemiology of Microbial Diseases, Yale School of Public Health, New Haven, CT, USA

Nancy H. Ruddle Department of Epidemiology of Microbial Diseases, Yale School of Public Health, New Haven, CT, USA

Laura A. Skrip Department of Epidemiology of Microbial Disease, Yale School of Public Health, New Haven, CT, USA

Jeffrey P. Townsend Department of Biostatistics, Yale School of Public Health, Yale University, New Haven, CT, USA

Rong Wang Department of Chronic Disease Epidemiology, Yale School of Public Health, New Haven, CT, USA

Abbreviations

$\beta_2 M$	β_2-Microglobulin
ABPA	Allergic bronchopulmonary aspergillosis
ADA	Adenosine deaminase
ADCC	Antibody-dependent cellular cytotoxicity
ADCI	Antibody-mediated cellular inhibition
ADRB	Antibody-dependent respiratory burst
AIDS	Acquired immunodeficiency syndrome
AIRE	Autoimmune regulator
ALL	Acute lymphoblastic leukemia
ALPS	Autoimmune lymphoproliferative syndrome
Als3p	Agglutinin-like sequence 3 protein
Alum	$KAl(SO_4)_2 \cdot 12H_2O$
AMA-1	Apical membrane antigen-1
AMD	Adult onset macular degeneration
AML	Acute myeloid leukemia
APC	Antigen-presenting cell
APCED	Autoimmune polyendocrinopathy-candidiasis-ectodermal dystrophy
APO BEC3	Apolipoprotein B mRNA editing enzyme catalytic polypeptide-like 3
APS-1	Autoimmune polyendocrine syndrome type 1
ART	Antiretroviral therapy
ASC	Apoptosis-associated speck-like protein containing CARD
BALT	Bronchial-associated lymphoid tissue
BCG	Bacillus Calmette-Guérin
BCR	B-cell receptor
BMI	Body mass index
BTK	Bruton tyrosine kinase
CAR	Chimeric antigen receptor
CCL	CC ligand
CCR5	C-C motif receptor 5 gene
CCR5Δ32	A 32-base pair deletion within the coding region of CCR5
CD	Cluster of differentiation
CD	Crohn's disease
cDC	Conventional dendritic cell
CDC	US Center for Disease Control and Prevention
CDR	Complementarity determining region

CGA	Candidate gene analysis
cGAMP	Cyclic GMP-AMP
CGD	Chronic granulomatous disease
CHMI	Controlled human malaria infection
CLP	Common lymphoid progenitor
CLR	C-type lectin receptor
CMC	Chronic mucocutaneous candidiasis
CMP	Common myeloid precursor
CMV	Cytomegalovirus
CoP	Correlate of protection
CpG	Cytosine phosphate guanine dinucleotide
CSA	Chondroitinsulfate A
C-section	Cesarean section
CSP	Circumsporozoite protein
CSR	Class switch recombination
cTEC	Cortical thymic epithelial cell
CTL	Cytotoxic T-lymphocyte
CTLA-4	Cytotoxic T-lymphocyte-associated protein 4
CVID	Common variable immunodeficiency disease
CXCL	CXC ligand
DAMP	Danger-associated molecular pattern
DC	Dendritic cell
DMARDS	Disease modifying antirheumatic drugs
dMN	Dissolvable microneedles
EBV	Epstein-Barr virus
ER	Endoplasmic reticulum
ERAP1	Endoplasmic reticulum aminopeptidase 1
ERBB2	Human epidermal growth factor receptor 2
ESN	Exposed seronegative
Fab	Fragment antigen-binding
Fc	Fragment crystallizable
FDA	Food and Drug Administration
FDC	Follicular dendritic cell
FDEIA	Food-dependent exercise-induced allergy
FHF	Familial Hibernian fever
FKS	Formalin-killed spherule
FMF	Familial Mediterranean fever
G6PD	Glucose-6-phosphate dehydrogenase
GAFFI	Global Action Fund for Fungal Infections
GALT	Gut-associated lymphoid tissue
GAP	Genetically attenuated parasite
GC	Germinal center
GI	Gastrointestinal tract
GIA	Growth inhibition assay
GLA	Glucopyranosyl lipid A
GM-CSF	Granulocyte monocyte colony stimulating factor
GWAS	Genome-wide association study
HAART	Highly active antiretroviral therapy

HbS	Sickling hemoglobin
HCT	Hematopoietic cell transplantation
HCV	Hepatitis C virus
HIGM	Hyper IgM syndrome
HLA	Human leukocyte antigen
HLH	Hemophagocytic lymphohistiocytosis
HMGB1	High-mobility group protein B1
HPV	Human papillomavirus
HSC	Hematopoietic stem cell
HSV	Herpes simplex virus
IBD	Inflammatory bowel disease
ICI	Immune checkpoint inhibitor
ICOS	Inducible T-cell costimulatory
IFN	Interferon
Ig	Immunoglobulin
ILC	Innate lymphoid cell
IMGT	International ImMunoGeneTics
iNKT	Invariant NKT cell
IPD	Immuno Polymorphism Database
IPEX	Immune dysregulation, polyendocrinopathy, enteropathy, X-linked
IRF3	Interferon response factor 3
IRIS	Immune reconstitution inflammatory syndrome
ISG	IFN-stimulated gene
ITAM	Immunoreceptor tyrosine-based activation motif
iTreg	Induced T regulatory cell
IVIg	Intravenous immunoglobulin
JAK	Janus kinase
KIR	Killer immunoglobulin-like receptor
LT	Lymphotoxin
LTNP	Long-term nonprogressor
LYST	Lysosomal trafficking regulator
M cell	Microfold cell
mAb	Monoclonal antibody
MALT	Mucosal-associated lymphoid tissue
MBL	Mannose binding lectin
mCoP	Mechanistic correlate of protection
MDR-TB	Multidrug-resistant tuberculosis
MEP	Megakaryocyte/erythroid progenitor
MetEnk	Methionine-enkephalin peptide
MHC	Major histocompatibility complex
MIF	Macrophage migration inhibitory factor
MIP	Macrophage inflammatory protein
MoDC	Monocyte-derived dendritic cell
MPL	3-O-desacyl-40-monophosphoryl lipid A
MPP	Multipotent progenitor
MS	Multiple sclerosis
MSP1	Merozoite surface protein 1

MSP2	Merozoite surface protein 2
MSP3	Merozoite surface protein 3
MTB	*Mycobacterium tuberculosis*
MTCT	Mother-to-child transmission
NAb	Neutralizing antibody
NALT	Nasal-associated lymphoid tissue
nCoP	Nonmechanistic correlate of protection
NCR	Natural cytotoxicity receptor
NEMO	Nuclear factor-κB essential modulator
NET	Neutrophil extracellular trap
NK cell	Natural killer cell
NLR	Nod-like receptor
NOS2A	Nitic oxide synthase 2A
NSAIDS	Nonsteroidal anti-inflammatory drugs
nTreg	Natural T regulatory cell
OR	Odds ratio
PACTG	Pediatric AIDS Clinical Trials Group
PAMP	Pathogen-associated molecular pattern
PD-1	Programmed death-1
pDC	Plasmacytoid dendritic cell
PDL-1	Programmed death-1 ligand-1
PfRH5	*Plasmodium falciparum* reticulocyte-binding protein homolog
PfSEA	*Plasmodium falciparum* schizont egress antigen
PGA	Poly(glutamic acid)
PID	Primary immunodeficiency disease
PLA	Poly(lactic acid)
PLC	Peptide loading complex
PLGA	D,L-lactide-co-glycolide
PML	Progressive multifocal leukoencephalopathy
PMN	Polymorphonuclear leukocyte
PMTCT	Promotion of prevention of MTCT
pNP	Polymeric nanoparticles
PROS1	Vitamin K-dependent plasma glycoprotein
PRR	Pattern recognition receptors
PtdSer	Phosphatidylserine
PTPN22	Lymphoid protein tyrosine phosphatase non-receptor type 22
PvDBP	*Plasmodium vivax* Duffy-binding protein
PVSRIPO	Polio-rhinovirus chimera
QS	*Quillaja saponaria*
R_0	R naught
RA	Rheumatoid arthritis
RAG	Recombination-activating gene
RANTES	Regulated upon activation normal T-cell expressed and secreted
RAS	Radiation-attenuated sporozoites
RESA	Ring-infected erythrocyte surface antigen
RFLP	Restriction fragment length polymorphism

RLR	Retinoic acid-inducible gene-1-like receptor
RRMS	Relapsing-remitting multiple sclerosis
RSV	Respiratory syncytial virus
RTK	Receptor tyrosine kinase
S1P	Sphingosine-1-phosphate
SAP	Signaling lymphocytic activation molecule/SLAM-associated protein
SCID	Severe combined immunodeficiency
SHM	Somatic hypermutation
SIP$_1$	SIP receptor
SIV	Simian immunodeficiency virus
SIVcpz	Immunodeficiency viruses infecting chimpanzees
SIVsmm	Immunodeficiency viruses infecting mangabeys
SLA	Second-generation lipid adjuvant
SLE	Systemic lupus erythematosus
SMFA	Standard membrane feeding assays
SNP	Single-nucleotide polymorphism
SS	Sjögren's syndrome
STAT1	Signal transducer and activator of transcription 1
STING	Stimulator of interferon gene
T1D	Type 1 diabetes
TAP	Transporter associated with antigen processing
TB	Tuberculosis
Tcm	Central memory T cell
TCR	T-cell receptor
TCR$\gamma\delta$ T cell	Gamma delta T-cell receptor
TdT	Terminal deoxynucleotidyl transferase
Tem	Effector memory T cell
Temra	Terminally differentiated effector memory cell
Tfh	T follicular helper cell
TGF	Transforming growth factor
TLR	Toll-like receptor
TNF	Tumor necrosis factor
Tpm	Peripheral memory T cell
TRA	Tissue-restricted antigen
TREC	T-cell receptor excision circles
Treg	Regulatory T cell
TRIM5α	Tripartite motif 5α protein
Trm	Tissue resident memory T cell
Tscm	Stem cell T memory cell
UDG	Uracil-DNA glycosylase
uNK	Uterine NK cells
WAS	Wiskott-Aldrich syndrome
WHO	World Health Organization
XLP	x-linked lymphoproliferative disease
ZFN	Zinc Finger Nuclease

Section I

INTRODUCTION

Introduction to Immunology, Epidemiology, and Immunoepidemiology

Linda M. Niccolai, Nancy H. Ruddle, and Peter J. Krause

1.1 Introduction

Immunology has traditionally focused on the immune system in the individual. Epidemiology focuses on populations. Advances in our knowledge of the interaction between the fields of epidemiology and immunology together form the new discipline of immunoepidemiology, the subject of this book. Here, we review key concepts of the two well-described fields and how their synthesis has created the new field of immunoepidemiology.

1.2 Immunology

1.2.1 Definition

Immunology is the study of that combination of cells and substances that protect multicellular organisms against foreign entities. All multicellular organisms survive in a world filled with microbes. In some cases the relationship is symbiotic, but in others the microbes cause pathogenic changes. To protect themselves from pathogens, multicellular organisms possess a variety of responses that together constitute the immune system. Teleologically, the immune system is thought of as a defense mechanism against microbial pathogens; in fact any protein, nucleic acid, or carbohydrate that is recognized as foreign has the potential to stimulate an immune response, such as pollen or a kidney transplant. Substances that elicit immune responses are known as *antigens*. The immune system plays

L. M. Niccolai
Department of Epidemiology of Microbial Diseases, Yale School of Public Health, New Haven, CT, USA
e-mail: linda.niccolai@yale.edu

N. H. Ruddle
Department of Epidemiology of Microbial Diseases, Yale School of Public Health, New Haven, CT, USA
e-mail: nancy.ruddle@yale.edu

P. J. Krause (✉)
Department of Epidemiology of Microbial Diseases, Yale School of Public Health and Departments of Medicine and Pediatrics, Yale School of Medicine, New Haven, CT, USA
e-mail: peter.krause@yale.edu

© Springer Nature Switzerland AG 2019
P. J. Krause et al. (eds.), *Immunoepidemiology*, https://doi.org/10.1007/978-3-030-25553-4_1

Table 1.1 The immune system is classically organized into innate and adaptive systems that work together in a coordinated response

Immune factor	Time of action	Type of action
Innate immunity		
Epidermis/mucosal surfaces	Immediate	Physical barrier
Macrophage	Minutes to hours	Phagocytosis and cytokine release
Dendritic cell	Minutes to hours	Phagocytosis and antigen presentation to lymphocytes
Neutrophil	Minutes to hours	Phagocytosis and cytokine release
Natural killer cell	Minutes to hours	Intracellular killing and cytokine release
Complement	Minutes to hours	Microbial killing and inflammation
Adaptive immunity		
B lymphocytes	Days	Antibody production and antigen presentation
T helper lymphocytes	Days	Cytokine release and cellular activation
T cytotoxic lymphocytes	Days	Intracellular killing and cytokine release

an important defensive role against microbial pathogens, parasites, and tumors. However, when immune dysfunction occurs, the system can target self tissue and cause autoimmune disease or an inappropriate response to foreign antigen and cause allergy. The system is beautifully set up to respond to a foreign substance, to eliminate it, and then to return to a baseline state. In some cases, the regulatory systems that govern the return to baseline are defective, resulting in chronic tissue damage.

The immune system is classically organized into *innate* and *adaptive* systems that work together in a coordinated fashion (Table 1.1). The innate system is present in all multicellular organisms, whereas the adaptive system is only present in jawed vertebrates. Immune cell populations of both innate and adaptive immune systems respond in diverse ways. Cells of the innate system include natural killer (NK) cells, monocytes, macrophages, and polymorphonuclear leukocytes, whereas the adaptive lymphoid system includes thymus-derived (T) and bone marrow–derived (B) lymphocytes and antigen-presenting cells. More recently, a class of cells called innate lymphoid cells have been described that possess some features of both the innate and adaptive systems. Cells of the immune system are found in the bone marrow, bloodstream, lymphatic vessels, lymphoid organs, and fixed tissues. Circulating immune cells are called leukocytes (white blood cells that distinguish them from red blood cells). The cells of the immune system are either derived from and/or are organized within specialized primary lymphoid organs such as the bone marrow and thymus or within secondary lymphoid organs that include tonsils, adenoids, lymph nodes, spleen, and Peyer's patches. They also may be found in organized but isolated lymphoid accumulations, particularly in the large intestine or in nonlymphoid tissues.

1.2.2 History

Historically, immunity was originally considered as humoral or cellular. This designation was based on the nature of the mediators that conferred defense. *Humoral immunity* is defined as protection from infection that can be transferred from one individual to another by means of serum, the acellular component of blood. This so-called called serum therapy was described by Emil Behring in 1891. We now know from the work of many scientists, including that of Paul Ehrlich in the late 1800s, that the serum constituents are antibodies, proteins that recognize foreign entities (antigens). *Cellular immunity* is defined as the ability of cells to provide defense, including transfer of immune reactivity from an immunized to a naïve individual. The terms "humoral" and "cellular" immunity are oversimplifications, however, because "humoral" antibodies are made by cells and antibodies can enhance cellular activity. The immune system also can be classified by its innate and adaptive components. Cells of the innate system recognize molecular structures that are common to various classes of pathogens, while those of adaptive system are more restricted and specific, each cell recognizing a unique part of the pathogen they target. The innate system provides immediate defense against pathogens, while the adaptive system requires days to become fully effective and coordinate with the adaptive immune system.

The most widely cited early innate immune system discovery was that of Ilya Ilyich Metchnikoff, who in the late 1880s discovered two types of white blood cells with the ability to engulf substances, including bacteria [1]. This was the first observation that once a microbe breached physical and chemical barriers, cells were involved in its elimination. These cells called *phagocytes* (Greek derivation: *phago* – eating; *cytes* – cells) express pattern recognition receptors, first postulated by Charles Janeway and described with his colleague Ruslan Medzhitov [2]. These receptors are located on the surface and some interior structures of immune cells and recognize microbial antigens. Bruce Beutler [3] and Jules Hoffman [4] are recognized for their characterization of these receptors and the roles these receptors play in recognizing pathogens. Once pathogens are recognized by these receptors, the cell is activated to ingest and kill the pathogen and to produce small molecular signal molecules called *cytokines* to activate other innate immune cells and alter body physiology to combat additional invading microbes [5].

As noted above, the adaptive immune system includes both cellular and humoral immune mechanisms. In contrast to the innate immune system, the adaptive system exhibits immunological memory, which is defined as the ability to mount a more robust (recall) response to a previously encountered antigen. This provides an evolutionary advantage, particularly to long-lived species such as humans who may encounter a pathogen multiple times. Immunological memory is the basis of vaccination whereby an individual is immunized with foreign antigen from an inactivated or attenuated pathogen or component of a pathogen. Vaccination does not cause disease but generates memory T and B cells against the pathogen that mount a vigorous defense when the pathogen is subsequently encountered.

A crucial role of the immune system is distinguishing tissue that is part of the host (self tissue) from nonhost (nonself tissue) and the related concept of self-tolerance. Ray Owen noted that healthy cattle with a nonidentical twin had circulating red blood cells from their twins, indicating they were tolerant of cells from another individual [6]. Frank Macfarlane Burnet and Peter Medawar tested the concept of tolerance in the 1950s. Macfarlane Burnet's contribution was predominately theoretical [7], whereas Medawar's was experimental [8]. The latter is considered the "father of transplantation" for his observation that skin or tumor grafts were rejected by mice if the tissue was from a genetically disparate donor. He then showed that mice could become "tolerant" of cells from another strain if they were exposed originally to those cells during fetal life. The tolerance of cells derived from the original strain was demonstrated by skin graft acceptance, leading eventually to the field of organ transplantation. The synergy between the two approaches embodies what is most useful in the field of immunology – a brilliant theory (Janeway/Burnet) confirmed in an experimental animal model (Medzhitov/Medawar) resulting in enormous benefit to humans. Jean Dausset, Baruq Benacerraf, and George Snell carried out groundbreaking work that characterized the crucial genetic differences that govern acceptance or rejection of foreign antigens (reviewed in [9]). A set of genes within the chromosomal region called the major histocompatibility complex (MHC) were found to be essential for determining whether or not a tissue graft was rapidly rejected. Transplants between individuals identical for those genes were tolerated unless they differed at other genetic regions called minor histocompatibility genes, in which case the graft would slowly be rejected. The MHC system is described more fully in Chap. 4.

In addition to MHC proteins on the surfaces of host cells, all host cells express tissue-specific "self" antigens. Individuals are tolerant of both their own MHC antigens and their tissue-specific antigens. The term "horror autotoxicus" was coined by Paul Erhlich to describe situations in which an individual reacted to self-antigens [10]. This loss of tolerance to self-antigens gives rise to autoimmune diseases in which the host mistakenly perceives its self-antigens as foreign and reacts against the tissues expressing those antigens. Examples of autoimmune diseases (and the antigens they target) include Type I diabetes (pancreatic β cells), multiple sclerosis (myelin sheath surrounding nerves), rheumatoid arthritis (proteins in joint tissue), and systemic lupus erythematous (DNA and RNA).

A tremendous variety of antibodies in any particular serum differ by which antigens they recognize based on the infectious history of the individual. They also possess other characteristics that group them into five subclasses (IgM, IgD, IgG, IgE, and IgA). For decades, immunologists grappled with the difficulty of understanding a mechanism that could give rise to pathogen-specific antibodies against millions of different potential pathogens that the individual had never before encountered. It was even more perplexing once it was realized that there were only about 21,000 genes in the genome that encoded for all proteins that needed to include antibodies. Insight into this problem came from Porter and Edelman who elucidated the structure of antibody molecules and later from Susuma Tonegawa who demonstrated that antibodies are formed by gene segments that can undergo a vast array of rearrangements [11]. The rearrangement of immunoglobulin gene segments is restricted to B cells and depends on the activity of a particular class of enzymes, RAG-1 and RAG-2, discovered in David Baltimore's group by David Schatz and Marjorie Oettinger [12].

Cellular immunity was recognized as the transfer of immune reactivity from an immunized to an immunologically naïve individual by means of cells, rather than antibodies. These cells were found in the blood, lymph nodes, and spleen and eventually came to be called T cells due to their development in the thymus, as discovered in the 1960s by Jacques Miller [13]. Bruce Glick described the importance of the bursa of Fabricius for antibody production in the chicken. Max Cooper, working with Robert Good, was able to separate out the roles of the thymus and bursa and the definition of another cell type that arises in the chicken bursa (hence the name B cells) or in the bone marrow or in the fetal spleen in other animals [14]). Attempts to understand the mechanism by which T cells recognize antigen were complicated by the fact that they do not secrete their receptor like B cells. Rather, the T cell receptor for antigen is only cell associated. The T cell receptor for antigen was almost simultaneously discovered by John Kappler and Pippa Marrack, Tak Mak, and Mark Davis [15]. The similarities of the T cell receptor to the B cell receptor were important; however, it was unclear if and how the T cell receptor bound to both foreign antigen and MHC protein. The X-ray crystallographic identification of MHC protein complexed to a peptide by Pamela Bjorkman and Donald Wiley provided critical insight into the mechanism of T cell recognition [16]. The MHC protein is located on an antigen-presenting cell. Antigen-presenting cells ingest a pathogen, digest it, and present fragments of the pathogen on MHC surface proteins. The T cell receptor is somewhat homologous to the B cell receptor in its antigen-binding structure and its ability to distinguish self from nonself; however, because it is not secreted, it does not provide effector functions.

Secreted molecules called cytokines mediate the effector functions of T cells. Although these molecules lack antigen specificity, their effector functions are mediated by binding to cytokine receptors on their target cells. The biologic activities of T cells include destruction of virus-infected cells, prevention of viral infection of cells, helping B cells to produce antibody, activating macrophages, and many others. Secretion of cytokine molecules is not limited to T cells. The first cytokines, discovered by Lindemann and Isaacs, were called interferons because they inhibited viral replication [17]. John David and colleagues [18] and Barry Bloom and Boyce Bennett [19] described macrophage migration inhibitory factor (MIF), which is produced by T lymphocytes after binding antigen and which inhibits macrophage migration. This was followed by the discovery of a cytotoxic factor by Nancy Ruddle and Byron Waksman [20] that was called lymphotoxin by Maury Granger and his group [21]. After these discoveries, there was an explosion of studies demonstrating a vast array of biologic activities found in the supernatant fluid of cells that contained newly discovered cytokines. There was considerable confusion in the field until molecular techniques allowed cloning of cytokine and cytokine receptor genes and further functional characterization. We now have a more comprehensive understanding of cytokines and their functions. Certain cytokines, such as GM-CSF, are routinely used therapeutically to restore granulocytes in cancer patients, while cellular and cytokine inhibitors are used for treatment of autoimmune diseases.

1.2.3 Major Concepts

A key tenet of the field of immunology is that the immune system can distinguish self from nonself, as well as recognize and respond to "foreign" entities. We are said to be "tolerant" of our self-components and reactive against foreign components. A fully functional immune system is dependent on both innate and adaptive components that interact and lead to responses appropriate for a particular pathogen. The evolution of memory provides a mechanism to generate a rapid response to previously encountered pathogens.

One way to consider immune system function is to think of it as acting in stages. A pathogen stimulates the host to defend itself. Multiple immune components, including individual immune cells, are organized to respond to a stimulus through recognition, signaling, and an effector response. This occurs through the recognition of the stimulus at the cellular level by a receptor that sends a signal to the cell to let it know that a foreign entity is present. The cell responds by producing effector molecules that activate the rest of the immune system. We call the stimulus a *ligand* and the recognition and responding element a *receptor*. The *effector* response varies according to the nature of the cell (Fig. 1.1). The ligand can be an antigen, the receptor can be a B cell receptor, and the effector can be a secreted antibody We will see many examples of this ligand–receptor interaction throughout this book.

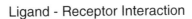

Ligand - Receptor Interaction

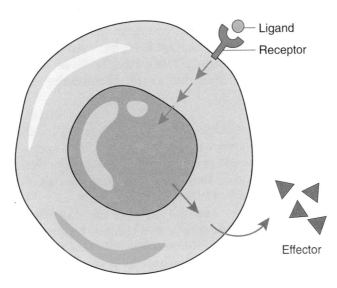

Fig. 1.1 Ligand–receptor interaction. A recurrent theme in immunology involves the interaction of a ligand with a receptor. This interaction occurs due to a recognition of a substance by a receptor. Once this occurs, a signal is transmitted from the receptor to the cell. This signal tells the cell to respond, which it does by releasing preformed molecules or synthesizing new ones. These molecules are called effector molecules. Examples of ligand–receptor interactions include antigen–B cell receptor and antibody synthesis and release, as well as antigen pattern recognition by Toll-like receptors and cytokine synthesis and release. (©Ruddle 2020)

1.3   Epidemiology

1.3.1   Definition

A common definition of epidemiology is the study of the occurrence, distribution, and determinants of health-related events, states, and processes in specified populations and the application of this knowledge to control relevant health problems [22]. A more concise definition for epidemiologic research is "the study of who gets sick and why at the population level."

1.3.2   History: Three Eras

1.3.2.1 The Beginning

The Greek physician Hippocrates may have been the first person to suggest that diseases were caused by behavioral and environmental factors rather than supernatural forces. In his published writings "On Airs, Waters, and Places" (circa 400 BCE) [23], he described how population health was likely affected by environmental factors such as climate and water quality:

"Whoever wishes to investigate medicine properly, should proceed thus: in the first place to consider the seasons of the year, and what effects each of them produces for they are not at all alike, but differ much from themselves in regard to their changes. Then the winds, the hot and the cold, especially such as are common to all countries, and then such as are peculiar to each locality. We must also consider the qualities of the waters, for as they differ from one another in taste and weight, so also do they differ much in their qualities. From these things he must proceed to investigate everything else. For if one knows all these things well … he will not be in doubt as to the treatment of the diseases."

He also provided examples of the health impacts of different climates. For example, he stated that in "a city that is exposed to hot winds … the heads of the inhabitants are of a humid and pituitous constitution, and their bellies subject to frequent disorders, owing to the phlegm running down from the head; the forms of their bodies, for the most part, are rather flabby…." He also described how water quality was important for health: "for water contributes much towards health. Such waters then as are marshy, stagnant … so that they are most apt to engender phlegm, and bring on hoarseness; those who drink them have large and obstructed spleens, their bellies are hard…" This attribution of health to behavioral and environmental factors was a novel concept during Hippocrates' time.

1.3.2.2 Early Modern Era

After Hippocrates, few (if any) epidemiologic advancements occurred for centuries. Then, beginning in the seventeenth century, individuals began to gather population-level data to identify patterns that could provide insight into causes of disease and death [24]. Perhaps one of the first to do this was John Graunt, a haberdasher and councilman in London, who published a landmark analysis of mortality data in 1662 titled, "Natural and Political Observations Mentioned in a Following Index and Made Upon the Bills of Mortality." Partly motivated by outbreaks of bubonic plague that afflicted the city, he used weekly counts of death to summarize and quantitatively describe patterns of disease occurrence. For example, he noted disparities between males and females, high infant mortality, and seasonal variation.

In the 1800s, William Farr engaged in similar work by systematically collecting and analyzing Britain's mortality and vital statistics. His work, published as a chapter "Vital Statistics" in 1837, sought to demonstrate that mortality was predictable and describable in mathematical terms. For example, one of his foci was on how marital status was associated with mortality, showing that married individuals had the longest life spans. Similar to Graunt, Farr contributed to the field of modern epidemiology by demonstrating how the systematic collection of individual-level data could be aggregated and summarized to describe associations at the population level to provide clues about determinants of health.

Fig. 1.2 Snow's map of the Broad Street pump area in London. Dr. John Snow mapped the locations of a cluster of 616 cholera deaths that occurred in London in 1854. Bars represent deaths that occurred in specific households. The map revealed that the majority of cases had proximity to a water pump on Broad Street. Further investigation of the drinking patterns of those who died revealed that a majority did in fact get their water from the Broad Street pump. This finding implicated a contaminated water supply rather than a "miasma" in the air that was the source of the outbreak: (*Source*: Courtesy of the Commonwealth Fund. In: Snow, J. *Snow on Cholera*. New York, NY; 1936).

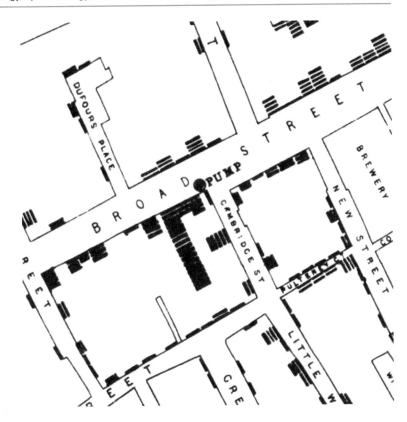

Working alongside Farr in London was John Snow, considered by many to be the father of modern epidemiology. He was a physician who practiced anesthesiology and studied the use of ether and chloroform gases [25]. He was also interested in cholera, as devastating epidemics had been occurring in London since the disease was first introduced in 1831. He is perhaps best known for the outbreak investigation he conducted in 1854. Snow had a hypothesis that cholera had a waterborne mode of transmission, in contrast to the prevailing belief that it was caused by "miasma" or something in the air. When a noticeable cluster of cholera deaths had occurred, Snow mapped their locations to reveal a pattern of proximity to a water pump on Broad Street (Fig. 1.2). Further investigation of the drinking patterns of those who died revealed that a majority did in fact get their water from the Broad Street pump. He also examined the drinking habits of populations who lived near the pump but were not affected by the epidemic and learned they often obtained water from other sources (e.g., workers at a nearby brewery drank their daily ration of malt liquor rather than water from the local pump). In this way, by comparing the drinking habits of groups of people (those who got cholera and those who did not), he was able to discern a pattern of disease that implicated the cause of the outbreak, water, obtained from the now famous Broad Street pump. Snow conducted other population-based studies to confirm that the source of cholera was contaminated drinking water. For example, in one study, he compared cholera mortality rates in neighborhoods of London that were served by different water companies. He found higher cholera mortality rates (nearly double) among persons living in areas served by Southwark and Vauxhall Waterworks Company that supplied its water from a contaminated part of the Thames River in contrast to residents of neighborhoods served by the Lambeth Waterworks Company that drew its water supply from a cleaner part of the river. In another study, he examined the mortality rates among households served by different water companies and observed a nearly tenfold increase in the death rate when households were served by Southwark and Vauxhall compared to Lambeth. Collectively, these population-level studies provided compelling evidence for the waterborne transmission of cholera. Though epidemiologic methods had not yet been formally described, Snow clearly demonstrated the use of population-based studies to identify risk factors for disease.

1.3.2.3 Contemporary Era

The twentieth century witnessed a prolific expansion of epidemiology education, writings, and methods that has continued to the present day. In the United States, the Welch–Rose Report of 1915 has been viewed as the basis for the critical movement in which the field of public health was recognized as distinct from medicine [26]. This resulted in the establishment of schools of public health supported by the Rockefeller Foundation. Some of the earliest programs were established at Tulane, Johns Hopkins, Columbia, Harvard, and Yale, all in place by the 1920s. Epidemiology textbooks began to be published in the 1930s. Into the twenty-first century, the depth and breadth of epidemiology have continued to advance by emerging technologies such as molecular diagnostics and statistical computing. Today, the field spans numerous topical areas such as infectious diseases, chronic illness, maternal health, and injuries. It uses a variety of approaches from molecular and genetic to social determinants. Emergent issues facing contemporary society such as climate change, emerging infections, bioterrorism, and gun violence can all be better understood and addressed through the application of epidemiologic methods. The common thread throughout this vast field and varied approaches is a focus on population health.

1.3.3 Major Concepts

Three major epidemiologic concepts relevant for immunoepidemiology are populations, causal inference, and basic reproduction number.

1.3.3.1 Populations

As described above, in both the definition and evolution of epidemiology, a key focus is on population health. Therefore, a key approach to studying the determinants (or risk factors) of health is achieved by comparing disease distributions between two or groups of people in a population. In its most simple form, the frequency of disease (outcome) is compared between two populations ("exposed" and "unexposed"), as depicted in the classic 2×2 table shown below (Table 1.2). Depending on the nature of the data collected, population-level measures of the frequency of disease may be prevalence, cumulative incidence, or incidence rates. For example, the prevalence of disease among those who are exposed to a particular risk factor may be calculated as $a/(a + b)$. Subsequently, by comparing measures of disease frequency between the groups in the population (exposed and unexposed), assessment of association can be made. For example, if the frequency of disease is higher among the exposed ($a/(a + b)$) than among the unexposed ($c/(c + d)$), then the relative measure of association (($a/(a + b)$)/($c/(c + d)$) would exceed the null value of 1, indicating a positive association between the exposure and the outcome, and one may conclude the exposure is possibly a risk factor. Again, the important tenet

Table 1.2 The "2×2" table in epidemiology

	Disease	No disease	Total
Exposed	a	b	$a + b$
Not exposed	c	d	$c + d$
Total	$a + c$	$b + d$	N

is that in epidemiologic research, disease frequencies are compared between groups of people in populations to learn about risk factors.

Key study designs used in epidemiologic research include cohort studies, randomized trials, case-control studies, and cross-sectional studies. Though their specific methods are distinct, they all share the fundamental approach of comparing disease frequencies in populations. For example, in a cohort study, a population of individuals who are classified as exposed or unexposed is followed over time for disease incidence which can then be compared as described above. Randomized trials are a special type of cohort study in which exposures are assigned by the investigators. In a case-control study, the comparison groups consist of those with and without disease, and the frequencies of previous exposures are compared. Cross-sectional studies are defined by the nature of data collection in that exposures and diseases are measured at the same point in time, but the fundamental comparisons between two (or more) groups in the population are the same as in the other designs. Thus, it can be seen in this very brief overview of measures of association and study design that all epidemiologic studies share the common feature of measuring the health of populations.

1.3.3.2 Causal Inference

Epidemiology is largely devoted to identifying causes of disease so that they can be prevented. While the goal of causal inference is likely intuitive to many people, what actually constitutes a "cause" has been, and continues to be, a matter of much discussion among scientists and philosophers. Much epidemiologic research has focused on examining associations between single exposures and single outcomes (e.g., smoking and lung cancer, a high-fat diet, and obesity). Methodological approaches have been developed to measure associations between these factors, with the goal of understanding which associations are likely to be actual risk factors or causal determinants of disease. It is now widely understood that most diseases have complex etiologies and that a multifactorial approach to understanding causes of disease is required. This is reflected in how approaches to causal inference have evolved over time with some illustrative examples presented in Table 1.3.

Most approaches that are invoked today are grounded in the earlier description of the web of causation that put forth the idea that causes of diseases result from multiple related factors. Important advancements have been made in the statistical approaches for modeling causal associations. For example, agent-based models, directed acyclic graphs, and marginal structural models are some of the sophisti-

Table 1.3 Examples of causal approaches in epidemiology

Henle–Koch postulates (1840) [27]	Focused on infectious agents and clinical diseases; a cause is one that satisfies the following three criteria: Organism occurs in all cases of disease Organism does not cause other diseases Organism can be isolated, grown, and induce disease in host
Web of causation (1960) [28]	Multicausal framework grounded in the belief that population patterns of health and disease can be explained by a complex web of numerous interconnected biological, behavioral, and social factors
Sir Austin Bradford Hill's guidelines (1965) [29]	Not a definition or model but rather a pragmatic approach of identifying causes using nine "criteria": Strength of association, consistency, specificity, temporality, gradient, plausibility, coherence, experiment, analogy
Sufficient-component causal model (1976) [30]	A sufficient cause of disease, in other words a complete causal mechanism, is a set of factors (components) that will inevitably produce disease. A given disease will have multiple causal mechanisms, and every causal mechanism involves the joint action of multiple components
Complex system approaches (2000s) [31]	Population health can be described by systems of interrelated factors (biological, behavioral, environmental, social) that are characterized by feedback loops (positive and negative), nonlinear relations, and emergent properties

cated approaches that are used today. It is clear that approaches to causal inference are increasingly complex and sophisticated but all are grounded in multilevel approaches that include both individual and population factors. These factors occur at multiple levels, including biologic/endogenous (e.g., genetic), individual/behavior (e.g., diet, education, psychological), environmental (e.g., built environments, air quality, food availability), and sociopolitical (e.g., social networks, cultural factors, and laws/policies).

1.3.3.3 Basic Reproduction Number

Of particular relevance for characterizing infectious disease transmission and dynamics is the key tenet of the basic reproduction number, which is sometimes called basic reproductive ratio, or basic reproductive rate, or "R naught" and denoted R_0. For diseases with person-to-person mode of transmission, this number refers to the expected number of new cases of disease that one case generates on average in an otherwise uninfected (susceptible) population [32]. The mathematical formula is as follows:

$$R_0 = \beta \times c \times d;$$

where, in general terms: β – transmission coefficient or risk (probability) of transmission per contact; c – number of contacts in population per unit time; and d – duration of infectiousness.

When $R_0 > 1$, each case will result in more than one additional case, resulting in epidemic spread. When $R_0 < 1$, each case will result in less than one additional case, resulting in epidemic die out. When $R_0 = 1$, each case will result in one additional case, resulting in a state of equilibrium. Conceptually, this is a very useful measure that provides a summary of several aspects of infectious disease. Of relevance for immunoepidemiology is that transmission dynamics of infectious diseases depend on both individual immunologic characteristics, including genetic susceptibility, immune status, and prior infections, as well as population characteristics such as mixing patterns among people and the immune status of the population.

1.4   Immunoepidemiology

1.4.1   Definition

Immunoepidemiology can be defined as the study of the diversity of immune responses in populations and the factors influencing this diversity. Our understanding of the components of the immune system and how they work together derives primarily from studies of the immune system in *individual* animal models and humans. In contrast, immunoepidemiology focuses on immune studies of animal and human *populations* over time, with considerable overlap between the two disciplines.

1.4.2   History

The field of immunoepidemiology arguably began in the late eighteenth century when Edward Jenner, the father of modern immunology and a country doctor, observed that milkmaids who developed cowpox were generally immune to smallpox. Jenner did not understand the immune mechanisms of protection but theorized that pus from cowpox lesions could protect against smallpox and used this material to develop an effective smallpox vaccine. His early training with great scientific investigators of the time provided the skills to publish his findings and to promote smallpox vaccination throughout his life.

The formal study of immunoepidemiology is thought to have begun in the early 1930s with the work of AC Fisher on human helminth *Schistosoma intercalatum* infections (shistosomiasis). He investigated the development of immunity to schistosomiasis in community settings in the Congo, addressing the central questions of how people develop protection against this infection and why it takes so long to

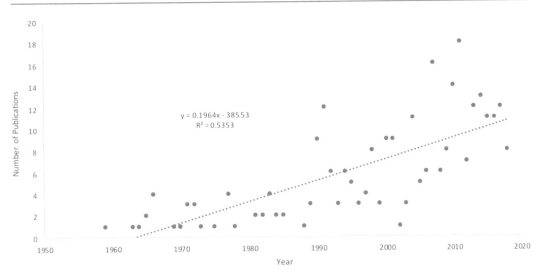

Fig. 1.3 Publications with the term "immunoepidemiology" in title or abstract 1959–2018. The publication numbers were calculated using a systematic review of the literature (see Methods and Fig. A1 in the Appendix). A linear regression model confirmed that the upward trend in publication number is statistically significant ($p < 0.0001$). (©Krause 2020)

achieve immunity [33]. He found that while immunity against *disease* occurred following initial infection, protection against *infection* took decades to develop. Immunity against disease means that a person can be reinfected with schistosomes but does not develop clinical symptoms, whereas immunity against infection means that reexposure to the pathogen does not result in infection or disease. Subsequent immunoepidemiologic studies have continued to focus more on helminth and other parasitic infections (especially malaria) than bacterial and viral infections, in part because animal models have been difficult to establish for many parasitic organisms. Basic information about the immunology of helminth infections have therefore inferred from immunoepidemiologic studies, often using modeling and seroepidemiologic tools [34]. Such studies also have led to an understanding of the effect of diminution or eradication of infections by host immunity. For example, the hygiene hypothesis theorizes that the relatively recent extermination of worms through antibiotics and public health measures in developed countries has contributed to the marked increase in hypersensitivity and autoimmunity in these populations [34].

Immunoepidemiology is an emerging field [35]. Since 1959, 279 papers have been published in English with the terms "immune epidemiology" or "immunoepidemiology" in the title or abstract. The number of publications has varied from year to year, but the overall trend has been upward (see Fig. 1.3, Appendix). Many other studies that address immunoepidemiologic issues have been published without the use of these terms because immunoepidemiology is not a well-recognized subfield of epidemiology or immunology. As far as we know, no textbook has been published on the subject. Further discoveries in immunoepidemiology will allow a better understanding of the role of immunity in determining epidemiologic patterns in human and wildlife populations and help in the planning of more effective diagnosis, treatment, and prevention of immunologic diseases.

1.4.3   Major Concepts

The primary tenant of immunoepidemiology is that the human immune system is highly complex with a vast array of diverse immune responses between individuals and populations. In fact, no two individuals have the same immune response to infection. Population immunity also is variable and depends on the genetic composition of the host population, its history of infection with pathogens, its general health status, and the availability of chemotherapy or vaccination. Although large numbers of people may die during epidemics, a population can survive because of the immunologic diversity of individuals within the population. Nonetheless, nonimmune populations may be decimated by the introduction of new diseases, as occurred with the introduction of measles and smallpox to native American populations by Europeans beginning in the fifteenth century.

The polymorphisms of genes in the major histocompatibility complex (MHC) provide a good example of how variability in the immune system affects individuals and populations. MHC proteins are located on all nucleated cell membranes and function to present microbial antigens to T lymphocytes. Such peptide presentation allows T cells to recognize and help destroy the invading pathogen. Each person has a unique set of MHC proteins that vary in their ability to present the antigens of different infectious pathogens. The MHC genotype of an individual will determine the various MHC proteins they express on their cell surfaces and the range of peptides that are presented by those proteins. The greater the variety of peptides from a pathogen that are presented to T cells, the greater the chance of an effective immune response. Therefore, at the population level, some individuals can be susceptible and others resistant to a given pathogen depending on their MHC genotype. This can also lead over time to changes in the frequencies of MHC alleles in a population, as susceptible individuals succumb to disease and others survive (See Chap. 7).

A more obvious example of immune variability that results in marked differences in disease outcome are people with clinically recognized inherited or acquired immunodeficiencies of varying severity, such as hypogammaglobulinemia, asplenia, AIDS, cancer, or immunosuppressive drug use. Each type of immunodeficiency adversely affects the outcome of infections differently. As just one example, a study of clinical response to the intraerythrocytic protozoal parasite *Babesia microti* showed that disease severity progressively worsened in people who were immunocompetent to immunocompromised to severely immunocompromised. Those who were immune intact experienced a mild-to-moderate febrile illness that cleared after a week of antiparasitic therapy. Those with a single immune deficiency such as asplenia suffered more severe disease that required hospital admission but ultimately resolved after a single course of antiparasitic therapy. A group with multiple immune deficiencies that included severe impairment of antibody function, such as B cell lymphoma with rituximab therapy, experienced severe acute babesiosis followed by multiple relapses of disease despite repeated courses of antibiotic therapy lasting as long as 2 years [36].

1.4.4 Immunoepidemiologic Study Objectives and Tools

The primary objectives of immunoepidemiology are to understand (i) the variable host immune responses to infection (and other foreign antigens) in individuals and populations, (ii) the genetic and environmental factors that influence this diversity, (iii) how the immune system evolves over time, and (iv) how immune dysfunction may arise or resolve in a population. These objectives can be achieved by *serosurveys* that measure antibodies to help determine the frequency of infection, *genetic studies* of specific alleles that code for a diverse set of specific immune cells, *immunologic function studies* of differences in a single type of immune cell between people, or *modeling* to predict and more fully understand immune differences within and between populations.

Immunoepidemiologic studies have provided an understanding of the causes, treatment, and prevention of numerous afflictions. The eradication of smallpox and the control of polio, cholera, plague, measles, and many other scourges of the past have been made possible in large part because of immunoepidemiologic research. Individuals with severe immunodeficiencies who experience repeated infections are readily identified, but we have not yet developed approaches that can routinely and prospectively identify more subtle immune defects. Periodic assessment of the immune status of healthy individuals are not performed by physicians, as is the case for yearly checks of weight, blood pressure, cholesterol, and lipid status [37]. Nor are regular immunologic surveys of populations performed by public health officials, as is the case for tobacco and alcohol use. Immunologic evaluation of individuals and populations could be very useful in the treatment and prevention of infection. This provides strong arguments for epidemiologists, immunologists, and general physicians to work more closely together to determine which immune characteristics would benefit from routine analysis and to develop such assays and screening procedures.

In this book, we examine how immunoepidemiologic studies provide an understanding of population differences in the frequency and severity of infection, cancer, and autoimmunity and how genetic and environmental factors have shaped immune function over time. We first provide a background of basic immunologic processes in the individual and then proceed to examine relevant topics in the field of immunoepidemiology.

Immunoepidemiological Tools

Researchers have used many tools in immunoepidemiologic investigations. Immunologists have elucidated strategies of defense against pathogens, offered insight into beneficial and harmful aspects of inflammation, and provided practical means of enhancing host defense, notably through vaccination. They also have developed tools to study the immunologic responses of populations. Both in vivo and in vitro immune assays are useful in defining the reactivity of a population to a particular antigen. In vivo assays include skin tests that consist of dermal scratch application or intradermal injection of an antigen. Individuals who are allergic to that substance may have an "immediate hypersensitivity" reaction mediated by antibody that occurs within 30 min (Fig. 1.4) [38]. Some antigens elicit a "delayed hypersensitivity" response that may take 48 to 72 h to develop due to immune cellular infiltration. These tests can be administered to groups of individuals and thus define exposure to pathogens such as mycobacteria (PPD test) or sensitivity to allergens. In vitro tests have proven to be even more useful. The types and specificities of antibody responses can be measured and characterized in populations. Seroepidemiologic testing identifies antibody to specific pathogens, which allows evaluation of the extent of infection by that pathogen in a population. More recently, serum cytokine testing has been used to characterize the immune status of populations.

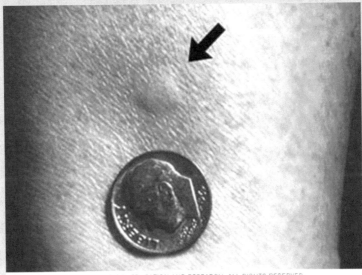

Fig. 1.4 Allergy skin testing. A small area of swelling with surrounding redness known as a wheal and flare is typical of a positive allergy skin test. (Used with permission of Mayo Foundation for Medical Education and Research. All rights reserved)

References

1. Kaufmann SH. Immunology's foundation: the 100-year anniversary of the Nobel Prize to Paul Ehrlich and Elie Metchnikoff. Nat Immunol. 2008;9(7):705–12. Epub 2008/06/20. https://doi.org/10.1038/ni0708-705.

2. Medzhitov R, Preston-Hurlburt P, Janeway CA Jr. A human homologue of the Drosophila toll protein signals activation of adaptive immunity. Nature. 1997;388(6640):394–7. Epub 1997/07/24. https://doi.org/10.1038/41131.

3. Poltorak A, He X, Smirnova I, Liu MY, Van Huffel C, Du X, Birdwell D, Alejos E, Silva M, Galanos C, Freudenberg M, Ricciardi-Castagnoli P, Layton B, Beutler B. Defective LPS signaling in C3H/HeJ and C57BL/10ScCr mice: mutations in Tlr4 gene. Science. 1998;282(5396):2085–8. Epub 1998/12/16

4. Lemaitre B, Nicolas E, Michaut L, Reichhart JM, Hoffmann JA. The dorsoventral regulatory gene cassette spatzle/toll/cactus controls the potent antifungal response in Drosophila adults. Cell. 1996;86(6):973–83. Epub 1996/09/20

5. Schreiber RD, Leonard W. Cytokines: Cold Spring Harbor. Woodbury, NY: Cold Spring Harbor Laboratory Press; 2018.

6. Owen RD. Immunogenetic consequences of vascular anastomoses between bovine twins. Science. 1945;102(2651):400–1. Epub 1945/10/19. https://doi.org/10.1126/science.102.2651.400.

7. Burnet FM, Fenner F. The production of antibodies. Melbourne: Macmillan; 1949.

8. Billingham RE, Brent L, Medawar PB. Actively acquired tolerance of foreign cells. Nature. 1953;172(4379):603–6. Epub 1953/10/03. PubMed PMID: 13099277

9. Klein G. The natural history of the MHC. New York: Wiley; 1986.

10. Mackay IR. Travels and travails of autoimmunity: a historical journey from discovery to rediscovery. Autoimmun Rev. 2010;9(5):A251–8. Epub 2009/11/04. https://doi.org/10.1016/j.autrev.2009.10.007.

11. Hozumi N, Tonegawa S. Evidence for somatic rearrangement of immunoglobulin genes coding for variable and constant regions. Proc Natl Acad Sci U S A. 1976;73(10):3628–32. Epub 1976/10/01. PubMed PMID: 824647; PMCID: PMC431171

12. Schatz DG, Oettinger MA, Baltimore D. The V(D)J recombination activating gene, RAG-1. Cell. 1989;59(6):1035–48. Epub 1989/12/22

13. Miller JF. Immunological function of the thymus. Lancet. 1961;2(7205):748–9. Epub 1961/09/30

14. Cooper MD, Raymond DA, Peterson RD, South MA, Good RA. The functions of the thymus system and the bursa system in the chicken. J Exp Med. 1966;123(1):75–102. Epub 1966/01/01. PubMed PMID: 5323079; PMCID: PMC2138128

15. Davis MM, Bjorkman PJ. T-cell antigen receptor genes and T-cell recognition. Nature. 1988;334(6181):395–402. https://doi.org/10.1038/334395a0. Epub 1988/08/04. PubMed PMID: 3043226

16. Bjorkman PJ, Strominger JL, Wiley DC. Crystallization and X-ray diffraction studies on the histocompatibility antigens HLA-A2 and HLA-A28 from human cell membranes. J Mol Biol. 1985;186(1):205–10. Epub 1985/11/05

17. Isaacs A, Lindenmann J. Virus interference. I. The interferon. Proc R Soc Lond B Biol Sci. 1957;147(927):258–67. Epub 1957/09/12

18. David JR, Al-Askari S, Lawrence HS, Thomas L. Delayed hypersensitivity in vitro. I. The specificity of inhibition of cell migration by antigens. J Immunol. 1964;93:264–73. Epub 1964/08/01

19. Bloom BR, Bennett B. Mechanism of a reaction in vitro associated with delayed-type hypersensitivity. Science. 1966;153(3731):80–2. Epub 1966/07/01

20. Ruddle NH, Waksman BH. Cytotoxicity mediated by soluble antigen and lymphocytes in delayed hypersensitivity. 3. Analysis of mechanism. J Exp Med. 1968;128(6):1267–79. Epub 1968/12/01. PubMed PMID: 5693925; PMCID: PMC2138574

21. Kolb WP, Granger GA. Lymphocyte in vitro cytotoxicity: characterization of human lymphotoxin. Proc Natl Acad Sci U S A. 1968;61(4):1250–5. Epub 1968/12/01. PubMed PMID: 5249808; PMCID: PMC225248

22. Last JM, editor. A dictionary of epidemiology. New York: Oxford University Press; 2001.

23. Hippocrates. On airs, waters, and places. Available at http://classics.mit.edu/Hippocrates/airwatpl.html.

24. Aschengrau A, George Seage III. Essentials of epidemiology in public health. 3rd ed. Burlington: Jones & Bartlett; 2014.

25. Johnson S. The ghost map: the story of London's Most terrifying epidemic–and how it changed science, cities, and the modern world. London: Penguin Books Ltd.; 2006.

26. Thomas KK. Cultivating hygiene as a science: the Welch-rose report's influence at Johns Hopkins and beyond. Am J Epidemiol. 2016;183:345–54.

27. Enans AS. Causation and Disease: The Henle-Koch Postulates Revisited. Yale J Biol Med. 1976;46:175–95.

28. MacMahon B, Pugh TF, Ipsen J. Epidemiologic methods. Boston: Little Brown & Company; 1960.

29. Hill AB. The environment and disease: association or causation? Proc R Soc Med. 1965;58:295–300.

30. Rothman KJ, Greenland S. Causation and causal inference in epidemiology. AJPH. 2005;95:S144–50.

31. Leischow SJ, Milstein B. Systems thinking and modeling for public health practice. Am J Public Health. 2006;96:403–5.

32. Thomas JC, Weber DJ, editors. Epidemiologic methods for the study of infectious diseases. New York: Oxford University Press; 2001.
33. Fisher AC. A study of schistosomiasis in the Stanleyville district of Congo. Trans R Soc Trop Med Hyg. 1934;28:277–306.
34. Woolhouse MEJ, Hagan P. Seeking the ghosts of worms past. Nat Med. 1999;5:1225–7.
35. Hellriegel B. Immunoepidemiology– bridging the gap between immunology and epidemiology. Trends Parasitol. 2001;17:102–6.
36. Krause PJ, Gewurz BE, Hill D, Marty FM, Vannier E, Foppa IM, Furman RR, Neuhaus E, Skowron G, Gupta S, McCalla C, Pesanti EL, Young M, Heiman D, Hsue G, Gelfand JA, Wormser GP, Dickason J, Bia FJ, Hartman B, Telford SR, Christianson D, Dardick K, Coleman M, Girotto JE, Spielman A. Persistent and relapsing babesiosis in immunocompromised patients. Clin Infect Dis. 2008;46:370–6.
37. Alpert A, Pickman Y, Leipold M, Rosenberg-Hasson Y, Ji X, Gaujoux R, Rabani H, Starosvetsky E, Kveler K, Schaffert S, Furman D, Caspi O, Rosenschein U, Khatri P, Dekker CL, Maecker HT, Davis MM, Shen-Orr SS. A clinically meaningful metric of immune age derived from high-dimensional longitudinal monitoring. Nat Med. 2019;25(3):487–95.
38. Pumphrey RS. Lessons for management of anaphylaxis from a study of fatal reactions. Clin Exp Allergy. 2000;30:1144.

Section II

IMMUNOLOGY BASICS

Organization and Cells of the Immune System

Paula B. Kavathas, Peter J. Krause, and Nancy H. Ruddle

2.1 Introduction

All organisms are subject to attack by microbial pathogens and therefore have developed immune mechanisms to combat infection. Even single-cell bacteria can be infected by viruses. In fact, one of the immune mechanisms discovered in bacteria has been exploited for a powerful gene editing technology called CRISPR. Innate immunity, also known as "natural immunity," has always existed for multicellular organisms. Innate defenses act immediately or within hours, react in the same manner to repeated pathogen exposure, and attack foreign invaders but not self-tissue. They also function in tissue repair and homeostasis. When the adaptive immune system appeared four to five million years ago in vertebrate animals, it developed in the context of the innate immune system so that the two systems are closely linked and work together in a coordinated fashion. The adaptive immune system also attacks foreign invaders, is slower to become activated (taking 5–7 days to weeks to fully develop), and becomes more effective with repeated pathogen exposure. While cells of the innate immmune system recognize classes of microbes, the adaptive immune system is more specific in that it recognizes individual microbes.

2.1.1 Surface Barriers and Mucosal Immunity

The first lines of innate immune defense are surface and mucosal barriers consisting of the skin and mucosal surfaces of the respiratory, gastrointestinal, oral cavity, and genitourinary tracts. The skin is made up of stratified epithelium and an underlying dermis that prevent pathogen entry. Mucosal surfaces consist of an epithelial barrier with a single-cell layer of cells forming tight junctions in the

P. B. Kavathas (✉)
Departments of Laboratory Medicine and Immunobiology, Yale School of Medicine,
New Haven, CT, USA
e-mail: paula.kavathas@yale.edu

P. J. Krause
Department of Epidemiology of Microbial Diseases, Yale School of Public Health and Departments of Medicine and Pediatrics, Yale School of Medicine, New Haven, CT, USA

N. H. Ruddle
Department of Epidemiology of Microbial Diseases, Yale School of Public Health, New Haven, CT, USA

© Springer Nature Switzerland AG 2019
P. J. Krause et al. (eds.), *Immunoepidemiology*, https://doi.org/10.1007/978-3-030-25553-4_2

gastrointestinal (GI) tract. The surfaces are covered with a viscous mucus lining secreted by specialized epithelial cells called goblet cells. This barrier functions to prevent pathogens from entering and is a first line of defense. Specialized cells in the GI tract called Paneth cells secrete antimicrobial peptides into the mucus layer that target bacteria or fungi. Expulsion of pathogens at the mucosal surface can occur through air (cough), liquid (defecation, urination), or ciliary action. The enzyme lysozyme in tears and saliva cleaves components of bacterial cell walls and the acidic environment of the stomach and the vagina create an inhospitable environment for some microbes. The skin and mucosal surfaces are richly enmeshed with blood and lymph vessels that can recruit large numbers of immune cells to a site of infection.

These barrier surfaces are colonized by trillions of bacteria, archaea, fungi, viruses, protozoa, and helminths collectively known as the "microbiota." The gut is home to the largest community of bacterial species (hundreds of species) with more than 100 trillion bacterial cells. Different microbes occupy different niches within the gut and altogether the ecological community is called the microbiome. An individual's microbiome plays an important role in their immune system and health. One of the most important functions is in colonization resistance. The microbiota can prevent the outgrowth of pathogenic enteric microorganisms such as *Salmonella*, *Shigella*, and pathogenic *E. coli*. Remarkably, the composition of the microbiome differs between people and is not static. It is influenced by diet, medical drugs, microbial exposure, host genetics, and other factors. Studies of the microbiome and its impact on disease is in its infancy. However, it is clear that differences between people with respect to their microbiome impact differences in disease susceptibility and outcome.

2.2 Cells of the Immune System

2.2.1 Overview

Cells in the blood that are not red blood cells are called white blood cells or leukocytes, from the Greek word "leukos" meaning "white" and cyte meaning "cell." These cells are constantly being generated in the body by the process known as hematopoiesis described below. The different cell types of the immune system can be thought of as members of the "immunological orchestra." While not a perfect metaphor, it is a useful comparison. Different instruments or cells play at different times depending on the type of music or the immunological response that is needed. There are major categories of instruments and of cell types and within each group there are subtypes. For instance, the categories of horns and winds have subgroups (i.e., French horn/trumpet, flute/piccolo). The same is true for the major categories of immune cells.

The metaphor of cell types with musical instruments breaks down, however, when it comes to the phenotypic plasticity of cells. While an instrument is static, cells of the immune system undergo changes during their development, upon activation, and in response to environmental alterations. Immune T cells have been described as naïve, activated, exhausted, anergic, or dying to indicate different states. Their cellular metabolism is rewired upon cell activation to facilitate cell growth, proliferation, and the production of effector molecules. Immune cells were initially categorized based on properties characteristic of either the innate or adaptive immune system and their ontogeny. As we learn more about these cells, we now know that a strict classification into "innate" or "adaptive" does not always apply.

Traditionally, the different immune cell types were defined by morphology and function. However, with advances in technology, they can be further subdivided according to their expression pattern of proteins. The pattern of cell surface proteins that a cell expresses is determined by mixing antibodies specific to a cell surface protein with immune cells; binding is detected using flow cytometry technology or mass cytometry. International workshops were held to provide a system for naming the cell surface proteins. Each protein was given a cluster of differentiation number (e.g., CD1), and there are now more than 300 different immune proteins with a CD designation. Single-cell RNA profiling is providing further insight into cell heterogeneity.

2.2.2 Cells of the Innate Immune System

One of the primary first responders during a bacterial infection is called a *macrophage* (Fig. 2.1). These cells arise from monocytes in the blood that differentiate into macrophages in the tissue or are seeded there during embryonic development. Macrophages residing in tissues are long-lived and

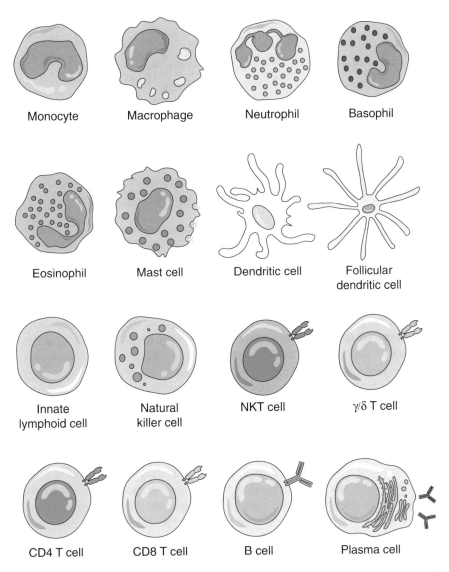

Fig. 2.1 Types of immune cells. Cells on the top two rows are innate immune cells. Granulocytes refer to the cell types with many granules and irregularly shaped nuclei (neutrophil, basophil, eosinophil, mast cell). The third row lists two cell types of the innate immune system (innate lymphoid cells (ILCs) and natural killer cells) and two cell types of the adaptive immune system with a relative invariant T cell receptor (NKT and γ/δ T cells). The last row has the two main subsets of T cells, a B cell and long-lived plasma cell producing antibody. (©Kavathas 2020)

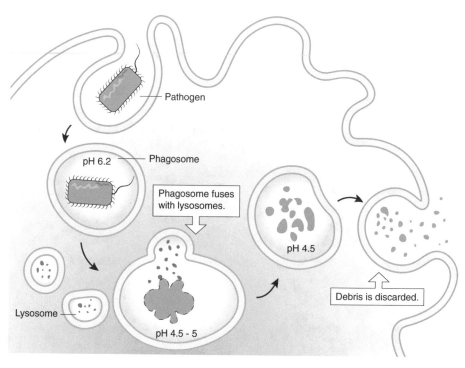

Fig. 2.2 Phagocytosis to engulf or "eat" and degrade a microorganism. A macrophage or neutrophil will engulf a microbe by the process of endocytosis. The endocytic vesicle called a phagosome will fuse with lysosomes in the cell in order to degrade the pathogen. The debris is released to the outside of the cell. (©Kavathas 2020)

function both in immunity and tissue homeostasis. When a pathogen enters the body, macrophages have receptors called pattern recognition receptors (PRR) that recognize some component of a microbe, the ligand, discussed in Chap. 3. The cells respond to bacteria by engulfing and internalizing the microbe within a membrane vesicle called a phagosome in a process called *phagocytosis* (Fig. 2.2). This term is derived from the Greek word "phago" or eat and "cytosis" or cell. A macrophage is therefore a macro or large eating cell. The phagosome subsequently fuses with a cytoplasmic vesicle called a lysosome that contains proteolytic enzymes and reactive oxygen species. These molecules kill and degrade the bacteria in the phagolysosome (Fig. 2.2). In order to communicate with or recruit other immune cells to help fight an infection, the macrophage secretes small molecules known as cytokines and chemokines that are described later in this chapter. Chemokines have chemoattractant properties that recruit other immune cells such as neutrophils and T lymphocytes to the area of infection.

Another important function of the macrophages is to remove dying host cells by phagocytosis. The ability of the macrophage to remove these cells is important for returning to homeostasis after an infection and when aging or dying cells need to be removed. Macrophages can also secrete molecules that enhance matrix tissue repair. Finally, macrophages located in certain tissues have specialized properties. Examples are microglial cells (brain), Kuppfer cells (liver), and Langerhans cells (skin). Macrophages can also take on inflammatory and anti-inflammatory properties based on certain signals they receive and have been referred to as M1 and M2 macrophages, respectively.

Fig. 2.3 NETosis to trap microbes. A neutrophil will release decondensed DNA and antimicrobial peptides to form a "neutrophil extracellular trap" or NET for microbes that cannot be phagocytosed such as filamentous yeast. The antimicrobial peptides function to induce pathogen death. (©Kavathas 2020)

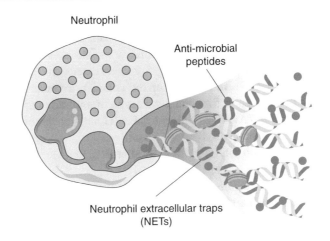

Neutrophil

Anti-microbial peptides

Neutrophil extracellular traps (NETs)

The *neutrophil* is another type of innate immune cell that is of central importance in killing pathogenic bacteria and fungi. They are the most abundant cell type in the blood (5×10^{10}/ml) and can be recruited to the site of infection in large numbers. Both neutrophils and macrophages kill pathogens by phagocytosis; however, unlike macrophages, which are found in tissues, neutrophils circulate in the blood and can move from the bloodstream to sites of infection. While spherical yeast cells of a pathogen like *Candida albicans* can be phagocytosed, the fungus can switch to a form producing large hyphae or filaments that invade tissue and are too large for phagocytosis. In this case, the neutrophil releases neutrophil extracellular traps (NETs), an extracellular mesh-like structure composed of decondensed DNA coated with antimicrobial effector molecules, which trap and kill pathogens (Fig. 2.3). The process is called *NETosis*. After an infection is cleared, the neutrophil can secrete molecules such as resolvins that promote healing. Neutrophils are short-lived cells surviving only a few days. Pus is composed of dead neutrophils and pathogens.

The *dendritic cell* (DC), another innate immune cell type, acts as a bridge between innate and adaptive immunity, alerting the adaptive immune system to the presence of a pathogen. These cells were named before their function was known because they had long extended processes that looked like the dendrites on neurons. Immature DCs are activated in the tissue upon encounter with a pathogen and undergo changes to become mature DCs. These cells migrate from the site of infection through lymphatic vessels to the nearest lymph node where they present antigen to T cells, a cell of the adaptive immune system. Their migration to the nearest lymph node can take 12–24 h or longer. There are three main subtypes of DCs. The conventional DCs (cDCs) are the professional antigen-presenting cells (APCs). The plasmacytoid DCs (pDCs) drive robust type I interferon responses, and the monocyte-derived DCs (MoDCs) drive tissue inflammation.

The *mast cell* is a long-lived, tissue-resident cell that is recruited from the blood to tissues. The cells mature under the influence of cytokines and growth factors in the local tissue microenvironment. These cells are located at boundaries of the body such as the gastrointestinal mucosa, respiratory mucosa, and skin as well as associated with blood vessels, nerve endings, and smooth muscle. They play an important role in host defense against helminth parasites but also impact bacteria, fungal, and viral infections. They can be activated when ligands bind to activating receptors leading to the release of pro-inflammatory and anti-inflammatory mediators present in stored granules. These include vasoactive amines (histamine and serotonin), proteoglycans, proteases, and cytokines. Mediators such as histamine cause contraction of smooth muscle that helps to expel parasites from the intestine by peristalsis. Coughing or sneezing is another mediator-generated response that helps expel parasites. Substances that can directly damage parasites also are released such as proteases. In the case of ectoparasites, which live on the outside of a host such as a tick, these mediators induce itching and scratching to help the host locate the tick and remove it. Inflammatory mediators such as cytokines released by mast cells help orchestrate antiparasitic defenses and promote expulsion of the parasites.

When antibodies evolved as part of the adaptive immune system, the mast cells evolved to express a surface receptor that bound one type of antibody named IgE. Mast cells can be coated with IgE binding to the antibody receptor, FcεR1, so that when sufficient antigen binds to the IgE, such that the receptor is cross-linked, a cell response occurs. The IgE is sometimes generated against innocuous substances leading to allergies. Mast cells are a major player in asthma and allergies discussed in later chapters.

Basophils and *eosinophils* are innate immune cells that play a major role in immunity against parasites, particularly helminths (worms). They generally circulate in the blood with a short half-life where they can be recruited into tissues in response to an appropriate inflammatory stimulus at the site of infection. Eosinophils, like mast cells, are resident in intestinal tissues. Since mast cells, basophils, eosinophils, and neutrophils all contain cytoplasmic granules with substances that are released after they are activated, they are all referred to as granulocytes. These cells (with the exception of mast cells) are also called polymorphonuclear leukocytes because they have multilobed nuclei.

Innate lymphoid cells (ILCs) play an important role in immune defense, inflammation, and tissue remodeling. They are located in tissues throughout the body. These cells are poised to respond to signals from barrier cells (epithelial cells) or from myeloid cells that secrete cytokines. The three groups of innate lymphoid cells are distinguished by their developmental program, mechanism of activation, their cell surface protein expression, and the cytokines they secrete. There are also subsets within each group. For instance, the group 1 ILCs include ILC1 and natural killer (NK) cells. NK cells circulate, whereas ILC1s are tissue-resident cells found in tissues such as the gut, liver, salivary gland, and uterus and are enriched in obesity (fat tissue). They play an important role against intracellular pathogens such as viruses as they produce a key cytokine in viral immune responses called interferon-γ (IFN-γ). Group 2 contains a single subset, ILC2 cells, that play a role in defense against helminths, the development of asthma and allergies, and the regulation of normal metabolism. They produce the cytokines and interleukins IL-5, IL-9, and IL-13, amphiregulin (stimulates epithelial cell repair), and the neurotransmitter/hormone methionine-enkephalin (MetEnk) peptides. The latter activates adipocytes, a cell type specialized for storage of fat, to induce lipolysis and increase energy expenditure to limit obesity. Group 3 ILCs are comprised of lymphoid tissue inducer cells (LTi), the natural cytotoxicity receptor (NCR)⁻ ILC3s, and NCR+ ILC3 cells. The tissue inducer cells promote lymphoid tissue organogenesis during fetal life and after birth by secreting the cytokines lymphotoxin α and β, as well as pro-inflammatory cytokines. The ILC3 cells produce the cytokines IL-17A and IL-22 that are important for killing extracellular bacteria and fungi at mucosal sites. They also regulate interactions between commensal bacteria and host immunity.

Natural killer cells (NK cells) are important in antiviral and tumor immunity. They comprise 5–20% of human peripheral blood lymphoid cells circulating throughout the body. They were originally described as cells that could kill tumor cells without priming. Activated NK cells respond by secreting inflammatory cytokines and killing infected cells or tumor cells. Normally, they do not kill host cells as they have inhibitory receptors on their surface (discussed in Chap. 3) that bind to MHC class I proteins expressed on all cells of the body. However, if (i) MHC class I proteins are reduced on infected or tumor cells, which then diminishes signals to inhibit the NK cells, and (ii) the infected/tumor cells express ligands for activating receptors, then the NK cells will become activated. Specialized uterine NK cells are critical for the formation of the placenta during pregnancy as discussed in Chap. 7. Heterogenous subsets of NK cells exist. In humans the two main types are

CD3⁻CD56^{dim} and CD3⁻CD56^{bright} cells. The dim cells (more mature) are predominant in the blood and the bright cells (less mature) are in the tissues. The CD56^{bright} NK cells produce high levels of IFN-γ in response to a target cell but have limited killing capacity, whereas the mature CD56^{dim} NK cells demonstrate a high level of cytotoxicity. Unlike other innate cell types, NK cells have the ability to form a memory-type cell which demonstrates a more robust response upon reencounter with the same antigen. This was shown in humans with CMV infections and is discussed in Chap. 3.

2.2.3 Cells of the Adaptive Immune System

T and B lymphocytes were initially thought to be uninteresting because most found in the blood had very little cytoplasm, so they seemed quiescent or inactive. However, after activation, these cells increase in size, change their metabolic state, and start producing large quantities of proteins. B and T lymphocytes circulate in the blood and lymph. They encounter foreign antigen in secondary lymphoid organs and differentiate into different effector cell subsets, and most cells then migrate into the tissues where the infection is located. Each B or T cell generally expresses one type of receptor for a specific antigen at roughly 10^5–10^6 copies/cell. One of the major differences between these two cell types is that once the B cell is activated, it secretes a soluble form of its receptor called an antibody. Antibodies have many different functions to be described later. In contrast, the T cell receptor functions solely for recognition and signaling and uses other mechanisms for fighting an infection such as secretion of cytokines.

There are multiple subsets of T and B cells. The two main T cell subsets are defined by the expression of the cell surface proteins CD4 and CD8, and two main subsets of B cells are B1 and B2. Traditionally, the CD4 cells were referred to as helper T cells and CD8 cells as cytotoxic cells. We now know there are multiple subsets within the CD4 and CD8 cell type. The characterization and function of the T and B cell subsets are discussed in Chap. 5. Another hallmark of these cells is the ability to differentiate into long-lived memory cells that show a more robust and rapid immune response upon reencounter with the same antigen.

2.3 Hematopoiesis

Hematopoiesis is the process by which pluripotent stem cells, located in the bone marrow in an adult and in the fetal liver, give rise to all the different cell types in the blood, including immune cells. Self-renewing, long-lived haematopoietic stem cells (HSCs) divide in the bone marrow to form daughter cells that either maintain their stem cell properties or become progenitor cells for different cell lineages (Fig. 2.4). There is a progressive continuum of restriction in differentiation potential as cells develop into different lineages. Master regulatory transcription factors influence cell fate decisions and changes in chromatin accessibility to these factors are observed during differentiation. The multipotent progenitor cell (MPP) gives rise to either the common myeloid precursor (CMP) or the common lymphoid progenitor (CLP). The CMP gives rise to either a granulocyte/monocyte progenitor (GMP) cell or the megakaryocyte/erythroid (MEP) progenitor. The MEP cell becomes either a megakaryocyte that forms platelets or a erythrocyte that forms red blood cells. The GMP progenitor gives rise to granulocyes (neutrophils, eosinophils, basophils, mast cells) and monocytes. Monocytes from the blood can enter tissue and become either macrophages or monocyte-derived dendritic cells. The CLPs differentiate into either innate lymphoid cells (ILCs), T or B lymphocytes, or dendritic cells. The innate lymphoid cells comprise three groups. The ILC1, ILC2, and ILC3 are subsets within group 1,2,3 respectively. Natural killer cells are a subset within group 1. Most of the cells developing in the

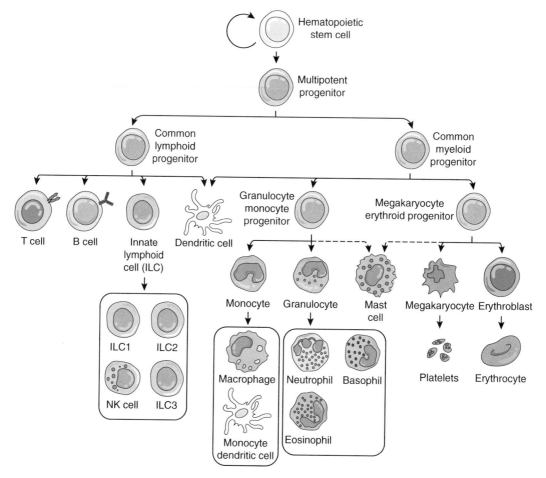

Fig. 2.4 Process of hematopoiesis. Pluripotent stem cells located in the bone marrow of adults give rise to all the different cell types in the blood including immune cells. These cells divide and either self-renew or give rise to the multipotent progenitor (MPP) which can either become the common myeloid progenitor (CMP) or the common lymphoid progenitor (CLP). As cells develop into different lineages of cells, the progenitor cells become more restricted in their differentiation potential until the final stage of development when the cells leave the bone marrow. The plasmacytoid DC (pDC) comes from either the CMP or CLP, whereas the classical DC is derived from the CMP. These are shown as dendritic cell in the diagram. (©Kavathas 2020)

bone marrow leave as mature cells. However, some continue to differentiate elsewhere such as the T cells in the thymus and the mast cell in tissues.

The pathways of differentiation lead to the production of the different cell types at rates appropriate for a healthy homeostatic state. However, the body can respond to perturbations such as infection or low oxygen. For instance, the production of monocytes and granulocytes can increase upon infection. On the other hand, in low oxygen conditions (e.g., top of a high mountain), the pathway producing more red blood cells is stimulated, thus allowing for flexible adaption to conditions that place stress on the system.

Not all immune cells are derived from the bone marrow HSC cells. For instance, during embryonic development, a bipotent erythroid/myeloid cell gives rise to red blood cells and tissue-resident macrophages such as microglia that reside in the brain. An innate type B cell called B1 also arises at this time.

2.4 Cytokines: Communication Signals Between Cells

2.4.1 Definition

Cytokines are low molecular weight proteins made by cells of the immune system that influence the behavior of other cells. Cytokines vary in their molecular weight from approximately 15 to 196 kDA, although some form multimers, resulting in even higher molecular weights. The word cytokine is derived from the Greek words cyto "cell" and kinesis "movement." Cytokines are produced by many cell types, not only those of the immune system. In this context, however, we will be concentrating on their production by cells of the immune system. Cytokines regulate the intensity and duration of the immune response by stimulating or inhibiting activation, proliferation, survival, migration, or differentiation of cells. They are secreted as part of the effector function of the innate and adaptive systems.

The nomenclature of the various cytokines is somewhat confusing, and in some cases based on the original discovery of a single biological activity, even though the factor was later discovered to possess several additional activites. For example, tumor necrosis factor (TNF) was named for its ability to kill tumors, but like most cytokines, it is *pleotropic*, that is, it exhibits many other activities, including inducing the production of other cytokines, killing target cells, and causing changes in endothelial cells lining blood vessels to allow other immune cells such as neutrophils and T cells to reach the site of infection. Other cytokines, called interleukins, were named in order of their discovery (IL-1 to IL-40) and were originally thought to be made by leukocytes to communicate with other leukocytes. However, other cell types can make or respond to interleukins, so this nomenclature is misleading. Other cytokines are members of the interferon (IFN) family. Some growth factors such as granulocyte-macrophage colony stimulating factor (GM-CSF) are also cytokines.

Cytokines can act on the cells that release them (*autocrine*) or on other nearby (*paracrine*) cells, as long as the target cells express the particular cytokine receptor on their cell surface. The absence of antigen specificity by cytokines and their high specific activity means they are very powerful and can be dangerous when released systemically, sometimes leading to disastrous consequences, such as hypotension, pulmonary edema, or shock. Thus, cytokine production is tightly regulated, so that both their mRNAs and proteins have short half-lives, ensuring that for the most part, they act for only a limited time period and over a short distance (Table 2.1).

2.5 Chemokines: Directional Signals

Chemokines are chemoattractant molecules ranging between 8 and 15 kDA that are produced constitutively or following cell activation and act over a concentration gradient. Chemokines signal through seven membrane-spanning G-protein-linked receptors that are expressed on various leukocyte cell types. These signals direct the target cells movement and induce changes in their activity. Chemokines were originally described by their biological activity, but the more recent nomenclature refers to their structure; CC chemokines have two adjacent cysteines near their amino terminus, whereas CXC chemokines have a single amino acid that interrupts the CC terminus. These CC ligands (CCL) or CXC ligands (CXCL) bind to and signal through respective CCLR or CXCLR receptors. Some chemokines are "promiscuous" in that they can signal through more than one receptor, and some receptors can bind more than one chemokine (Fig. 2.5). Examples of constitutive chemokines that have an organizing function in lymphoid organs (see below) include CCL19 and CCL21. These chemokines guide T cells and DCs by their expression of CCR7, the receptor for CCL19 and CCL21, to the parafollicular areas of lymph nodes and maintain them at these specific sites within the lymph node. On the other hand, B cells, expressing CXCR5, are directed to their location in the lymph node by CXCL13.

Table 2.1 Cytokines. This is a partial list of the cytokines. They are grouped as families based on their receptor usage

Family name	Examples	Receptors	Activities/Characteristics
Type I interferons	IFN-α, IFN-β, IFN-κ, IFN-ω	IFNAR	Antiviral; immune response modulation
Type II interferon	IFN-γ	IFGNGR	Inflammation; Th1 cytokine; macrophage activation
Type III interferon	IFN-λ	IFNLR	Antiviral, inflammation
Colony stimulating factors	G-CSF; GM-CSF; M-CSF	G-CSFR; CD116; CSF-1R	Neutrophil development; myelomonocytic cell differentiation; monocytic lineage growth
Immediate TNF	TNF (TNF-α), LT-α (TNF-β); LTβ, LTα1β2	TNFRI or TNFRII, HVEM; LTβR	Genes linked within MHC complex; roles in Inflammation; cytotoxicity; lymphoid organ development and many more;
Extended TNF	CD40L, FasL, APRIL and BAFF, LIGHT, TRAIL	CD40, Fas, TACI or BCMI, HVEM or LTβR; DR4 or DR5, DCR1, DCR2 or OPG	A few of the 19 ligands and 29 receptors of this family whose genes are located throughout the genome; roles in killing, B cell activation and survival, bone remodeling and many more
Interleukin-1	IL-1α, IL-β, IL1-Rα; IL-18, IL-33	IL-1R1	Fever; IFN-γ induction, TH1 activation; TNF induction
Interleukin--2	IL-2; IL-3, IL-4, IL-5; IL-7; IL-12; IL-13; IL-15; IL-21, IL-23	Common γ chain	T cell growth; B cell activation; T cell maintenance, pre-B and pre-T cells; NK activation and Th1 polarization; B cell growth and activation IgE; T memory; B, T, NK cell
Interleukin-6	IL-6, IL-11, IL-27, LIF, OSM, CNTF, CLC, CT-1	gp130	Acute phase reaction, B cell stimulation, balance between Tregs and Teffs, metabolic regulation, neural functions
Interleukin-17	IL-17 (IL-17A), IL-17B, IL-17C, IL-17D, IL-17F		Neutrophil recruitment, inflammation, some autoimmune diseases
Migration inhibitory factor	MIF	CD74-CXCR4	macrophage migration inhibition; Induces steroid resistance, macrophage activation,
Transforming growth factor	TGF-β	TGFβR	Anti-inflammation; switch to IgA

Fig. 2.5 Chemokine receptor and ligand pairings. Chemokine receptors belonging to each of the chemokine families (C, CC, CXC, and CX3C) are represented around the outer ring of the wheel; their chemokine ligands are shown along the wheel spokes. Receptors with a single known ligand are shown in the area of the circle shaded yellow. (Reproduced with permission (Fig. 1 from Gemma et al. [22].))

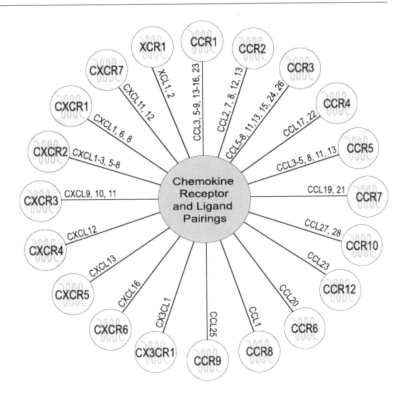

Chemokines are induced by inflammatory cytokines, such as TNF, from stromal cells. For example, a chemokine such as CCL2 (MCP-1) is induced by TNF from an activated macrophage, which then recruits additional monocytes, expressing CCR2 to the site and again amplifying the immune response.

2.6   The Lymphatic System and Lymphoid Organs

2.6.1   Definition

The *lymphatic system* is comprised of a series of vessels that connects lymphoid organs with each other, the bloodstream, and the rest of the body (Fig. 2.6). The lymphatic system serves three purposes: fluid homeostasis, lipid transport, and antigen and lymphoid cell transport. The earliest function of the lymphatic system in evolution was to return fluid leaking out of blood vessels into tissues back into the blood. The fluid in tissues is first collected in thin-walled, blind-ended lymphatic capillaries. These are made up of cells with spaces between them so that extracellular fluid can enter the vessel. The fluid, called lymph, then moves into larger lymphatic collecting vessels and is eventually returned to the blood. In primitive animals, such as zebra fish that have no lymphoid organs, per se, the major function of lymphatic vessels is to maintain fluid equilibrium by regulating fluid volume. In humans, 8–12 liters of fluid and protein per day from the extravascular compartments are returned to the blood through the lymphatic system.

This system subsequently evolved to have an additional role in *immune surveillance*. Higher organisms acquired lymph nodes that are connected to lymphatic vessels. The lymph from tissues moves through lymphatic vessels into lymph nodes, which serve to filter the lymph and help remove pathogens. In addition to transporting particulate antigens, soluble antigens, and microorganisms to the

Fig. 2.6 The lymphoid system. The lymphoid system consists of primary lymphoid organ (thymus and bone marrow) and secondary lymphoid organs (lymph nodes, spleen, Peyer's patches, tonsils, adenoids), connected by lymphatic vessels that connect to the blood circulation at the right and left subclavian veins. (©Ruddle 2020)

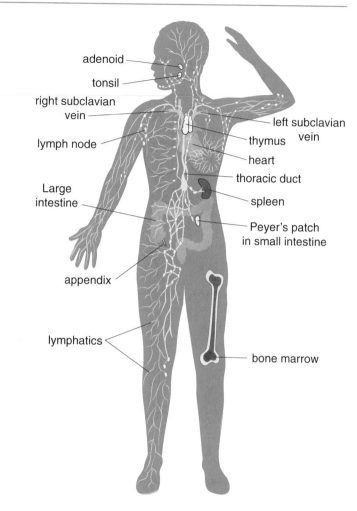

lymph node, the lymph also serves to transport antigen-presenting cells, including dendritic cells. Activated DCs migrate to lymph nodes and encounter T cells of the adaptive immune system to alert them to the presence of a pathogen. Lymph even has some polymorphonuclear leukocytes but does not contain red blood cells or platelets and thus does not clot and has a milky white appearance. The lymph node closest to an infected site that receives lymph fluid, antigen, and antigen-presenting cells is called the draining lymph node. In addition, fat from the gut is absorbed into the lymphatics for transport to the blood.

Unlike the blood circulatory system in which fluid is propelled by the heart, the lymphatic system lacks a pump. A combination of extrinsic and intrinsic forces moves lymph against a hydrostatic pressure gradient in most regions of the body. A driving force of fluid movement is compression of the vessel by skeletal muscle contractions. Furthermore, collecting lymphatic vessels are endowed with an intrinsic pumping activity. *One-way valves* within the lymphatic vessels facilitate movement of lymph in one direction, eventually entering the bloodstream. Lymph collects in the large *thoracic duct* from lymphatic vessels in the trunk of the body and then enters into the left *subclavian vein* through a connection of lymphatic and blood vessels and enters the bloodstream. Similarly, lymph from the head and upper body enters through the right subclavian vein (Fig. 2.6). Thus, the physical interconnection of blood and lymphatic systems allows constant recirculation and access of lymphocytes and antigen throughout the body.

2.6.2 Lymphatic System Pathology

Not only do immune cells travel through the lymphatic system, but cancer cells that have metastasized can also move through the lymphatic vessels far from where the tumor first appeared. For many types of solid tumors, this is a common pathway of metastasis representing a more advanced stage of the cancer. For instance, in breast and other cancers, tumor cells can sometimes be found in lymph nodes that are then surgically removed along with the tumor. As a result, between 6% and 30% of patients undergoing breast cancer surgery experience tissue swelling (lymphedema). *Lymphedema* is a patho-logical condition that occurs when there is impaired lymphatic drainage that leads to interstitial accu-mulation of proteins and associated fluid. Lymphedema may also be caused by a hereditary defect that blocks lymphatic vessel development. In filariasis, a mosquito-transmitted infection, parasitic nema-todes or roundworms reside in the lymphatic system, disrupt vessel and fluid transport, and cause severe swelling in the lower extremities. This condition is also known as elephantiasis because severe swelling of the affected leg resembles an elephant's leg.

2.6.3 Primary Lymphoid Organs

The two primary or central lymphoid tissues where immune cells develop and mature are the bone marrow and the thymus. The *bone marrow* is the site of hematopoiesis and differentiation of all leu-kocytes beginning with the hematopoietic stem cell (HSC). Partially mature T lymphocytes (pre-T cells) leave the bone marrow and migrate to the thymus where they complete their differentiation and selection. The *thymus*, an organ over the heart, is divided into a cortex and medulla. Pre-T lympho-cytes enter through blood vessels and pass through the parenchyma of the thymus where they encoun-ter cells and signals that sustain their development into mature, naïve (foreign-antigen inexperienced) T cells. These will leave the thymus and populate secondary lymphoid organs (Fig. 2.6).

2.6.4 Secondary Lymphoid Organs

Secondary or peripheral lymphoid organs, the sites of antigen encounter with T and B cells, include the spleen, lymph nodes, tonsils, appendix, adenoids, Peyer's patches, and mucosal-associated lym-phoid tissue (MALT) such as bronchial (BALT), nasal (NALT), and gut (GALT). These are sites where mature T and B lymphocytes are activated to respond to pathogens. All secondary lymphoid organs are compartmentalized into regions rich in either T or B cells. T and B cells are guided to their locations by means of chemokine receptors on their surfaces that respond to chemokines produced by stromal cells in the lymphoid organs.

Lymph nodes are encapsulated kidney bean–shaped organs at defined regions throughout the body (Fig. 2.7). They are compartmentalized into B cell–rich follicles and T cell–rich paracortical regions. Antigen enters lymph nodes through afferent lymphatic vessels as soluble protein or transported by dendritic cells. Soluble antigens percolate into the lymph node through the capsule and can be pre-sented on the surface of follicular dendritic cells to B cells or continue through conduits to the T cell zone. Activated mature DCs in peripheral tissues migrate to the paracortical region of the lymph node under the influence of chemokines CCL21, and CCL19 produced by stromal cells and postcapillary venules termed *high endothelial venules* (HEVs). There they can activate antigen-specific T cells.

Naïve T cells that circulate in the bloodstream express LFA-1, CCR7, and L-selectin (CD62L), which allow interactions with their respective ligands, ICAM-1, CCL19 or CCL21, on the HEV vessels that lead into the lymph node. This chemokine action facilitates migration across the blood vessel into the

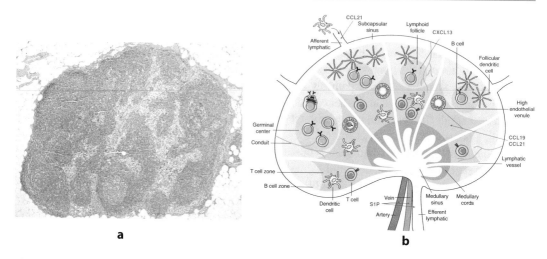

Fig. 2.7 (**a**) Lymph node organization. Hematoxylin and eosin staining of a normal human lymph node. Photograph courtesy of Dr. David Hudnall, Yale School of Medicine. (**b**) Lymph node organization. A diagrammatic rendering of a normal human lymph node demonstrating the chemokine-mediated compartmentalization of T and B cells and their antigen-presenting cells. Antigen and dendritic cells enter through the afferent lymphatic vessels. Naïve lymphocytes enter the LN through arterioles and enter the parenchyma via HEVs and leave through efferent lymphatic vessels or veins. (©Ruddle 2020)

lymph node parenchyma in order to localize in the T cell zone. Those T cells with a specific receptor for a particular antigen from the invading pathogen are activated after antigen presentation by DCs. Activation causes the T cells to multiply and change their surface receptors, by reducing CCR7 and upregulating SIP_1, the receptor for the chemokine SIP which is at high levels in blood and lymph. This allows them to migrate out of the lymphoid organ via efferent lymphatic vessels. These vessels lead to the thoracic duct which in turn connects to the bloodstream and eventually to the site of infection.

B cells also enter through HEVs, but their expression of the CXCR5 receptor allows them to travel to another site in the lymph node known as the B cell follicle, a source of the chemokine CXCL13. B cells that encounter their specific antigen in follicles are activated to become antibody-secreting cells (plasma cells). These cells migrate to the medullary cords and leave the lymph and migrate to the bone marrow (Fig. 2.6). B cells that have not encountered antigen can migrate from the lymph node via efferent lymphatics.

The *spleen* is a bean-shaped organ located in the left side of the abdomen. It is about 4 inches in length and is divided into red pulp and white pulp (Fig. 2.8). It expands when an infection occurs. The red pulp functions as a source of red blood cells during fetal development. Macrophages in the red pulp serve primarily as a filter to remove red blood cells that are senescent, damaged, or infected with malaria, babesia, or other pathogens. The white pulp shares anatomical similarities with lymph nodes having T lymphocyte and B lymphocyte sectors, although antigen enters the spleen through the bloodstream rather than lymphatic vessels. The spleen is the first line of defense against blood-borne pathogens through macrophage activity and activation of B and T lymphocytes.

Peyer's patches are accumulations of lymphoid cells in the submucosa of the small intestine. Their structure is similar to that of lymph nodes with T and B cell compartments and their respective antigen-presenting cells, as well as HEVs for the entrance of naïve lymphocytes from the blood into the parenchyma (Fig. 2.9). Peyer's patches lack afferent lymphatic vessels and thus antigen is introduced in a different manner. Interspersed through the epithelial layer of the gut lumen are specialized micro-

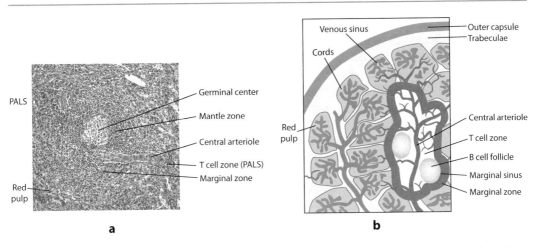

Fig. 2.8 (**a**) Spleen organization. Hematoxylin and eosin staining of a normal human spleen, demonstrating red and white pulp. Photograph courtesy of Dr. David Hudnall, Yale School of Medicine. (**b**) Spleen organization. A diagrammatic rendering of the white pulp of the spleen demonstrating the site of cell entry through the central arteriole. T cells are located in the periarteriolar lymphoid sheath (PALS), B cells in follicles. (©Ruddle 2020)

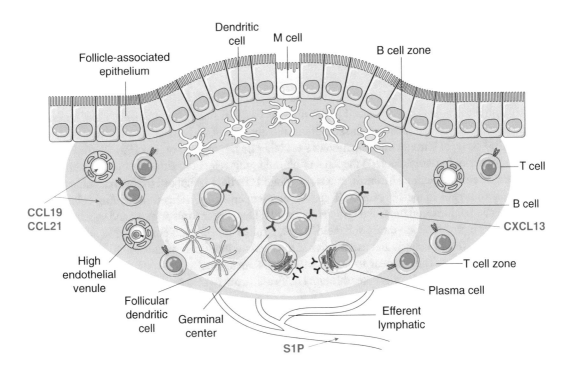

Fig. 2.9 Peyer's patch organization. Antigen enters through M cells where it encounters dendritic cells. T and B cells are compartmentalized as in the lymph nodes. Lymphocytes leave via the efferent lymphatic vessels that direct cells to mesenteric lymph nodes. (©Ruddle 2020)

folded (M) cells that are capable of taking up substances from the gut, both by transcytosis and by their expression of specific receptors for certain microbial pathogens. Foreign antigens enter Peyer's patches and are transported below the epithelial layer where they may encounter additional antigen-presenting cells such as macrophages and dendritic cells that further transport antigens to the B cell follicles and T cell interfollicluar zone. Naïve lymphocytes enter through HEVs. After encounter with antigen, immune cells leave Peyer's patches and migrate to mesenteric lymph nodes through efferent lymphatic vessels.

Tonsils and adenoids provide defense at the entrance to the gastrointestinal tract and the lungs. Humans are equipped with adenoid tissue and several tonsils. All are organized in a manner similar to lymph nodes with regard to their T and B cell compartmentalization, HEVs, and antigen-presenting cells. They also are equipped with crypts to capture invading pathogens and specialized M (multifold) cells that can take up pathogens and transport them to conventional antigen-presenting cells.

Mucosal-associated lymphoid tissues (MALT) are dispersed throughout the body near mucosal tissue. Due to their location at sites of antigen entrance, they can be considered an early line of defense. They are found in the nose, throat, lungs, and gut and are highly influenced by their local environments and subjected to constant stimulation. The appendix is a tubal protrusion at the junction of the small and large intestine in humans. Its function is unknown.

Bronchus-associated lymphoid tissues (BALT) are located in the lungs. They are the least organized of lymphoid tissues and the most subject to the environment. That said, they are critical sites of early antigen encounter and markers of inflammation.

2.6.5 Tertiary Lymphoid Tissues

Tertiary lymphoid tissues, also known as ectopic lymphoid tissues, tertiary lymphoid structures, or tertiary lymphoid organs are organized accumulations of cells. In contrast to primary and secondary lymphoid organs that are specified in fetal life in the absence of exogenous antigen, they arise after birth in the course of chronic inflammation at sites other than lymphoid organs (Fig. 2.10). Examples of tertiary lymphoid tissues include the sites of chronic graft rejection, chronic hepatitis virus infection in the liver, autoimmune diseases, and some tumors. Tertiary lymphoid tissues resemble secondary lymphoid organs in their organized T and B cell compartments, antigen-presenting cells, HEVs, lymphoid chemokines, conduits, and lymphatic vessels. They differ from primary and secondary lymphoid organs in that they are rarely surrounded by a stromal capsule, are embedded in another organ (e.g., the brain, the pancreas), and can resolve if the original inductive stimulus (e.g., microbe, auto-antigen) is removed. They appear to possess functions analogous to those of secondary lymphoid organs in that naïve T and B cells enter through HEVs and are activated by antigen. This can be beneficial in localized defense against microbes or tumors or detrimental in autoimmune diseases.

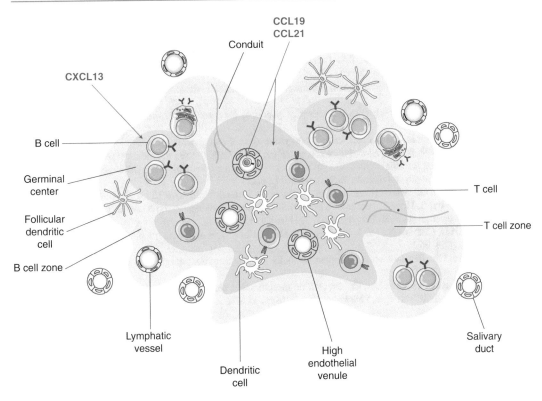

Fig. 2.10 Tertiary lymphoid tissue/organ. A diagrammatic rendering of an organized lymphoid accumulation resembling a secondary lymphoid organ in the salivary gland of an individual affected with Sjogren's syndrome, an autoimmune condition. There are T and B cell compartments, HEVs, chemokines, and lymphatic vessels. However, tertiary lymphoid tissues rarely have a stromal capsule. (©Ruddle 2020)

References

1. Akirav E, Truman LA, Ruddle NH. Lymphoid tissues and organs. In: Paul WE, editor. Fundamental immunology. 7th ed. Philadelphia: Lippincott, Williams, and Wilkins; 2012.
2. Blander JM, Longman RS, Iliev ID, Sonnenberg GF, Artis D. Regulation of inflammation by microbiota interactions with the host. Nat Immunol. 2017;18(8):851–60.
3. Bonilla FA, Oettgen HC. Adaptive immunity. J Allergy Clin Immunol. 2010;125(2 Suppl 2):S33–40.
4. Boudreau JE, Hsu KC. Natural killer cell education in human health and disease. Curr Opin Immunol. 2018;50:102–11.
5. Buenrostro JD, Corces MR, Lareau CA, Wu B, Schep AN, Aryee MJ, et al. Integrated single-cell analysis maps the continuous regulatory landscape of human hematopoietic differentiation. Cell. 2018;173(6):1535–48 e16.
6. Collington SJ, Williams TJ, Weller CL. Mechanisms underlying the localisation of mast cells in tissues. Trends Immunol. 2011;32(10):478–85.
7. Drayton DL, Liao S, Mounzer RH, Ruddle NH. Lymphoid organ development: from ontogeny to neogenesis. Nat Immunol. 2006;7(4):344–53.
8. Eisenbarth SC. Dendritic cell subsets in T cell programming: location dictates function. Nat Rev Immunol. 2019;19(2):89–103.
9. Freud AG, Mundy-Bosse BL, Yu J, Caligiuri MA. The broad spectrum of human natural killer cell diversity. Immunity. 2017;47(5):820–33.
10. Frossi B, Mion F, Tripodo C, Colombo MP, Pucillo CE. Rheostatic functions of mast cells in the control of innate and adaptive immune responses. Trends Immunol. 2017;38(9):648–56.

11. Iwasaki A, Medzhitov R. Control of adaptive immunity by the innate immune system. Nat Immunol. 2015;16(4): 343–53.
12. Lam VC, Lanier LL. NK cells in host responses to viral infections. Curr Opin Immunol. 2017;44:43–51.
13. Palm NW, de Zoete MR, Flavell RA. Immune-microbiota interactions in health and disease. Clin Immunol. 2015;159(2):122–7.
14. Randolph GJ, Ivanov S, Zinselmeyer BH, Scallan JP. The lymphatic system: integral roles in immunity. Annu Rev Immunol. 2017;35:31–52.
15. Reddy KV, Yedery RD, Aranha C. Antimicrobial peptides: premises and promises. Int J Antimicrob Agents. 2004;24(6):536–47.
16. Robinson JP, Roederer M. History of science. Flow cytometry strikes gold. Science. 2015;350(6262):739–40.
17. Rosen CE, Palm NW. Functional classification of the gut microbiota: the key to cracking the microbiota composition code: functional classifications of the gut microbiota reveal previously hidden contributions of indigenous gut bacteria to human health and disease. BioEssays. 2017;39(12)
18. Spitzer MH, Nolan GP. Mass cytometry: single cells, many features. Cell. 2016;165(4):780–91.
19. Turner MD, Nedjai B, Hurst T, Pennington DJ. Cytokines and chemokines: at the crossroads of cell signalling and inflammatory disease. Biochim Biophys Acta. 2014;1843(11):2563–82.
20. Vivier E, Artis D, Colonna M, Diefenbach A, Di Santo JP, Eberl G, et al. Innate lymphoid cells: 10 years on. Cell. 2018;174(5):1054–66.
21. Wilk AJ, Blish CA. Diversification of human NK cells: lessons from deep profiling. J Leukoc Biol. 2018;103(4): 629–41.
22. White GE, Iqbal AJ, Greaves DR. CC chemokine receptors and chronic inflammation. Therapeutic opportunities and pharmacological challenges. Pharmacol Rev. 2013;65(1):47–89. https://doi.org/10.1124/pr.111.005074.

Innate Immunity: Recognition and Effector Functions

3

Paula B. Kavathas, Peter J. Krause, and Nancy H. Ruddle

3.1   Introduction

A major question in the field of immunology was the nature of the mechanism by which microorganisms that have invaded the body are detected. It was critically important to be able to distinguish between microbes that could cause disease and an innocuous substance that enters the body such as a plant seed that is not harmful. The late Dr. Charles Janeway had noted that in order to generate a strong antibody response to a protein antigen after injection into a mouse, you needed to add killed bacteria. He called this "the immunologists' dirty little secret." The microbial stimulus served as an adjuvant, a substance to enhance an immune response. The initial discovery of a receptor that would detect a microbial ligand, or the presence of "danger," was made in studies using *Drosophila melanogaster* and independently in studies using mice. The story of the discovery in flies is described below to illustrate how studies in a variety of organisms can illuminate important principles applicable to humans. A description of the different types of receptors and what they recognize is an example of how the immune system is able to detect a variety of ligands from lipids, carbohydrates, and proteins to nucleic acids. This allows the immune system to detect a range of microbes from extracellular bacteria and fungi to intracellular viruses and bacteria. Each receptor transmits a signal upon ligand binding that evokes a response that is appropriate and protective against the type of infecting pathogen. This is a remarkable system.

P. B. Kavathas (✉)
Departments of Laboratory Medicine and Immunobiology, Yale School of Medicine, New Haven, CT, USA
e-mail: paula.kavathas@yale.edu

P. J. Krause
Department of Epidemiology of Microbial Diseases, Yale School of Public Health and Departments of Medicine and Pediatrics, Yale School of Medicine, New Haven, CT, USA

N. H. Ruddle
Department of Epidemiology of Microbial Diseases, Yale School of Public Health, New Haven, CT, USA

© Springer Nature Switzerland AG 2019
P. J. Krause et al. (eds.), *Immunoepidemiology*, https://doi.org/10.1007/978-3-030-25553-4_3

3.2   Pattern Recognition Receptors

A major distinguishing feature of innate from adaptive immunity is the recognition of pathogens using germ line-encoded receptors that bind conserved molecular patterns associated with groups of similar pathogens. These are referred to as *pathogen-associated molecular patterns* (PAMPs). The receptors that recognize PAMPs are called *pattern recognition receptors* (PRRs). In humans there are approximately 60 PRRs, comprising several families. PAMPS represent the major targets of innate immune recognition and have several common characteristics:

(i)   PAMPs are relatively invariant structures shared by large groups of microorganisms. This property of PAMPs allows a limited number of germ line–encoded receptors of the host to recognize a wide variety of microorganisms.
(ii) PAMPs are produced only by microbes and not by the host organism. In other words, PAMPs are chemically distinct from any structure synthesized by the host cells. This property prevents innate immune attack against self-tissue.
(iii) PAMPs generally are molecules essential for the survival of the microbes. Mutations in PAMPs are likely to be lethal or to reduce the fitness of the microbe. This increases the likelihood that a microbe will not be able to alter the structure of its PAMP molecules and thereby escape recognition by the innate immune system.

The best-characterized family of pattern recognition receptors is the *Toll-like receptor (TLR)* family. The first TLR was identified in 1988 as a homologue of the *Drosophila melanogaster* Toll receptor, which regulates fly development and immunity. The laboratory headed by Christiane Nüsslein-Volhard, a German developmental biologist and Nobel Prize winner, found that a mutation in a certain gene had a profound effect on fly development. She used the word "Toll" which means "cool" or "awesome" in German to describe the mutant phenotype. The gene that encoded a transmembrane protein was therefore called the Toll receptor. The interior cytoplasmic domain of the Toll receptor has a region homologous to a domain in the receptor for the interleukin 1 cytokine, called *Toll–interleukin receptor (TIR)* homology domain. This suggested a potential role for the Toll receptor in fly immunity. To test this hypothesis, the Toll protein was disrupted in adult flies; they died of fungal infection. This resulted in the discovery of the first pattern recognition receptor (PRR).

The TLR family of receptors localizes either to the outer plasma membrane or interior endosomal membranes (Fig. 3.1). There are ten human TLRs. Each receptor is specific for a different set of microbial products. For instance, TLR2 binds to lipoproteins in the cell walls of gram-positive bacteria and TLR4 binds to lipopolysaccharides in the membrane of gram-negative bacteria. Fungi have unique sugars in their cell walls that serve as targets for TLR6. Another major category of TLR receptors are nucleic acid sensors, which are particularly important for recognition of viruses that are produced within host cells (Fig. 3.1). Given that different viruses have either RNA or DNA genomes, it is important that there are sensors for both types of nucleic acids. The TLR sensor for DNA is TLR9, while those for RNA include TLR3 for double-stranded RNA and TLR7 and TLR8 for single-stranded RNA. These TLRs are localized on endosomes within the cell. TLR9 detects unmethylated CpG nucleic acid typically found in bacterial DNA. Following receptor–ligand binding, TLR receptor dimerization is induced and signaling is initiated through association with one of two adaptor proteins: the MyD88 (myeloid differentiation factor 88) adaptor molecule used by most TLRs, except for TLR3 that uses the TRIF (TIR-domain-containing adaptor-inducing IFNβ factor) adaptor. These adaptors activate distinct signaling pathways resulting in activation of the transcription factor NF-κB or interferon-regulatory factors resulting in cellular changes, such as secretion of cytokines/chemokines, antimicrobial peptides (described below), and type I interferons.

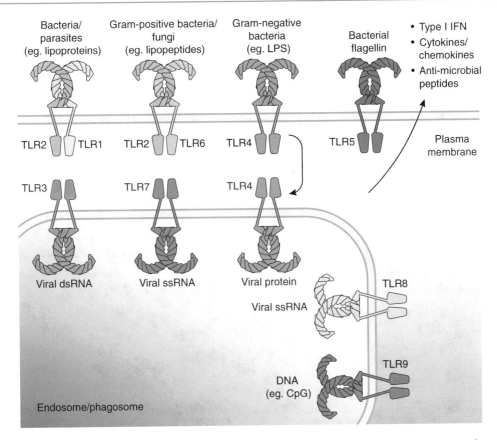

Fig. 3.1 Toll-like receptors (TLRs). The TLR receptors in humans are located either on the plasma membrane or on the endosome. Ligands bind to the receptors and induce receptor dimerization and signaling. Membrane TLRs bind structures on extracellular pathogens and TLRs on the endosome bind ligands for intracellular microbes. When TLR-4 is endocytosed, it can also bind ligands. Elicited responses include secretion of type I interferons, other cytokines and chemokines, and antimicrobial peptides (TLR-10 is not shown as it is less well characterized). (©Kavathas 2020)

Another family of receptors called the *C-type lectin receptors* (CLR) also detect cell wall components of bacteria or fungi. *Lectins* are proteins that bind to sugar molecules. Examples include the *dectin-1* receptor which binds to β-glucan on fungi or the *mannose receptor* binding the sugar mannose on bacteria. The multitude of types of pattern recognition receptors increases the probability of detecting a variety of pathogens. Another advantage of different PRRs recognizing the same pathogen is that microbes that have evolved an evasion strategy for one type of PRR (so that its PAMP is altered and no longer binds) will be recognized by a different PRR.

The *NOD-like receptors* (NLRs) are another family of PRRs that are intracellular so as to detect pathogens that are located inside a cell. NLRs have a nucleotide-binding oligomerization domain (NOD) and C-terminal leucine-rich repeats (LRR). There are 23 members of this family subdivided into three groups based on domains within their proteins. The *NOD 1 and 2 receptors* detect fragments of bacterial peptidoglycans from intracellular bacteria such as *Mycobacterium tuberculosis* or *Chlamydia trachomatis*. NOD2 recognizes a muramyl dipeptide (MDP) structure found in almost all bacteria. Activation of NLRs results in several biological effects including induction of inflammatory cytokines and type I interferons. This activation can also lead to stimulation of *autophagy* whereby host membranes surround a pathogen and form a vesicle that then fuses with lysosomes to kill the

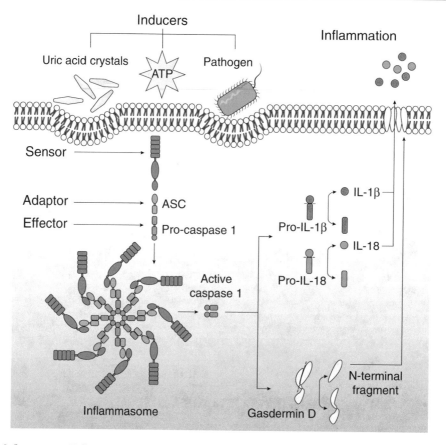

Fig. 3.2 *Inflammasome*. Inflammasomes are supramolecular complexes formed by assembly of a sensor (pattern recognition receptor), an adaptor (ASC, apoptosis-associated speck-like protein containing CARD), and an effector (such as caspase-1). Assembly is triggered by inducers that can either be microbial products or DAMPs (damage-associated molecular patterns). Two classes of sensors are NOD-like receptors (NLRs) and AIM2-like receptors. Ligand binding to the receptor induces receptor dimerization and formation of the complex. Pro-caspase-1 is cleaved into its active form functioning as a cysteine protease. It cleaves the pro-forms of the cytokines IL-1β and IL-18 leading to their secretion. The protein gasdermin D is cleaved and one of the fragments oligomerizes and inserts in the plasma membrane forming a ring-shaped pore. (©Kavathas 2020)

pathogen. Autophagy is an evolutionarily conserved normal host mechanism for recycling and degradation of cytoplasmic constituents that is stimulated in the presence of a pathogen.

Some intracellular NLR family members lead to the formation of a complex called the *inflammasome* (Fig. 3.2). For instance, *AIM-2* is an NLR receptor for double-stranded (ds) DNA which is capable of detecting poxviruses such as *Vaccinia* virus whose genome is dsDNA. When the receptor binds its ligand, it dimerizes and interacts with the adaptor protein *ASC* (apoptosis-associated speck-like protein containing CARD) to form a multimeric signaling complex called the inflammasome. This leads to activation of *caspase-1*, a cysteine protease that cleaves a pro-form of the cytokines IL-1β and IL-18 into their bioactive forms. The IL-1β and IL-18 cytokines are released leading to further inflammation. Caspase-1 also cleaves the cytosolic protein *gasdermin D* causing it to oligomerize into a ring-shaped pore that inserts in the plasma membrane of the infected cell. The pore causes ionic imbalance that leads to osmotic lysis and a form of cell death called *pyroptosis* that leads to inflammation (see Cell Death text box).

The NLRP3 inflammasome formed with the NLRP3 receptor, ASC, and pro caspase-1 is an example of a global sensor that is activated by both microbial products (PAMPs) and host damage-associated molecular patterns (DAMPS) (Fig. 3.2). Tissue damage or metabolic stress creates DAMPs that are recognized by the NLRP3 inflammasome. Recognition of DAMPS is a mechanism to indirectly sense that something is amiss such as when a pathogen has caused damage to a cell. For example, in certain metabolic disorders, uric acid crystals form in joints. These are taken up by cells such as macrophages by micropinocytosis and are transported to lysosomes. They damage the lysosome by rupturing its membrane releasing its contents into the cytoplasm. This causes activation of the NLRP3 inflammasome and joint inflammation resulting in *gout*. The elucidation of this pathway suggested a target for therapy, that is, blocking the IL-1 cytokine released as a result of NLRP3 inflammasome activation. Asbestos particles can also lead to activation of the NLRP3 inflammasome inducing lung inflammation and *asbestosis*. These are modern diseases caused by alterations in diet, lifestyle, and environment. Mutations in the NLRP3 gene are present in some individuals with autoinflammatory diseases such as *Muckle–Wells syndrome*.

RNA viruses that replicate in the cytosol are recognized mainly by the RNA sensors *retinoic acid–inducible gene-1-like (RLR) receptors* located in the cytoplasm (Fig. 3.3). These include RIG-1 that detects double-stranded RNAs containing a 5′ triphosphate or diphosphate found in RNA viruses such as influenza and *Ebola*. Another receptor MDA5 binds long, double-stranded RNAs (>2 kb). The receptors signal through the adaptor protein MAVS located on the surface of mitochondria and lead to activation of the transcription factor IRF-3/7. This leads to the synthesis and secretion of type I interferons, as well as the NF-κB transcription factor that induces proinflammatory cytokines.

The *cGAS–STING pathway* is an evolutionarily conserved detection system that senses nucleic acids of DNA viruses, retroviruses, and bacterial DNA (Fig. 3.4). This intracellular sensing pathway detects DNA of approximately 25 bp. The cGAS enzyme (nucleotidyltransferase) binds to DNA via its sugar backbone and thus is not sequence specific. This catalyzes the synthesis of cyclic GMP-AMP (cGAMP), a 2′,3′-linked GMP-AMP dinucleotide that binds to the transmembrane adapter protein in the endoplasmic reticulum (ER) called STING (stimulator of interferon genes). This leads to phosphorylation of the transcription factor IRF3 (interferon response factor 3) and production of type I interferons, IFNα and IFNβ. The existence of intracellular nucleic acid sensors raises the fundamental question of how to distinguish nonself DNA vs. self DNA in order to avoid autoimmunity. These details are still being worked out.

Some specialized innate immune cell types, such as dendritic cells, macrophages, and other myeloid cells, express most of the PRR receptors, whereas other cells such as epithelial cells lining mucosal surfaces or endothelial cells lining blood vessels express only a subset of receptors. Each receptor can trigger different signaling pathways inside the cell so that the innate immune response is appropriate for the type of pathogen and the site of infection. The inducible gene expression activated by some TLRs can be "wired" differently depending on cell type. For instance, activation of TLR7 and TLR9 in conventional dendritic cells and macrophages leads to secretion of proinflammatory cytokines, while these TLRs in plasmacytoid dendritic cells trigger secretion of type I interferons.

3.3 Principles of Receptors and Signal Transduction

The molecule that binds to a receptor and causes a signal to be initiated is called a ligand. The steps in signal transduction can be categorized as (1) *initiation* with ligand binding to the receptor, (2) *signal transduction* with propagation and amplification of the signal through activation of internal signaling pathways, and (3) *termination* of the signaling response. Some receptors bind ligand but do not

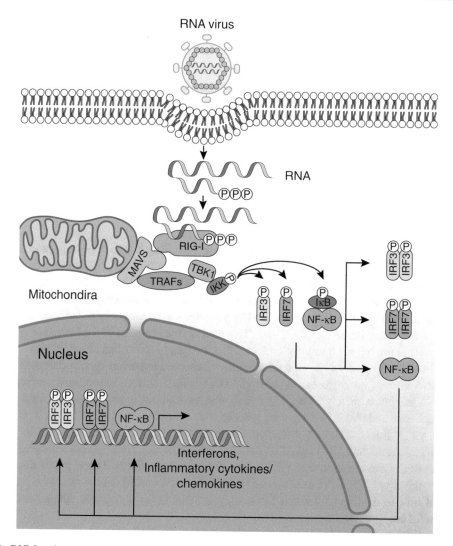

Fig. 3.3 RIG-I pathway. The RIG-I receptor binds viral dsRNA with a terminal 5′-triphosphate in the cytosol. Upon ligand binding, the receptor undergoes a conformational change to recruit the adapter molecule MAVS (mitochondrial antiviral signaling) protein. This leads to the recruitment of additional proteins leading to the activation of the transcription factors NF-κB and IRF3 and IRF7. NF-κB is normally held in the cytoplasm by binding with the protein IκB. When it is phosphorylated, it disassociates and NF-kB can move into the nucleus. The IRF3 (interferon response factor 3) and 7 proteins are phosphorylated and dimerize so that they then move into the nucleus. These factors induce expression of the potent antiviral proteins IFN-α and IFN-β as well as other cytokines and chemokines. (©Kavathas 2020)

directly transmit a signal. Instead they are associated with additional transmembrane protein(s) that provides the signaling function following receptor–ligand binding. Receptors can send a signal that is either activating or inhibitory. The ability of immune cells to interact with other cells through receptor–ligand interactions or by products secreted by one cell, such as a cytokine, facilitates communication between cells of the body.

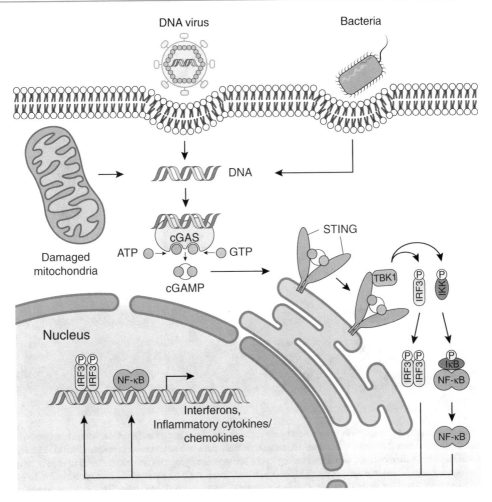

Fig. 3.4 cGAS–STING Pathway. The cGAS enzyme (nucleotidyltransferase) binds to dsDNA of about 25 base pairs. This catalyzes the synthesis of the cyclic dinucleotide GMP-AMP which then binds to STING (stimulator of interferon genes) located in the endoplasmic reticulum. This leads to phosphorylation and dimerization of the transcription factor IRF3 (interferon response factor 3) and activation of the transcription factor NF-κB which enter the nucleus. This leads to the production of type I interferons as well as other cytokines and chemokines. (©Kavathas 2020)

3.4 Responses Elicited by Pattern Recognition Receptors

3.4.1 Inflammation

Following the recognition and binding of a ligand to a PRR of an innate immune cell, a series of bio-chemical signals are generated within the cell. The production of certain cytokines, called inflamma-tory cytokines, leads to the induction of *acute inflammation* occurring within minutes or hours (Fig. 3.5). Let's imagine that a person has scraped their knee and that bacteria have invaded the dam-aged skin. The receptor on a macrophage in the skin that recognizes that class of bacteria will bind to the bacterium and send signals resulting in initiation of phagocytosis and secretion of cytokines and chemokines by the macrophage within minutes as well as protein synthesis within hours. The chemo-kines help to recruit additional immune cells, such as neutrophils, from the blood to the site of infec-

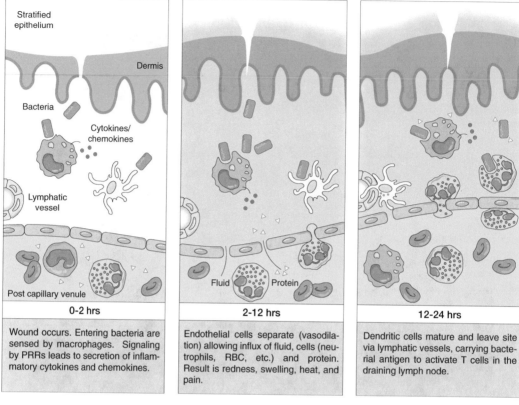

Fig. 3.5 Inflammation. Inflammation is initiated by an inducer such as a microbe, in this illustration a bacterium that enters the host. It is sensed by innate immune cells through their pattern recognition receptors (PRRs). Macrophages located underneath the skin become activated leading to the secretion of cytokines and chemokines to induce inflammation. Changes include recruiting cells from the blood into the tissue such as neutrophils and vasodilation to increase blood into the area. The four signs of inflammation are redness, swelling, heat, and pain. This process occurs in post-capillary venules. If the microbe is not cleared by innate immune cells, activated dendritic cells will migrate to the draining lymph node, carrying foreign antigen, where they can activate T cells of the adaptive immune system. (©Kavathas 2020)

tion. Certain cytokines (e.g., TNF-α, IL-1, IL-6) induce adhesion molecules to be expressed on the endothelial cells lining postcapillary venules allowing the neutrophils to stick to the vessel walls. These cytokines cause endothelial cells in the vicinity of infection to separate from each other, allowing immune cells and increased fluid into the site of infection. These changes allow neutrophils to move into the infected tissue.

There are four characteristics of inflammation:

- *Swelling* is due to fluid and cells entering the tissue. Clotting proteins form a fibrin mesh to wall off the damaged cells from healthy tissue.
- *Pain*: Swelling is sensed by nerves and inflammatory chemicals. This results in less movement and forces the injured individual to rest, facilitating the healing process.
- *Heat and redness*: The increased blood flow to the area leads to redness and heat.

The cytokines IL-1, IL-6, and TNF-α produced by macrophages help orchestrate the inflammatory response. They also act on temperature-control sites in the hypothalamus and on muscle and fat cells, altering energy mobilization to generate heat. This causes a rise in body temperature producing fever. Acute inflammation induces *sickness behaviors* to maximize resources for fighting an infection to the immune system. For instance, fatigue/lethargy, loss of appetite, social withdrawal, cessation of grooming, and suppression of libido are some of the changes that occur. The cytokines IL-1 and IL-6 travel through the blood and bind to specific cytokine receptors on liver hepatocytes causing the secretion of *acute phase proteins* that enter the circulation. One such protein, *C-reactive protein*, binds to bacterial surfaces promoting their phagocytosis. Measuring the presence of C-reactive protein in the blood is used clinically for diagnosing infections or inflammatory diseases.

Inflammation can also occur as a result of tissue injury and release of mediators such as high-mobility group box 1 (HMGB1) protein normally found in the nucleus of cells. Once HMGB1 is outside the cell, it can function as an alarmin or DAMP. This is referred to as sterile inflammation. In addition, excessive inflammation due to the overproduction of cytokines, as may occur when bacteria invade the blood stream (sepsis), can lead to organ damage and death.

Once there is clearance of a pathogen that has provoked an inflammatory response, an active process to stop inflammation and heal tissue damage is initiated (Fig. 3.6). Specialized pro-resolving mediators such as lipoxins, resolvins (resolution–phase interaction products), protectins, and maresins (macrophage mediators in resolving inflammation) are made and secreted. For example, during inflammation, the activated neutrophil produces leukotriene B4, a potent chemoattractant. During resolution of inflammation, neutrophils switch to produce lipoxins as a stop signal to limit further neutrophil recruitment. Interestingly, resolvins are produced from essential fatty acids from marine oils or other sources in the human diet. There are different mechanisms to induce resolution. During a response to a helminth infection, a tissue repair program is induced in macrophages in the presence of IL-4, IL-13, and apoptotic cells. Thus, returning the host to a state of homeostasis after inflammation is not only because of a reduction in inflammatory mediators but there are cellular and molecular mechanisms to resolve inflammation. Such mechanisms involve both the immune and neurologic systems.

An alternative outcome of resolution and return to homeostasis after inflammation is a state of chronic inflammation. If the inducer of acute inflammation is not successfully eliminated, the system then switches to a state of chronic inflammation (Fig. 3.6). The inducer is either sequestered, such as granuloma formation in tuberculosis and/or there is an adaptation. One goal of adaptation is to minimize tissue damage by reducing inflammation. Formation of tertiary lymphoid organs is also observed

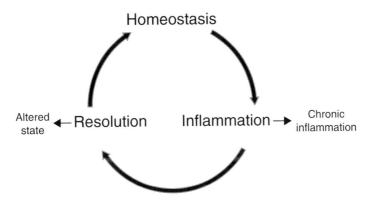

Fig. 3.6 States of tissues. Normally tissues are at homeostasis. A microbial invasion can result in inflammation. Usually, this is resolved by an active process when the pathogen is cleared, returning the tissue to the state of homeostasis. However, sometimes chronic inflammation results. Also, if there is sufficient tissue damage, fibrosis may develop and the tissue never returns to the original state of homeostasis. (©Kavathas 2020)

in chronic inflammation. In some cases, the inducer is gone, but there is sufficient damage and fibrosis so that the tissue does not return to homeostasis but rather assumes an altered state.

3.4.2   Antimicrobial Responses

Antimicrobial peptides are made and secreted during bacterial infections. Over a thousand different antimicrobial peptides involved in host defense exist in plants and animals. The two main families are called *defensins* and *cathelicidins*. Insertion of a *defensin* into the membrane of a gram-negative bacterium leads to its death. Defensins form a pore in the membrane of the microbe causing permeabilization of the membrane and cell death. Many antimicrobial peptides have dual functions and can also act as chemoattractants to recruit immune cells to the sites of infection. Some are constitutively made by specialized epithelial cells in the gastrointestinal tract called Paneth cells to ensure an antimicrobial peptide presence in the gut at all times. They produce large amounts of α-defensins and other antimicrobial peptides.

A major response to a viral infection is the production of type I interferons (IFN) by cells expressing the PRR for detection described above. Once secreted, they bind IFN receptors on the same immune cell (autocrine) or neighboring cells (paracrine) and trigger expression of 300–1000 genes known collectively as *IFN-stimulated genes* (ISGs). These genes encode proteins that "interfere" with the pathogen by inhibiting viral replication and/or boosting adaptive immunity. Type I interferons also bind to NK cells and stimulate their proliferation and activation.

Toll-like receptor signaling can induce the expression of noncoding RNAs, such as the microRNAs miR-155 or miR-146a/b. MicroRNAs (miR) repress gene expression by inhibiting translational initiation and/or by degrading RNA. On average each miR binds about 200 different mRNAs. Altering microRNA expression can thus modulate both innate and adaptive immune responses.

Phagocytosis is another important response by macrophages and neutrophils whereby they engulf and degrade a microbe such as a bacterium or single-cell yeast (Chap. 2). Neutrophils also perform NETosis to trap and destroy bacteria such as *Salmonella* and filamentous fungi (Chap. 2).

3.5   Natural Killer (NK) Cell Recognition and Response

Natural killer cells represent a bridge between innate and adaptive immune cells functioning as innate cells or cooperating with the adaptive immune system. They have mechanisms to kill virus-infected cells or tumor cells even if they have not previously encountered the pathogen. They therefore were named natural killer cells. NK cells can be activated by the cytokines IL-15 and IL-2 or IL-15 and IFNγ. They integrate signals from activating or inhibitory receptors; their response depends on the balance between these signals. The cells are heterogenous with regard to the pattern of receptors expressed on each cell. In order not to kill host cells and preserve tolerance, NK cells have inhibitory receptors that detect MHC class I present on normal cells of the body (Fig. 3.7).

There are two types of NK receptors that sense the presence of MHC class I. First, the CD94:NKG2A inhibitory receptor binds the non-polymorphic HLA-E MHC class I protein on all cells of the body (Fig. 3.7). In order for HLA-E to be on the surface, it must bind peptides derived from the leader sequence of HLA-A, HLA-B, and HLA-C; without this peptide HLA-E does not fold properly and so cannot be expressed. Thus, HLA-E expression correlates with levels of the other MHC class I proteins. Changes in HLA expression regardless of the type of HLA will potentially affect HLA-E expression. The second way NK cells sense MHC class I is through their killer immunoglobulin-like receptors (KIRs) which bind epitopes on proteins encoded by certain genes in the MHC complex

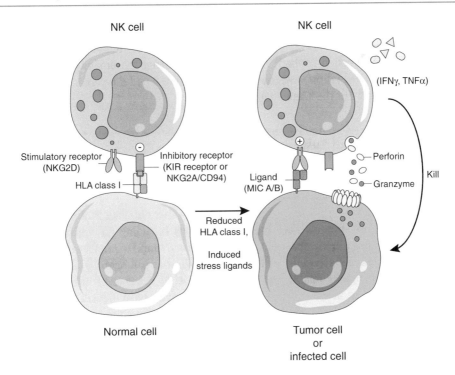

Fig. 3.7 NK cells and HLA missing self. Natural killer cells are normally in a quiescent state as they express inhibitory receptors, KIRs or NKG2A/CD94, that bind to HLA class I molecules present on all tissues in the body except red blood cells. However, upon infection or in the presence of a tumor cell that has reduced MHC class I, the inhibitory signal is greatly reduced allowing for activation of the NK cell if ligands are present that bind to activating receptors. For example, the NKG2D activating receptor binds MICA/B, a stress-induced ligand sometimes found on virus-infected or tumor cells. (©Kavathas 2020)

described in Chap. 7. The KIR receptors and their MHC class I ligands can vary for each individual as both gene systems are highly polymorphic. Both the KIR and CD94:NKG2A receptors ensure that NK cells do not react to cells expressing normal levels of MHC class I. However, if cells have reduced MHC class I, the inhibitory signals from either set of receptors are diminished making it easier for the NK cells to be activated. Host cells that have lost HLA expression because of infection (i.e., certain herpesviruses block expression), malignancy, or damage can be detected as "missing self-HLA class I" and be killed by NK cells.

For the NK cells to kill target cells, one or more activating receptors must be activated. The activating receptor NKG2D binds to the proteins *MIC-A* and *MIC-B* and *ULBP* family members that are induced on virus-infected cells and some tumor cells (Fig. 3.7). These are known as *stress-induced ligands*. In the presence of cytokines such as IL-2 and IL-15, the expression of the activating natural cytotoxicity receptors (NKp30, NKp44, and NKp46) and NKG2D are increased. NK cells kill target cells by releasing the contents of granules (perforin and granzymes) leading to apoptosis. NK cells also secrete proinflammatory cytokines, such as IFNγ and TNFα, which affect both innate cells such as dendritic cells, macrophages, and neutrophils, as well as adaptive CD4 and CD8 T cells.

An activating receptor found on NK cells with memory properties is the NKG2C receptor. The receptor was shown to recognize HLA-E which presents a peptide from a protein made by the cytomegalovirus (CMV), thus providing specificity for CMV. The levels of NKG2C are elevated on the memory NK cells which increases the avidity for binding the ligand.

NK cells can cooperate with the adaptive immune system because they express an Fc receptor for IgG antibody. When antibody binds to a virus-infected cell, NK cells bind the antibody and kill the infected cell in a process called antibody-dependent cell-mediated cytotoxicity (ADCC) (Chap. 5). This is an example of coevolution whereby an innate cell developed a receptor for interaction with antibody, a key component of the adaptive immune system.

3.6   The Complement System

3.6.1   Definition

The complement system consists of more than 50 proteins that circulate in the blood, lymph, and extracellular fluids. These proteins have multiple functions including (i) attaching to the surface plasma membrane of pathogenic microbes (including bacteria and fungi) to kill them directly; (ii) attaching and serving as a "handle" (*opsonin*) to facilitate ingestion of pathogen by phagocytic cells; and (iii) releasing chemical signals that attract phagocytic cells to the area of infection. Complement proteins are primarily made in the liver but many cell types synthesize them. The elucidation of the function of individual complement proteins has been revealed through the susceptibility to infection of individuals deficient in particular complement proteins in the serum.

Activation of the complement system by antibody that is adherent to a microbial pathogen is known as the *classical pathway* because it was the first to be discovered. In the *classical activation pathway* (Fig. 3.8), the first component of complement (C1) is activated after it binds to an antibody molecule that is specifically attached to the surface of a microbe exposing a binding site for C1. When C1 binds, it undergoes a conformational change and becomes a serine protease that cleaves two other complement proteins, C2 and C4, into fragments called C2a, C2b, C4a, and C4b. The C2a and C4b combine to form *C3 convertase*, a serine protease enzyme that splits the C3 complement protein into C3a and C3b. The same sequential cascade of complement protein cleavage and fragments of complement components combining into a single new protein that acts as an enzyme to lyse yet another complement protein continues until a *membrane attack complex* (MAC) is formed on the surface of a bacterium. The membrane attack complex consists of the combined set of C5b, C6, C7, C8, and C9 molecules and creates a hole in the plasma membrane of the microbe disrupting its osmotic integrity that then leads to microbial lysis and death (Fig. 3.8).

The complement cascade can be activated through two other pathways, the alternative pathway and the lectin pathway. Each of these pathways is initiated by a bacterial infection before the classical pathway is activated because they are not dependent on antibody production which takes a week or more to develop. The *alternative pathway* is activated when C3 is hydrolyzed spontaneously on a microbial surface to C3b (Fig. 3.8). When the C3b protein binds to factor B, it is now susceptible to cleavage by a protein called factor D. The Bb fragment bound to C3b (C3b–Bb) acts as the C3 convertase of the alternative pathway system and enzymatically breaks down more C3 amplifying the generation of C3b. The subsequent complement cascade is identical to the classical pathway. Because C3 can potentially be hydrolyzed on the surface of normal host cells, these cells have regulatory proteins that interfere with C3b binding and thus prevent activation of the complement cascade and damage to these cells. The *lectin pathway* of complement activation occurs when mannose-binding lectin (MBL) binds to a mannose sugar on a microbial surface, such as a bacterium or fungus. This lectin, a protein that recognizes mannose sugars on microbial surfaces, is secreted by the liver after receiving signals from cytokines during infection. The structure of MBL resembles a component of C1 in the classical pathway. The MBL transforms C2 and C4 to C2 a and b and C4 a and b. C2a and C4b join together as C3 convertase that then breaks down more C3. This starts a cascade that is the same as the

Activation

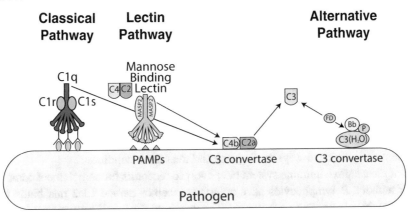

Later Steps/Outcome

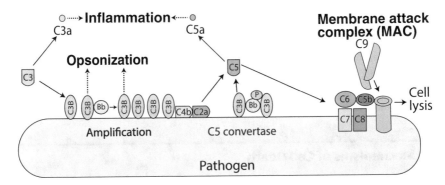

Fig. 3.8 Pathways of complement activation and effector function. (A) Complement activation occurs when complement proteins attach to (i) a pathogen surface followed by the spontaneous hydrolysis of C3 (alternative pathway), (ii) antibody that is attached to the pathogen surface (classical pathway), or (iii) mannose-binding lectin that is attached to the pathogen surface (lectin pathway). (B) Later steps in the complement cascade result in effector functions. These include attachment to pathogen surfaces that enhance microbial ingestion by phagocytes (C3b), attraction of inflammatory cells such as neutrophils (C3a and C5a), enhancement of B cell activation (C3d), and formation of a membrane attack complex that forms a pore in the surface membrane of the pathogen and destroys it (C5a, C6, C7, C8, and C9). (Adapted from West et al. [23]) (©Krause 2020)

classical and alternative pathways. Thus, the three complement activation pathways have different starting points, but all three produce C3 convertase with the identical subsequent activation process.

The three complement pathways provide redundant mechanisms to ensure complement activation in case one or the other pathways fail to be activated. They also provide an amplification mechanism for complement activity. In general, the membrane attack complex is most effective against gram-negative bacteria and less so against gram-positive bacteria and fungi. Certain pathogenic microbes such as K1 *Escherichia coli, Haemophilus influenzae* type b, *Neisseria meningitidis, Streptococcus pneumoniae*, group A and B streptococci, and some salmonella serotypes have a sialic acid or a polysaccharide capsule that covers their plasma membrane and inhibits complement binding. Mammalian cells have surface sialic acid to inhibit complement activation. Those microbes with sialic acid have evolved the same strategy to inhibit complement activation. While they are resistant to the alternative or lectin pathway attack mechanisms, they are susceptible to the classic pathway because antibody molecules can traverse these barriers and initiate the complement cascade.

As with any component of the immune system, there are regulatory processes to prevent uncontrolled immune activation. As previously mentioned, mammalian cells produce regulatory proteins on their surface that impede the activation of complement components. Several regulatory proteins produced by mammalian cells inhibit activation at various steps in the complement cascade. These include *C1 inhibitor*, *C4-binding protein*, and *protectin (CD59)* and factor H, each of which can prevent the formation of the membrane attack complex. Insufficient regulation or excessive activation of the complement system, as can occur with sepsis or trauma, can lead to widespread tissue damage. Much current complement research is focused on a better understanding of the scope of excessive complement activation and ways to diagnose and treat these conditions.

Cells of the adaptive immune system have evolved receptors for complement components to facilitate their activity. B lymphocytes have a surface receptor named CR2 that binds the complement protein C3d which is bound to a pathogen. The threshold for B cell activation is lowered when the B cell receptor binds antigen and the CR2 receptor binds C3d that is bound to pathogen. Complement also interacts with the adaptive immune system by keeping antigen–antibody complexes small and soluble, which helps prevent immune complexes from depositing in organs and causing tissue damage that leads to arthritis, nephritis, and vasculitis. C1 binds to immune complexes, activating the Classical pathway. The subsequent formation of C3b then binds covalently with immune complexes and prevents their deposition. People with inherited serum deficiencies of classical complement components such as C1q, C2, C3, and C4 not only have a higher incidence of infection with certain microbial pathogens but also a higher incidence of immune complex disease than the general public. Thus, while complement is part of the innate immune system, it can modulate and be modulated by the adaptive immune system in ways that enhance protection against infection.

3.7 Mechanisms of Cell Death

Cell death is a (paradoxically) crucial aspect of life. There are several different mechanisms of cell death. How a cell dies affects the immune response to that event. Some forms of death result in inflammation and in other forms the dead cells are eliminated by macrophages without inflammation. For instance, the normal turnover of cells results in dying or senescent cells. In this case inflammation does not occur and would not be beneficial. However, cell death can be triggered by injury or by pathogen infection and in these cases inflammation will be induced. Such inflammation allows removal of the pathogen and also contributes to wound healing after damage. The three main mechanisms of cell death are apoptosis, necrosis, and pyroptosis.

Programmed cell death, as originally defined by Wylie, Kerr, and Currie, is a process whereby in the course of normal development, cells die by a defined, orderly process that results in nuclear condensation, release of DNA and cell fragments, and uptake and removal of the cell fragments by phagocytic cells, with little accompanying inflammation. This process was termed apoptosis, from the Greek for "petals falling off." Many examples of this process occur in normal development, including resorption of the tadpole tail, digit formation, and the difference between the extremities of chickens (claws) and ducks (webs). Horvitz and Sulston began the unraveling of the mechanism of apoptosis by carefully delineating the orderly progression of cell death in the development of the worm, *C. elegans*. This was shown to be dependent on the products of a series of well-defined cellular genes. Cytotoxic cells induce the same process via a similar mechanism through members of the TNF family (FasL, TNF, LTα). This process generally does not induce inflammation.

Pyroptosis is also a form of programmed cell death that is induced through stimulation by bacterial PAMPs or DAMPS creating a complex called the inflammasome that results in the secretion of inflammatory cytokines and in cell death induced by the enzyme caspase-1 activating gasdermin to form a cell pore, releasing the cell contents. The cell is disrupted, and it releases its own "danger" molecules and cytokines, including IL-1β and IL-18, inducing inflammation.

Necrosis is a process by which cells are killed by mechanical injury, a variety of toxins, chemicals, or cellular factors that results in lysis and release of cellular contents. This process can be induced by antibody and complement or by cells of the immune system (cytotoxic T cells, NK cells) through perforin delivery of cytotoxic molecules, such as granzymes. Necrosis results in accumulation of inflammatory cells and release of additional inflammatory cytokines such as IL-1, IL-6, and TNF.

References

1. Bosurgi L, Cao YG, Cabeza-Cabrerizo M, Tucci A, Hughes LD, Kong Y, et al. Macrophage function in tissue repair and remodeling requires IL-4 or IL-13 with apoptotic cells. Science. 2017;356(6342):1072–6.
2. Boxberger N, Hecker M, Zettl UK. Dysregulation of inflammasome priming and activation by MicroRNAs in human immune-mediated diseases. J Immunol. 2019;202(8):2177–87.
3. Broz P, Dixit VM. Inflammasomes: mechanism of assembly, regulation and signalling. Nat Rev Immunol. 2016;16(7):407–20.
4. Chen Q, Sun L, Chen ZJ. Regulation and function of the cGAS-STING pathway of cytosolic DNA sensing. Nat Immunol. 2016;17(10):1142–9.
5. Crowl JT, Gray EE, Pestal K, Volkman HE, Stetson DB. Intracellular nucleic acid detection in autoimmunity. Annu Rev Immunol. 2017;35:313–36.
6. Dantzer R, Kelley KW. Twenty years of research on cytokine-induced sickness behavior. Brain Behav Immun. 2007;21(2):153–60.
7. Evavold CL, Kagan JC. How inflammasomes inform adaptive immunity. J Mol Biol. 2018;430(2):217–37.
8. Foster SL, Medzhitov R. Gene-specific control of the TLR-induced inflammatory response. Clin Immunol. 2009;130(1):7–15.
9. Goldberg EL, Asher JL, Molony RD, Shaw AC, Zeiss CJ, Wang C, et al. Beta-hydroxybutyrate deactivates neutrophil NLRP3 inflammasome to relieve gout flares. Cell Rep. 2017;18(9):2077–87.
10. Hendricks DW, Balfour HH Jr, Dunmire SK, Schmeling DO, Hogquist KA, Lanier LL. Cutting edge: NKG2C(hi)CD57+ NK cells respond specifically to acute infection with cytomegalovirus and not Epstein-Barr virus. J Immunol. 2014;192(10):4492–6.
11. Ivashkiv LB. IFNgamma: signalling, epigenetics and roles in immunity, metabolism, disease and cancer immunotherapy. Nat Rev Immunol. 2018;18(9):545–58.
12. Kawai T, Akira S. Toll-like receptors and their crosstalk with other innate receptors in infection and immunity. Immunity. 2011;34(5):637–50.
13. Kieser KJ, Kagan JC. Multi-receptor detection of individual bacterial products by the innate immune system. Nat Rev Immunol. 2017;17(6):376–90.
14. Kotas ME, Medzhitov R. Homeostasis, inflammation, and disease susceptibility. Cell. 2015;160(5):816–27.
15. Liu Y, Olagnier D, Lin R. Host and viral modulation of RIG-I-mediated antiviral immunity. Front Immunol. 2016;7:662.
16. Maeda K, Caldez MJ, Akira S. Innate immunity in allergy. Allergy. 2019;00:1–15.
17. Magna M, Pisetsky DS. The role of HMGB1 in the pathogenesis of inflammatory and autoimmune diseases. Mol Med. 2014;20:138–46.
18. O'Neill LA, Golenbock D, Bowie AG. The history of Toll-like receptors - redefining innate immunity. Nat Rev Immunol. 2013;13(6):453–60.
19. Parham P, Guethlein LA. Genetics of natural killer cells in human health, disease, and survival. Annu Rev Immunol. 2018;36:519–48.
20. Ram S, Lewis LA, Rice PA. Infections of people with complement deficiencies and patients who have undergone splenectomy. Clin Microbiol Rev. 2010;23(4):740–80.
21. Ricklin D, Barratt-Due A, Mollnes TE. Complement in clinical medicine: clinical trials, case reports and therapy monitoring. Mol Immunol. 2017;89:10–21.
22. Serhan CN, Levy BD. Resolvins in inflammation: emergence of the pro-resolving superfamily of mediators. J Clin Invest. 2018;128(7):2657–69.
23. West EE, Kolev M, Kemper C. Complement and the regulation of T cell responses. Annu Rev Immunol. 2018;36:309–38.

Adaptive Immunity: Antigen Recognition by T and B Lymphocytes

4

Paula B. Kavathas, Peter J. Krause, and Nancy H. Ruddle

4.1 Introduction

The adaptive immune response evolved in vertebrates to provide an additional system for fighting infections after physical barriers were breached and the innate immune response failed to eliminate the invading pathogen. The two main cell types of the adaptive immune system are T and B lymphocytes. While cells of the innate immune system recognize classes of pathogens, cells of the adaptive immune system evolved to be much more specific. Instead of recognizing an invasion by a gram-negative bacterium that has lipopolysaccharide in its membrane, the adaptive immune system recognizes exactly which gram-negative bacterium is present (e.g., *Chlamydia trachomatis*). The adaptive immune system mounts an immune response that is especially effective against intracellular pathogens because of its ability to recognize and destroy infected host cells.

A major question in the field of immunology was how the adaptive immune cells could have receptors with the potential to specifically recognize millions of different microbes. Even more perplexing was the fact that there are only approximately 21,000 genes in the human genome making it possible to have millions of different antigen receptors. The distinctive mechanism used by T and B cells to create millions of different receptors with one type of receptor per cell, was discovered by Dr. Susumu Tonegawa who won a Nobel Prize in Medicine for his unexpected and novel finding. In this chapter, we will discuss how this happens.

Another important feature of the adaptive immune system is the ability of naïve T and B cells to develop into memory cells. Think of your advantage as you navigate this world with your ability to "remember." Memory T and B cells are advantageous as they are able to fight reinfection more effectively than naïve cells are able to fight an initial infection. Naïve T and B cells become activated and

P. B. Kavathas (✉)
Departments of Laboratory Medicine and Immunobiology, Yale School of Medicine,
New Haven, CT, USA
e-mail: paula.kavathas@yale.edu

P. J. Krause
Department of Epidemiology of Microbial Diseases, Yale School of Public Health and Departments of Medicine and Pediatrics, Yale School of Medicine, New Haven, CT, USA

N. H. Ruddle
Department of Epidemiology of Microbial Diseases, Yale School of Public Health, New Haven, CT, USA

© Springer Nature Switzerland AG 2019
P. J. Krause et al. (eds.), *Immunoepidemiology*, https://doi.org/10.1007/978-3-030-25553-4_4

begin combating pathogens within 5–10 days after the onset of infection. In contrast, memory T or B cells respond more rapidly within 1–2 days. The accelerated response is especially relevant for long-lived individuals such as humans who can reencounter the same pathogen multiple times during their lifetime. This principle is also the basis for the use of vaccines that induce the creation of memory cells against a specific pathogen without the need to experience a serious infection.

4.2   Cells of the Adaptive Immune System

Naïve T and B lymphocytes circulate between the bloodstream and the lymphatic vessels until they encounter antigen and conditions for activation in secondary lymphoid organs. Activation of the T and B cells leads to clonal proliferation so that what begins as low numbers (10–100 s) of antigen-specific B or T cells expands to 10^5–10^6 cells to keep pace with the expanding amount of pathogen. Cell size increases dramatically, protein production increases, and metabolism changes. Some cells will become effector cells that fight the infection, while others will become memory cells. B cells can also differentiate into long-lived antibody-producing cells called plasma cells that reside in the bone marrow. An individual plasma cell produces an antibody of a single specificity.

4.2.1   T Cells

The majority of T cells have a T cell receptor composed of an alpha and beta polypeptide (Fig. 4.1) that recognizes peptide–MHC complexes. The two main lymphocyte subsets express either the CD4 or CD8 cell surface co-receptor proteins. The CD4 T lymphocytes are known as helper cells because they "help" with the function of other immune cells such as macrophages, to kill ingested microbes, or B cells, to make antibody. The CD4 T cell subsets were first identified as either T helper I (Th1) or T helper II (Th2) cells. When it was later realized that there were other CD4 subsets, they were named based on their functions, the predominant cytokine they produced, and their pattern of cytokine secretion. These include Th9 (IL-9), Th17 (IL-17 cytokine), Th22 (IL-22), and T follicular helper cells (Tfh) cells (IL-21), which help B cells produce antibody. The T regulatory cell or Treg (IL-10) is an important CD4 subset that maintains tolerance to self-antigens and prevents autoimmune disease. The characteristics and functions of these T cell subsets will be discussed in Chap. 5. CD8 T cells are known as the cytotoxic T cells because they identify and destroy tumor cells and cells infected by an intracellular virus or bacterium. We now know that it is possible for a CD4 cell to have cytotoxic function and a CD8 cell to have a regulatory function, so the original categorization of the CD4 as a helper cell and the CD8 cell as a cytotoxic cell has exceptions.

4.2.2   B Cells

The two major categories of B cells are B1 and B2 cells. They both express an immunoglobulin receptor, but the B1 cells are considered as innate-like cell and the B2 cells are usually just referred to as B cells of the adaptive immune response. The latter normally require help from the CD4 helper cells in order to be activated, but T-independent activation can occur as discussed in Chap. 5. The B cell immunoglobulin receptor can bind to proteins, lipids, carbohydrates, and small molecular groups including DNA and RNA. One of the main functions of B cells is to secrete antibody (a soluble form of the B cell receptor) after activation (Fig. 4.1). They also can serve as antigen-presenting cells to T cells and can secrete cytokines.

Antibody

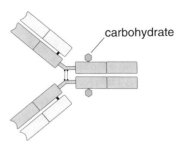

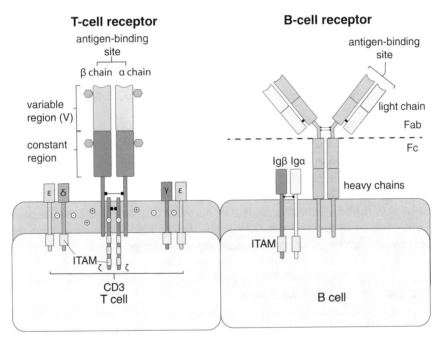

Fig. 4.1 Structure of the B cell and T cell receptors. Lymphocyte antigen receptors consist of the *T cell receptor* (TCR) on the T cell surface, the *B cell receptor* (BCR) on the B cell surface, and the *secreted antibody molecule*. The antibody lacks the transmembrane domain of the BCR. The antibody can be cleaved by papain and reduction of the disulfide bonds in the hinge region results in (i) two fragment antigen-binding (Fab) components and (ii) one fragment crystallizable (Fc) component (the effector moiety of the antibody molecule). The TCR contains α and β chains that bind antigen, but signals are transmitted by the associated CD3 complex of proteins (εδ, γε, and ζ ζ). Interaction between proteins is in part mediated by positive and negative charges within the transmembrane domains. Immunoreceptor tyrosine-based activation motifs (ITAMS) are motifs in the cytoplasmic tail that interact with adaptor proteins for signal transduction. The Igα and Igβ chains interacting with the BCR contain ITAMS as do CD3 proteins. (©Krause 2020)

The B1 cells are a bridge cell between innate cells and adaptive cells that respond within hours in contrast to T and B cells that respond around 5–10 days. The B1 cells have increased expression of the TLR pattern recognition receptors and do not require CD4 T cell help to develop and be activated. A number of B1 cells express an autoreactive BCR that cross-reacts with antigens common to many pathogens such as phosphocholine.

4.3 B Cell Receptors (BCRs), Antibody, and T Cell Receptors (TCRs)

4.3.1 Structure of B Cell Receptor and Antibody

Antigen receptor molecules on B and T cells consist of two components, a variable domain involved in antigen recognition and a number of constant domains of a similar size that are required for structural integrity (Fig. 4.1). The receptors are noncovalently attached to other cell membrane proteins that deliver activation signals to the interior of the B or T cell (Fig. 4.1).

The B cell receptor (BCR) consists of four polypeptide chains, two identical heavy chains and two identical light chains. The heavy chains are attached to each other by a disulfide bond and contain one variable domain and three or four constant domains. Each domain consists of approximately 100 amino acids. The light chain contains one variable and one constant domain. Each light chain is attached to a heavy chain by a disulfide bond. The secondary structure of each domain is composed of two sheets of β-strands that are connected to each other by short segments of amino acids that form loops. Antigen contact is made with amino acids in three loops, named CDR1, 2, and 3 (complementarity determining region) in the variable domains of the heavy and light chains (Fig. 4.1). The strength of the antibody–antigen binding is called the *affinity of binding* and is determined both by the chemical properties and size of the binding site

The B cell receptor and antibody (secreted form of the receptor) is a Y-shaped molecule. The antibody molecule can be cut with an enzyme called papain. Under reducing conditions, two identical fragments are produced that are able to bind antigen and so are named Fab or fragment antigen binding. The Fab region consists of an entire light chain and the variable and first constant domain of a heavy chain. The relatively invariant part of the antibody molecule consisting of the constant domains of the heavy chains is named Fc because it can be crystalized (fragment crystallizable). A hinge region located between the two Fab regions and the Fc region keeps the complex together and provides flexibility to accommodate antigen of various sizes.

4.3.2 Structure of the T Cell Receptor

The T cell receptor (TCR) is a membrane-bound protein composed of two polypeptide chains (α and β) with one variable and one constant domain each (Fig. 4.1). Two major differences between T cell and B cell receptors are (i) TCRs are not produced in a secreted form after activation and (ii) the nature of their ligands is different. The TCR recognizes and binds peptide antigens presented on the cell surface by major histocompatibility complex (MHC) proteins, while B cell receptors bind antigen independently of MHC molecules.

4.4 The Major Histocompatibility Complex (MHC): Antigen Processing and Presentation

4.4.1 Definition

The human MHC gene complex comprises a group of linked genes located on chromosome 6p in humans that encode the cell surface proteins MHC class I and MHC class II. The MHC gene complex also contains many additional genes that encode molecules used to execute diverse functions associated with immune responses such as the complement proteins C2 and C4, the cytokines of the immediate LT/TNF family (Fig. 4.2) and proteins involved in antigen processing. In the early 1950s, the

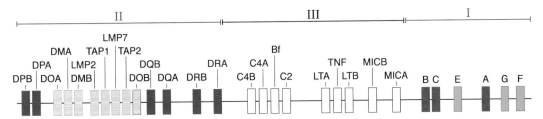

Fig. 4.2 Simplified map of the human MHC region. The MHC region, called HLA in humans, is located on chromosome 6p spanning about 4 kb. The genes encoding the MHC class I genes (HLA-A, HLA-B, HLA-C) and nonclassical MHC class I genes (HLA-E, HLA-F, HLA-G) are closely linked (region I). The MHC class II genes (HLA-DR, HLA-DQ, HLA-DP) are linked to genes for the peptide transporter (TAP), the proteasome components (LMP), and the DO and DM genes involved in peptide loading of MHC II. Other immune-related genes that are clustered in region III include complement proteins (C4A, C4B, Bf), cytokines (TNF, LTα, LTβ), and stress-induced proteins (MICB, MICA). (©Kavathas 2020)

MHC genetic region was found to be important in mice for skin graft acceptance or rejection. If two animals were not genetically identical for the MHC region, then the skin graft was rejected rapidly (7–10 days), whereas mismatch at some other genetic regions led to very slow rejection. Therefore, this region was called the "major histocompatibility complex" with "histo" meaning tissue compatibility and "major" indicating the importance of this region for matching. In the late 1950s and early 1960s, investigators were studying cell surface proteins named human leukocyte antigens (HLA). These turned out to be the human counterpart of the murine MHC proteins. The genes for these proteins are highly polymorphic (see Chap. 7). A gene is polymorphic if at least 1% of the population has an alternative allele or form of the gene encoding a protein with a different amino acid sequence. There are hundreds of different alleles for the HLA genes. Matching for HLA proteins turned out be critical in organ transplantation.

Dr. Rose O. Payne was a key figure in the discovery of the HLA genes. She studied antibodies found in serum that formed in patients after blood transfusions and from multiparous women who had reacted to the paternal HLA antigens expressed by the fetus. These antibody reagents were used for genetic analysis of the HLA system. She and (Sir) Walter Bodmer described the first three alleles of the HLA system. In humans there are three MHC class I proteins whose genes are named HLA-A, HLA-B, and HLA-C (Fig. 4.2). The three MHC class II proteins are dimers with an alpha and beta chain and corresponding genes named HLA-DRα and β, HLA-DQα and β, and HLA-DPα and β. The HLA genes are the most polymorphic genes in the human genome. Much less polymorphic are the nonclassical MHC I genes HLA-E, HLA-F, and HLA-G.

It took almost 30 years after the initial discovery of MHC and HLA to determine how the proteins encoded by these genes worked. An important discovery was made by Peter Doherty and Rolf Zinkernagel in 1975 who demonstrated that cytotoxic T cells from one individual infected with a certain viral pathogen could kill host-infected cells but not cells from another individual that was infected by the same virus but had a different MHC type. The requirement for the T cell receptors to see self-MHC as well as foreign antigen was referred to as *MHC restriction*. They were awarded the Nobel Prize for this discovery. A critical discovery to understanding the mechanism for how MHC functions was the elucidation of the crystal structure of an HLA protein by Pamela Bjorkman and Don Wiley in 1987. Dr. Bjorkman spent many years as a graduate student solving this incredibly challenging problem, but ultimately, she made an amazing discovery. The crystal structure showed that the MHC protein had a groove formed by two parallel α-helices with β-strands forming the base of the groove (Fig. 4.3). Inside the groove was a peptide of roughly 8–11 amino acids in length.

It was subsequently discovered that MHC molecules made in the endoplasmic reticulum (ER) are loaded with a peptide and then transported to the cell surface. The T cell receptor contacts both an

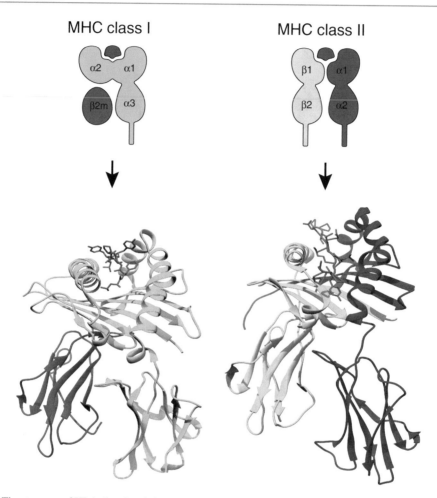

Fig. 4.3 The structure of HLA class I and class II. A schematic of HLA class I and II is shown on the top panel and a ribbon diagram of the structure determined by X-ray crystallography on the bottom panel. (i) The HLA class I molecule, HLA-A2, is a heterodimer of a 43-kDa membrane protein associated with β_2-microglobulin (12 kDa). The outer two domains of HLA class I (α1 and α2) form a peptide-binding cleft or groove with two α-helices forming the sides of the cleft and beta-pleated sheets forming the floor. A peptide of nine amino acids (LFGYPVYV) is depicted in the groove. The membrane proximal immunoglobulin-like domain, α3, is relatively conserved. (ii) The HLA class II molecule, HLA-DR1, is composed of two transmembrane glycoproteins alpha (34 kDa) and beta (29 kDa) that are noncovalently associated. The N-terminal regions of each chain forms a peptide-binding cleft or groove, similarly to HLA class I. A binding peptide of 15 amino acids is depicted. In contrast to the HLA class I groove, the ends of the MHC II groove are open thus being able to accommodate longer peptides of about 15–25 amino acids. Structures are from the PDB database (HLA-A2, ID:1DUY), (HLA-DR1, ID:3L6F). (©Kavathas 2020)

MHC protein and the peptide within its groove. If the groove carries a peptide from a protein of a pathogen or an abnormal protein, it is recognized by the T cell as nonself or foreign. Thus, the function of the MHC protein is to bring peptides to the cell surface for presentation to and recognition by T cells in order to detect the "health state" of the cell.

4.4.2 MHC Class I and MHC Class II Proteins

The two types of MHC proteins, MHC class I and MHC class II, differ both structurally and in the source of peptides that they present to T cells. The MHC class I protein is a single polypeptide on the cell surface that is associated with a soluble protein named β_2-microglobulin (β_2M) (Fig. 4.3). The MHC class I protein is present on the surface of all cells of the body with the exception of mature red blood cells. In contrast, the MHC class II protein is a dimer of alpha and beta polypeptide chain (Fig. 4.3) expressed on the subset of immune cells called professional antigen-presenting cells (APC) that include dendritic cells (DC), macrophages, and B cells. MHC class II is also present on cortical epithelial cells in the thymus where T cells develop and can be induced on the surface of other cells in the presence of cytokines such as interferon gamma (IFN-γ) or on activated CD4 and CD8 T cells. MHC class I expression increases in the presence of IFN-γ as well. Also, HLA-C is expressed at one-tenth levels of HLA-A and HLA-B and is important for NK cell responses (see Chap. 7) as well as for T responses. The nonclassical HLA proteins HLA-E, HLA-F, and HLA-G are structurally similar to HLA class I proteins but have more limited tissue expression and are relatively invariant.

The HLA proteins are expressed codominantly so that an individual heterozygous at HLA-A, HLA-B, and HLA-C can express six different HLA class I proteins. Because the MHC class II proteins are formed with an alpha and beta chain, the alpha chain encoded on one chromosome can theoretically pair with the beta chain encoded on the other chromosome (trans) or with the linked beta chain (cis). For HLA-DR the alpha chain is conserved so a heterozygous individual for DRβ would express only two HLA-DR proteins. Assuming that different DQα chains pair with similar efficiency with DQβ chains and the same for DPα and DPβ, there are four possible HLA-DP and HLA-DQ proteins in a heterozygous individual.

4.4.3 Antigen Processing and Presentation

MHC class I and MHC class II proteins acquire and bind peptides in different cellular compartments. These MHC class I peptides are derived from either host proteins or proteins made from microbes that infect cells. An organelle in the cell called the proteasome degrades host or foreign intracellular proteins into short peptides of roughly 10–20 amino acids and deposits them into the cytosol of the cell. This is called *antigen processing* (Fig. 4.4). The peptides are either degraded further into amino acids which can be reused or they are transported into the endoplasmic reticulum (ER) by two transporter proteins, TAP1 and TAP2 (the transporter associated with antigen processing) located in the membrane of the ER. Some peptides are trimmed in the ER by resident aminopeptidases (ERAP1,2) to allow them to fit into the MHC binding groove. The peptide loading complex (PLC) consists of three chaperones initially associated with MHC class I and β_2M to facilitate peptide loading onto the MHC groove. Once a peptide of roughly 8–11 amino acids binds with sufficient affinity, the PLC complex dissociates and the MHC–peptide complex is transported to the Golgi and then to the cell surface. Normally the MHC class I proteins are loaded with peptides derived from normal cellular proteins. This process of loading peptides onto MHC molecules for display on the cell surface where they can be recognized by CD8 T cells is called *antigen presentation* (Fig. 4.4).

The peptides that are presented by MHC class I vary depending on the particular HLA protein and the amino acid sequence of its groove. Most peptides have either a hydrophobic or a basic residue near their ends that interact with binding pockets in the bottom of the MHC class I groove. For example, some 9-mer peptides have relatively invariant amino acids at positions P2 and P9, as they contact

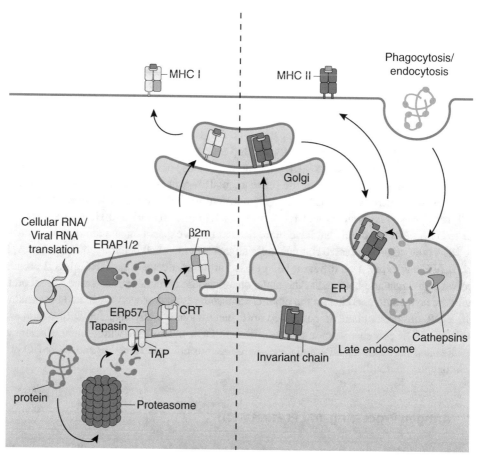

Fig. 4.4 Antigen processing and presentation pathways for HLA class I and II. The *left* panel is the MHC class I pathway in which peptides from intracellular proteins are degraded into peptides by the proteasome, transported into the ER by the TAP transporters, further processed by ERAP1/2, and then loaded into the MHC class I groove/cleft. The peptide loading complex (CTS, ERp57, tapasin) then dissociates and the p-MHC I moves to the cell surface via the Golgi. The *right* panel is the MHC class II pathway in which extracellular proteins are transported into the cell in a vesicle which fuses to a vesicle carrying MHC class II from the ER. The invariant chain blocks loading of peptide in the ER to the MHC-II groove. In the late endosome, it is degraded and peptides processed from proteins by enzymes such as cathepsins. The p-MHC II protein is then transported to the cell surface to present peptides to T cells. (©Kavathas 2020)

amino acids within the binding pocket. These are called anchor residues. The other amino acids can vary and most of them are available to contact the TCR. The positions of the anchor residues can vary for different peptides. Thus, each MHC molecule can present peptides from many different proteins.

The MHC class II molecules expressed on "professional" antigen-presenting cells (APC) acquire their peptides from proteins from outside the cell (Fig. 4.4). Proteins are internalized by phagocytosis (dendritic cells and macrophages) or by endocytosis (B cells) so that they are sealed off from the cytosol in endocytic vesicles. The internalized antigens are degraded into peptides by enzymes in the endocytic vesicles. When the MHC class II molecules are synthesized in the ER, a protein called the invariant chain binds to the peptide binding groove of MHC class II so that it cannot acquire a peptide in the ER. The invariant chain also targets vesicles containing MHC class II for transport to endosomes. The vesicle transporting MHC class II fuses with an endocytic vesicle carrying internalized foreign protein antigen. The invariant chain is removed from MHC class II by proteolysis, leaving a small peptide called CLIP in the groove that can be substituted with peptides generated from the internalized protein antigens. An MHC class II molecule named HLA-DM that cannot bind peptides instead facilitates dissociation of CLIP and binding of other peptides in the endocytic vesicle. The size of the peptides ranges from 15 to 25 amino acids, and because the grove for MHC class II is open at both ends, the peptides can extend out from the groove. Normally, in the absence of extracellular antigen, the MHC class II molecules are occupied with peptides from cellular membrane proteins or internalized serum proteins undergoing lysosomal degradation. The MHC class II–peptide antigen complex moves to the surface of the antigen-presenting cells for potential interaction with the TCR of the antigen-specific CD4 T cell.

Professional antigen-presenting cells have the capacity to internalize proteins from the outside of the cell and present their peptides by MHC class I molecules in a process called *cross-presentation*. This is important for killing of intracellular pathogens like viruses. Because some viruses do not infect antigen-presenting cells, it would be difficult for a dendritic cell to present a viral peptide on MHC class I proteins to CD8 T cells if it were not for cross-presentation. In the cytosolic pathway of cross-presentation, large protein fragments exit the endosome containing foreign antigen and are processed into peptides by the proteasome in the cytoplasm, transported into the ER by the TAP transporters, and loaded onto MHC class I. The other less efficient pathway is the vesicular pathway by which MHC class I in vesicles fuses with the endosome and picks up peptides of the correct size that are then transported to the cell surface.

4.5   T Cell Co-receptors CD4 and CD8

The main roles of the CD8 and CD4 cell surface glycoproteins are to serve as co-receptors with the TCR for binding an MHC–peptide complex and subsequently transmitting a signal inside the T cell that results in cellular changes. The T cell receptor generally has low affinity for peptide–MHC; the co-receptors help strengthen and stabilize the interaction as CD8 binds MHC class I and CD4 binds MHC class II (Fig. 4.5). The TCR interacts with the top of the MHC groove containing the peptide, whereas the CD4 and CD8 co-receptors bind to the same MHC + peptide but at a different site (Fig. 4.5). CD8 binds to the α3 immunoglobulin-like domain of MHC I and the underside of the groove (α2 domain). CD4 binds to the immunoglobulin-like domains of both alpha and beta chains of the MHC class II dimer. With co-receptors, the T cell can be activated with small numbers of specific peptide–MHC complexes. Without the co-receptors, higher numbers of specific peptide–MHC complexes on antigen-presenting cells are required in order for the T cell to be activated. In addition, the T cell receptor can recognize similar peptides presented by the same MHC protein. This phenomenon is called cross-reactivity. The number of cross-reactive peptides that are potentially recognized is greatly increased when co-receptors are present. The intracellular region of the co-receptors binds a tyrosine kinase called p56^{lck}, important for signal transduction, that is activated upon co-receptor interaction with MHC.

The main functions of the CD4 and CD8 T cells differ because MHC class I presents peptides from intracellular pathogens and binds CD8, whereas MHC class II presents peptides from extracellular pathogens and binds CD4. Therefore, the CD8 T cells are poised to eliminate cells infected with an intracellular pathogen presenting foreign peptides on MHC class I. In contrast, the CD4 T cell provides help to B cells, macrophages, and other cells fighting extracellular pathogens after recognition by its TCR of peptides from extracellular pathogens presented by MHC class II. This is discussed in more detail in Chap. 5.

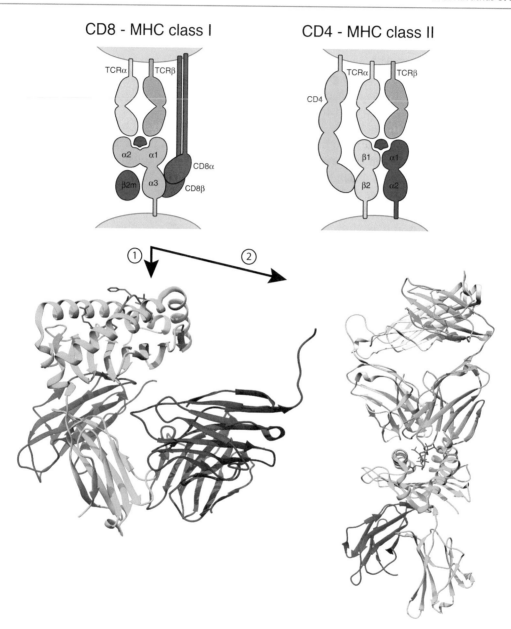

Fig. 4.5 The CD8 and CD4 co-receptor interactions with MHC class I and class II and the TCR with MHC class I. Top is schematic of CD8αβ, TCRαβ, and MHC class I complex (left) and CD4, TCRαβ, and MHC class II complex (right). Below are ribbon diagrams of the crystal structure of (1) murine CD8αβ with MHC class I (CD8-MHCI; ID, 3DMM) and (2) human TCR with MHC class I from the PDB database (TCR-MHCI; ID, 6DKP). (©Kavathas 2020)

4.6   Generation of B and T Cell Receptors

4.6.1   Introduction

The development of B and T cells with receptors that can recognize virtually any invading microbe or tumor is a remarkable feat. Instead of a single gene encoding each receptor as occurs with innate immune cell receptors, both the B cell receptor (BCR) and T cell receptor (TCR) genes are assembled from gene segments and diversity is generated by using different combinations of gene segments. This process occurs in all B and T cells as they mature in the bone marrow (B cells) or in the thymus (T cells). The antigen receptor loci for each chain of the B and T cell receptors, containing all the different gene segments, can be quite large, spanning as much as several megabases of DNA.

4.6.2 Generating a B Cell Receptor: V(D)J Recombination and Combinatorial Diversity

There are multiple gene segments called variable (V), diversity (D), and joining (J) segments in the immunoglobulin heavy chain locus. For the heavy chain, there are roughly 50 V segments (varies among individuals), 23 D segments, and 6 J segments. The sequence of the variable domain of the BCR is created by linking a single V, D, and J segment together. This occurs by a process of somatic recombination so that the segments that are initially far apart on the chromosome become linked together in the DNA. In the case of the heavy chain, a D and J segment are first joined by rearranging the DNA (Fig. 4.6). A V segment is then joined with the DJ rearrangement. For the

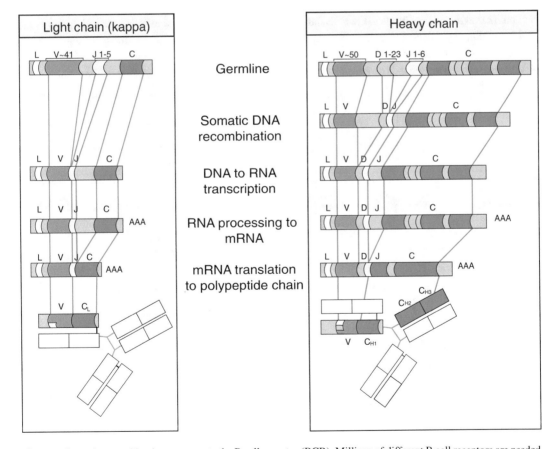

Fig. 4.6 Somatic recombination to generate the B cell receptor (BCR). Millions of different B cell receptors are needed to recognize the enormous number of pathogens. B lymphocyte genes that encode for the B cell receptor are comprised of many segments that randomly assort to create a receptor protein that differs from all other B cell receptor proteins. The B cell receptor is made up of light and heavy chain components. For the κ light chain, there are approximately 41 different variable (V) gene segments and 5 joining (J) segments and for the λ light chain approximately 30 and 4 gene segments, respectively. Final V and J segments of the variable region of the antibody are joined together and then joined to a constant region gene. A similar gene assortment and joining occurs among the 50 V segments, 23 D segments, and 6 J segments of the heavy chain. (Adapted from Parham [15]) (©Krause 2020)

light chain, V and J segments are directly joined; there are no D segments. In humans there is a kappa light chain with about 41 V segments and 5 J segments and a lambda light chain with 29–33 V and 5 J segments. The number of V, D, and J segments determine how many different possible recombination events can occur and the potential diversity for that chain. There are about a million possible VDJ combinations. The various steps in VDJ combination are shown in Fig. 4.6.

Once the VDJ (heavy chain) or VJ (light chain) DNA region has formed, it is closely linked to a genetic region encoding the constant domain on the same chromosome. Therefore, the variable encoding DNA is transcribed along with the constant domain DNA into a single mRNA that is subsequently spliced to remove introns and link the exons together to encode the heavy or light chain protein. Further somatic recombination on the other chromosome stops so that each B cell produces an IgM and IgD antibody with a single specificity. This is called *allelic exclusion*.

4.6.3 Mechanisms Generating B Cell Receptor Diversity

The rearrangement of all V, D, and J gene segments is guided by short, flanking DNA sequences called recombination signal sequences (RSS). To initiate the process of linking different gene segments, the recombination machinery binds to the RSS flanking the two participating gene segments and then cuts the DNA immediately adjacent to each gene segment (Fig. 4.7). The two ends next to the gene segments are joined to form a coding joint. The DNA in-between is lost. The proteins that do this, called RAG1 and RAG2, are only expressed in lymphocytes so that this process for creating the BCR only occurs in B cells.

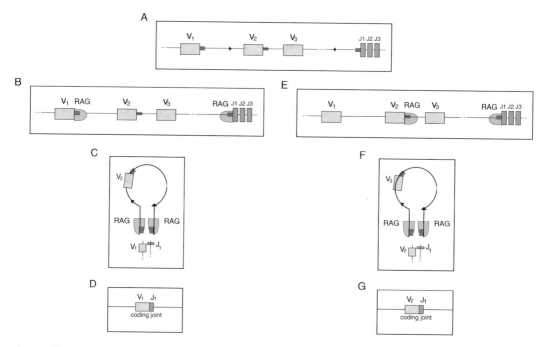

Fig. 4.7 Process of somatic recombination to generate the BCR. *A.* Gene segments in the light chain gene of an immature B cell in the bone marrow. *B and E.* Attachment of recombination-activating proteins (RAG-1 and RAG-2) to different sections of the light chain gene. The RAG proteins bind to noncoding parts of DNA that are adjacent to the V and J sequences known as recombination signal sequences and shown as horizontal purple rectangles. The same process occurs in heavy chain and T cell receptor formation. *C and F.* The two RAG complexes adhere to one another creating a DNA hairpin and these enzymes splice the DNA and hold it in place as other enzymes join the broken ends. *D and G.* The action of RAG proteins creates a coding joint which encodes a segment of the B cell receptor protein; the coding joint of D and G differ and will produce a B cell receptor that differs from the other. (Adapted from Parham [15]) (©Krause 2020)

All of the CDR loops that bind antigen show a great deal of sequence variability. In the case of CDR1 and CDR2, the variability results from which V segment is used. The V segments differ in their sequence that encodes the CDR1 and 2 loops. In contrast, the sequence for the CDR3 loop is much more variable because the sequence of the loop is encoded by the end of a V segment and the short D and J segments for the heavy chain and the J segment for the light chain. Different combinations of heavy- and light-chain V regions pair to form the antigen-binding site contributing to additional diversity. Thus, the antigen binding site consists of 3 variable loops from the heavy chain and 3 from the light chain (6 in all).

4.6.3.1 Junctional Diversity

Additional variability occurs at the joints between the different V, D, and J segments as a result of the addition or subtraction of nucleotides during the recombination process. The enzyme, terminal deoxynucleotidyl transferase (TdT), adds nucleotides, while exonucleases delete nucleotides during the joining process. When nucleotides are added or subtracted, they can disrupt the reading frame of the coding sequence leading to either a nonfunctional or functional protein. Thus, junctional diversity is achieved at the expense of some nonfunctional proteins. These contributes to additional sequence diversity in the CDR3 loop.

4.6.4 Generation of T Cell Receptors

The T cell receptor genes are formed from gene segments in a process similar to that used by B cells (Fig. 4.8). The TCRαβ receptor has an alpha chain resulting from combining of different V (variable) and J (joining) segments and the beta chain from combining V, D, and J segments. There are 70–80 Vα segments and 61 Jα segments for the alpha chain and 52 Vβ1 segments, 2 Vβ2 segments, 13 Jβ

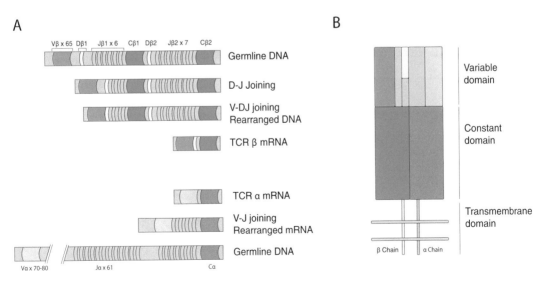

Fig. 4.8 Somatic recombination to generate the α-, β-, T cell receptor (TCR). The VDJ recombination mechanism used for creating B cell receptor diversity (Fig. 4.6) is used for creating T cell receptor diversity. Instead of light and heavy chains found in the B cell receptor, the T cell receptor is composed of alpha (α) and beta (β) chains or in a subset of T cells, gamma (γ) and delta (δ) chains. Panel A shows the transition from germline DNA with many possible V, D, and J segments for the beta chain and V and J segments for the alpha chain to a single VJ or VDJ sequence in TCR mRNA of the α and β chains, respectively. This occurs through somatic recombination in a T lymphocyte during development. Panel B shows the TCR that is created from the TCR mRNA and how each protein component of the TCR has been encoded from a specific V, D, or J gene segment. The variable region is responsible for antigen binding while the constant region is embedded in the T cell surface. (Adapted from DeSimone et al. [8]) (©Krause 2020)

segments for the beta chain. A small subset of T cells (<10% of T cells in the thymus) are called TCRγδ cells (Chap. 2). They have a TCRγδ receptor that is relatively invariant. It is formed by somatic recombination with eight V, two D, and three J segments for the delta chain and seven V and two J segments for the gamma chain. Because the genes encoding the T cell receptor delta (δ) gene segments are located within the TCRα chain locus, when the alpha-chain gene segments are rearranged, the δ locus is deleted so that T cells will not express both TCRαβ and TCRγδ receptors.

4.7   Structural Variation in Immunoglobulin Constant Regions

Five types of antibody classes (or isotypes) exist, each with distinct physical, biologic, and effector properties: IgA, IgD, IgE, IgG, and IgM. These isotypes differ in the amino acid sequence of the constant domains of their heavy chains and have different effector functions as described in Chap. 5. Naïve B cells that have not encountered antigen have membrane-bound IgM and IgD. B cells are activated after antigen stimulation and initially produce primarily IgM antibody. They can later change their isotype so that the variable domain is linked to the constant domains of either IgG, IgA, or IgE, in the presence of particular cytokines secreted by the CD4 Tfh cell. This process called isotype (class) switch is described in Chap. 5. While the structure of the receptor for each antibody isotype has a Y shape on the surface of the B cell (Fig. 4.9), the secreted forms of the IgM and IgA antibody are different as described below.

IgM Instead of three Ig constant domains, IgM has an extra Ig constant domain (four total). Three of the domains on one heavy chain interact with the same domains on the other heavy chain (dimer). A larger structure is formed by linking five of these dimers into a pentamer. The dimers are linked to together by a polypeptide called the J chain, for joining chain. IgM antibodies dominate early in immune responses and therefore their individual antigen-binding sites have low affinity. However, pentamerization leads to the formation of a high *avidity* structure with ten antigen-binding sites. *Avidity of binding* refers to the overall strength of binding between antibody and antigen. Because IgM is so large, it is mainly found in the blood and, to a lesser extent, the lymph.

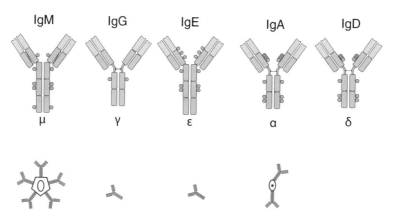

Fig. 4.9 Structure of antibody isotypes. Individual antibody isotype structures are shown. Differences exist in the number of heavy chain constant domains, the presence or absence (about 1–2% of IgG proteins) of a hinge region, the location of disulfide bonds, and the number and distribution of carbohydrate groups (shown as circles). The figures below show the structure of antibody isotypes as they are found in vivo (monomers, dimers, or pentamers). (©Krause 2020)

IgG IgG is a monomeric, divalent form of antibody that predominates in the blood and extracellular fluid. It is a major component of late and memory responses. In humans there are four subclasses of IgG (IgG1, 2, 3, 4) with different biological properties. The antigen-binding site generally has high affinity for antigen, resulting from somatic hypermutation and affinity maturation described in Chap. 5. IgG crosses the placenta so that babies are born with maternal IgG in their circulation. This is a form of protective immunity transferred from mother to baby.

IgA IgA is a monomeric, tetravalent form of antibody in which two IgA dimers are joined by a J chain which is a separate protein, generating a secretory IgA. The major function of IgA is to protect mucosal surfaces, and it is the main antibody secreted into the gut, respiratory tract, and maternal milk. Because it operates mainly in locations where complement and phagocytes are not normally present, it functions chiefly as a "neutralizing" antibody. For instance, it can neutralize toxins produced by pathogenic gut bacteria or block viral infection.

IgE A monomeric antibody produced in response to macroscopic parasites such as worms and is the predominant isotype of the allergic response. It is present only at very low levels in blood or extracellular fluid, because it is bound avidly by high-affinity IgE receptors on mast cells, basophils, and activated eosinophils. These cells are coated with IgE on their surface.

IgD Found on the membrane of mature B cells and is involved in B cell activation. Minute quantities are found in serum. Not much is known about its role.

4.8 T Cell Subsets with Relatively Conserved T Cell Receptors

4.8.1 Invariant NK T Cells (iNKT)

Given that the CD4 and CD8 T cells recognize peptide–MHC class I complexes, it is useful to have lipid-reactive T cells. The iNKT cells have this function as they respond to lipid antigens presented by a class I-like nonpolymorphic cell surface protein called CD1d. The iNKT cells have a semi-invariant T cell receptor composed of an invariant TCR α-chain and a TCR β-chain formed from a limited number of TCRβ variable gene segments. iNKT cells are distinguished from peptide–MHC class I-reactive T cells in that they are tissue-resident cells. They respond very rapidly to TCR and/or cytokine signals with an immediate and copious production of cytokines that trigger cells of the innate and adaptive immune system. They are also capable of directly lysing tumor cells.

4.8.2 Gamma Delta T Cells (TCR$\gamma\delta$ T Cells)

These T cells have a T cell receptor formed by two different chains, called gamma and delta. They are located primarily in the tissues but can be present in the blood at low levels. They have been referred to as innate-like cells because their functional potential is developmentally preprogrammed so that when activated they can respond rapidly to infection or tissue dysregulation in synchrony with the innate response. Interestingly, these T cells have a predominant TCR$\gamma\delta$ specific to their tissue location, suggesting that the ligands for the TCR$\gamma\delta$ are expressed in the tissue, though most are unknown. One possibility is that loss of the ligand after stress can be sensed as loss of "normality." Members of the 11-member family of butyrophilin (BTN) and butyrophilin-like molecules comprise another class of cell surface ligands that are modified upon cell stress. Low molecular weight phosphoantigens can bind BTNs causing a conformational change that is likely to be the active form of the ligand. The BTNA31 is essential for TCR-dependent activation of human peripheral blood Vγ9Vδ2+ T cells. The TCRγδ cells have receptors that are also found on conventional NK cells whose ligands, MICA and B, are induced on the surface of stressed cells. Therefore, these cells play an important role in tissue surveillance.

4.9 T and B Cell Development and Central Tolerance

4.9.1 Introduction

An overall goal of lymphocyte development is the generation of T and B lymphocytes with functional receptors that can recognize foreign pathogens but that do not react to self, that is, are tolerant to self. Both B and T cells arise in the bone marrow from hematopoietic stem cells. B cells complete their development in the bone marrow, whereas pre-T cells that lack an antigen receptor travel to the thymus where they mature and acquire a receptor. For both B and T cells, central tolerance mechanisms eliminate self-reactive cells during development. Once the cells circulate in the body, autoreactivity is prevented by peripheral tolerance mechanisms to be discussed in later chapters.

4.9.2 Education of T Cells in the Thymus, Positive and Negative Selection, and Central Tolerance

The goal of T cell development is the generation of CD8 and CD4 T cells with a diverse repertoire of antigen receptors that interact with foreign peptide in the context of self-MHC I or MHC II but no longer recognize self-MHC alone or self-MHC plus self-tissue-specific antigens. These events occur in the thymus before birth and before encounter with foreign invaders and result in the death of approximately 99% of the T cells in the thymus. The 1% of naïve T cells that do exit from the thymus (a primary lymphoid organ) into the periphery, seed tonsils, lymph nodes, and spleen (secondary lymphoid organs). In humans this occurs by 24 weeks of gestation.

T cells with a receptor-binding peptide-MHC class I or peptide-MHC class II are selected in the cortex of the thymus (Fig. 4.10). Pre-T double-negative (DN) (i.e., lacking the CD4 and CD8 co-receptors) cells enter the outer or cortical region of the thymus from a blood vessel. Once in the cortex, gene rearrangement events occur, as described above, as the cells go from DN1, to DN2, and to DN3. At the DN3a stage, the cells differentiate either to TCRγδ T cells or DN3b cells expressing a preTCRβ with an invariant preTCRα chain. They then mature to the DN4 stage and finally to cells expressing a complete TCRαβ as well as CD4+ and CD8+ called double-positive cells (DP). Cortical thymic epithelial cells (cTECs) express both MHC class I and class II, compared to epithelial cells in other parts of the body that only express MHC class I. At this point a "Goldilocks" phenomenon occurs; those T cells with TCRs with a very low affinity for MHC class I or II die by neglect. Those with very high affinities for MHC on cTECs die by programmed cell death or apoptosis. This process is termed negative selection. Those T cells whose TCRs have a moderate affinity for MHC class II receive a survival signal from cTECS to become CD4+ (SP) cells. Similarly, T cells with moderate affinities for MHC class I survive as CD8+ cells (positive selection). Once these events occur, the

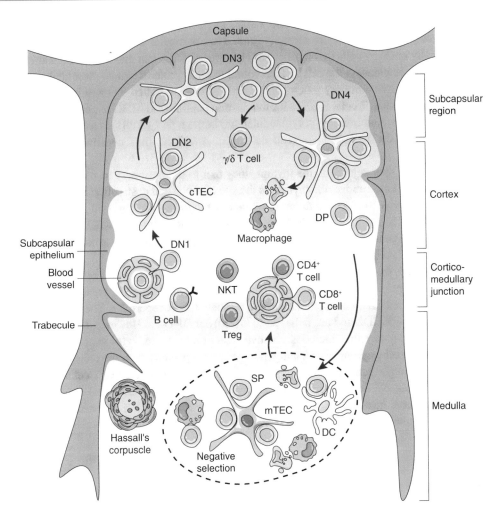

Fig. 4.10 T cell development in the thymus. Pre-T cells enter the thymus at the corticomedullary junction and travel through the cortex as DN1, DN2, and DN3 cells as their TCR genes undergo rearrangement. At the DN3 stage, some T cells differentiate into γδ T cells. Others continue as DN4 cells, eventually expressing an αβ TCR and CD4 and CD8 (DP cells). DP cells interact with cortical thymic epithelial cells cTECs expressing class I and class II MHC and differentiate into CD4+ or CD8+ (SP) cells (positive selection). If they do not interact with cTECs or their TCR reacts with too high affinity, they die and are taken up by macrophages. SP T (CD4 or CD8) cells enter the medulla and react with AIRE expressing medullary TECs. They also encounter a small population of B cells at the cortical medullary junction. SP cells are eliminated if their TCR recognizes a tissue-specific antigen (negative selection). The fully mature naïve cells leave via venules and enter into the circulation. Roughly 1% of the thymocytes survive the process to exit the thymus. Hassall's corpuscles that are regions of cornified epithelial cells, macrophages, and some dying T cells produce thymic hormones and cytokines. (©Ruddle 2020)

thymocytes express high levels of the chemokine receptor, CCR7, and migrate to the source of its ligands (CCL19 and CCL21) in the medulla.

The medulla is the site of elimination of autoreactive cells that have the potential to cause autoimmunity. After rearrangement to create a TCR, some T cells express a receptor that binds strongly to self-peptide plus MHC, a dangerous situation. Negative selection, a process to eliminate such autoreactive cells, occurs in the medulla or inner part of the thymus. A subset of medullary thymic epithelial cells (mTECs) express MHC class I and high levels of MHC class II as well as the transcriptional regulators, AIRE (autoimmune regulator) and Fezf2. These regulators induce expression of tissue-restricted self-antigens (TRA) that are normally limited to a particular tissue. Insulin, one example of a TRA, is normally made by cells in the pancreas. However, mTECs can make very small amounts of this protein. Insulin peptides on the cell surface bound to HLA proteins can be presented by mTECs directly or picked up by medullary macrophages or DCs and presented to maturing T cells. Such antigen presentation causes T cells specific for that insulin peptide plus MHC to undergo apoptosis or programmed cell death. Autoimmune polyglandular syndrome type 1 (APS1) is an autoimmune condition exhibited by individuals with genetic defects in *AIRE* and thus negative selection and is described in Chap. 6.

After T cells finish their sojourn in the thymus, they exit to the periphery as naïve cells, ready to encounter antigen. As noted above, the thymus is the site of much cell destruction and fewer than 1% of the thymocytes survive to leave the thymus. While most thymic emigrants will never react to self, some can still respond to peptides from TRAs that are not under the control of AIRE or Fezf2 and thus not expressed in the thymus. Therefore, additional mechanisms are required to avoid reactivity to self. This is the purview of peripheral tolerance, to be discussed in Chap. 6.

Two other cell types that develop in the thymus are the invariant NKT (iNKT) cells and natural T regulatory cells (nTreg). The NKT cells recognize glycolipid antigens presented by a non-polymorphic MHC molecule, CD1d, and exhibit a restricted TCR repertoire. They can be CD4$^+$ or express neither CD4 nor CD8 and are believed to arise from DP cells. However, they have a different developmental pathway that includes positive selection by thymocytes instead of by cortical epithelial cells. This pathway imparts an antigen-experienced phenotype to the cells as they exit the thymus so that they can be activated more rapidly compared to peptide reactive T cells. Regulatory T cells that have the transcription factor Foxp3$^+$ arise in the medulla. Their TCRs recognize tissue-restricted self-antigens. Instead of dying, they receive a survival signal. These cells play a role in preventing autoimmunity. Naïve T cells that have exited the thymus can also give rise to Tregs name iTregs described in Chap. 5.

4.9.3 Education of B Cells in the Bone Marrow and Central Tolerance

Central B cell tolerance is a combination of both positive and negative selection. B cell development progresses from the pro-B to the pre-B cell (Fig. 4.11). The heavy (H) chain genes undergo DJ and then VDJ rearrangements and the RAG genes are active. Then the H chains pair with a surrogate light chain and the RAG genes are inactive. The RAG genes again become active and the light chain genes undergo VJ rearrangements (Fig. 4.11). During this process, the B cell has several chances to produce a functional BCR. That is, the H chain genes are first rearranged from one parental chromosome. If this is unsuccessful, the B cell can then use the genes from the other parental chromosome. If successful, a signal is sent to cease rearrangement. In a similar manner, the light chain genes are rearranged, with kappa genes undergoing rearrangement first and then lambda genes if kappa is unsuccessful. The immature B cell expresses IgM, and at that stage a positive "tonic" signal from the B cell receptor turns off RAG expression, stops somatic recombination, and mediates B cell survival.

In the course of cell development, because generation of the BCR is random, some B cells are autoreactive. The goal of further development is to eliminate such autoreactive cells by negative selection while retaining reactivity to foreign antigens. Two checkpoints exist to prevent B cell reactivity with self-antigens and subsequent pathology. These checkpoints are in the bone marrow (central tolerance) or in the spleen and lymph nodes (peripheral tolerance). In the course of central tolerance, B cells with a high affinity for self-antigens are eliminated by apoptosis. Those whose BCRs have an intermediate affinity may become anergic or can undergo a process termed receptor editing in which

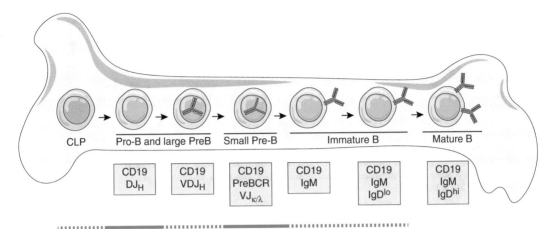

Rag1 and Rag2 expression and activity

Fig. 4.11 B cell development in the bone marrow. B cell development takes place in the bone marrow in a series of steps. In the first step, RAG1 and RAG2 expression are high in order to allow rearrangement of the heavy chain genes. Once successful rearrangement has occurred, the RAG genes are inactive so that the pre-B cells can proliferate. A pre-BCR, located in the cytoplasm, includes a surrogate light chain (dotted line) and a rearranged heavy chain. The RAG genes are active once more so that the light chain genes can rearrange. The BCR in the form of surface IgM and surface IgD are produced and the naïve B cell proceeds to the periphery. (©Kavathas 2020)

secondary recombination events in light gene segments occurs, generating a new BCR. If that BCR retains self-reactivity, the cell may again be eliminated by apoptosis or, if not autoreactive, it can leave the bone marrow. Nevertheless, some autoreactive B cells do emerge from the bone marrow. Peripheral tolerance is designed to prevent autoreactive T and B cells in the periphery from causing autoimmunity. This is discussed in Chap. 6.

References

1. Adams EJ, Gu S, Luoma AM. Human gamma delta T cells: evolution and ligand recognition. Cell Immunol. 2015;296(1):31–40.
2. Anderson MS, Su MA. AIRE expands: new roles in immune tolerance and beyond. Nat Rev Immunol. 2016;16(4):247–58.
3. Bjorkman PJ, Saper MA, Samraoui B, Bennett WS, Strominger JL, Wiley DC. Structure of the human class I histocompatibility antigen, HLA-A2. Nature. 1987;329(6139):506–12.
4. Blander JM. The comings and goings of MHC class I molecules herald a new dawn in cross-presentation. Immunol Rev. 2016;272(1):65–79.
5. Blum JSW, Pamela A, Cresswell P. Pathways of antigen processing. In: Paul WE, Littman DR, Yokoyama WM, editors. Annual review of immunology, Annual reviews, Palo Alto, California USA. vol. 31; 2013. p. 443–73.
6. Bodmer J, Bodmer W. Rose Payne 1909-1999. With personal recollections by Julia and Walter Bodmer. Tissue Antigens. 1999;54(1):102–5.
7. Crosby CM, Kronenberg M. Tissue-specific functions of invariant natural killer T cells. Nat Rev Immunol. 2018;18(9):559–74.
8. De Simone M, Rossetti G, Pagani M. Single cell T cell receptor sequencing: techniques and future challenges. Front Immunol. 2018;9:1638.
9. Flajnik MF. A cold-blooded view of adaptive immunity. Nat Rev Immunol. 2018;18(7):438–53.
10. Golstein P, Griffiths GM. An early history of T cell-mediated cytotoxicity. Nat Rev Immunol. 2018;18(8):527–35.
11. Jung D, Giallourakis C, Mostoslavsky R, Alt FW. Mechanism and control of V(D)J recombination at the immunoglobulin heavy chain locus. Annu Rev Immunol. 2006;24:541–70.
12. Kumar BV, Connors TJ, Farber DL. Human T cell development, localization, and function throughout life. Immunity. 2018;48(2):202–13.

13. Meffre E, Wardemann H. B-cell tolerance checkpoints in health and autoimmunity. Curr Opin Immunol. 2008;20(6):632–8.
14. Munoz-Ruiz M, Sumaria N, Pennington DJ, Silva-Santos B. Thymic determinants of gammadelta T cell differentiation. Trends Immunol. 2017;38(5):336–44.
15. Parham P. The Immune System. Garland Science, 3rd edition. 2009, chapter 4.
16. Roth DB. V(D)J recombination: mechanisms, errors, and fidelity. Microbiol Spectr. 2014;2:1–11.
17. Rowley B, Tang L, Shinton S, Hayakawa K, Hardy RR. Autoreactive B-1 B cells: constraints on natural autoantibody B cell antigen receptors. J Autoimmun. 2007;29(4):236–45.
18. Schatz DG, Swanson PC. V(D)J recombination: mechanisms of initiation. Annu Rev Genet. 2011;45:167–202.
19. Schroeder HW Jr, Cavacini L. Structure and function of immunoglobulins. J Allergy Clin Immunol. 2010;125(2. Suppl 2):S41–52.
20. Takaba H, Takayanagi H. The mechanisms of T cell selection in the thymus. Trends Immunol. 2017;38(11):805–16.
21. Trowsdale J, Knight JC. Major histocompatibility complex genomics and human disease. Annu Rev Genomics Hum Genet. 2013;14:301–23.
22. Vantourout P, Laing A, Woodward MJ, Zlatareva I, Apolonia L, Jones AW, et al. Heteromeric interactions regulate butyrophilin (BTN) and BTN-like molecules governing gammadelta T cell biology. Proc Natl Acad Sci U S A. 2018;115(5):1039–44.
23. Wang R, Natarajan K, Margulies DH. Structural basis of the CD8 alpha beta/MHC class I interaction: focused recognition orients CD8 beta to a T cell proximal position. J Immunol. 2009;183(4):2554–64.
24. Wardemann H, Yurasov S, Schaefer A, Young JW, Meffre E, Nussenzweig MC. Predominant autoantibody production by early human B cell precursors. Science. 2003;301(5638):1374–7.
25. Wencker M, Turchinovich G, Di Marco Barros R, Deban L, Jandke A, Cope A, et al. Innate-like T cells straddle innate and adaptive immunity by altering antigen-receptor responsiveness. Nat Immunol. 2014;15(1):80–7.
26. Zhao X, Sankaran S, Yap J, Too CT, Ho ZZ, Dolton G, et al. Nonstimulatory peptide-MHC enhances human T-cell antigen-specific responses by amplifying proximal TCR signaling. Nat Commun. 2018;9(1):2716.
27. Zinkernagel RM, Doherty PC. Immunological surveillance against altered self components by sensitised T lymphocytes in lymphocytic choriomeningitis. Nature. 1974;251(5475):547–8.
28. Zoete V, Irving M, Ferber M, Cuendet MA, Michielin O. Structure-based, rational design of T cell receptors. Front Immunol. 2013;4:268.

Adaptive Immunity: Effector Functions, Regulation, and Vaccination

5

Paula B. Kavathas, Peter J. Krause, and Nancy H. Ruddle

5.1 Introduction

A key feature of the adaptive immune response is its ability to respond effectively and appropriately to invasion by a microbe. An analogy would be the varied response a person would exhibit depending on whether a raccoon or a fly entered their room. The response to an infection by a helminth must be different than the response to a viral infection. Naïve CD4 T cells that are activated by an antigen-presenting cell (APC) will differentiate into subsets that have effector functions appropriate for the pathogen encountered. Cytokines secreted by the APCs play an important role in determining the type of CD4 effector cell that develops. Similarly, activated B cells that initially secrete antibody of the IgM isotype will later secrete antibody of a different isotype with an effector function best suited for the type of pathogen. When an inappropriate CD4 effector cell is generated in response to a pathogen, pathology may ensue.

While activation of immune cells is critical, it is also important to downregulate immune responses. Therefore, there are multiple mechanisms designed to inhibit the immune response. One such mechanism is the expression of inhibitory receptors. Both activating and inhibitory receptors exist on the surface of immune cells to regulate their responses. The correct magnitude of response requires a balance between activating and inhibitory signals to both clear the pathogen yet avoid tissue pathology. When the immune system is unable to clear a pathogen and enters a state of chronic inflammation, immune T cells can acquire a state of "exhaustion," whereby they are alive but not functional. In this case they express multiple inhibitory receptors. This reduces the damage caused by chronic inflammation. Therapies that block inhibitory receptors are now used in the clinic for cancer immunotherapy allowing previously blocked or "exhausted" CD8 cytotoxic cells to kill the tumor (Chap. 16).

P. B. Kavathas (✉)
Departments of Laboratory Medicine and Immunobiology, Yale School of Medicine, New Haven, CT, USA
e-mail: paula.kavathas@yale.edu

P. J. Krause
Department of Epidemiology of Microbial Diseases, Yale School of Public Health and Departments of Medicine and Pediatrics, Yale School of Medicine, New Haven, CT, USA

N. H. Ruddle
Department of Epidemiology of Microbial Diseases, Yale School of Public Health, New Haven, CT, USA

© Springer Nature Switzerland AG 2019
P. J. Krause et al. (eds.), *Immunoepidemiology*, https://doi.org/10.1007/978-3-030-25553-4_5

5.2   T Cell Activation

5.2.1   Activation by Antigen-Presenting Cells

Once naïve T cells leave the thymus, they circulate throughout the body between the lymphatic and vascular systems and eventually enter the secondary lymphoid organs through high endothelial venules (HEVs). They are guided to T cell zones in the lymph nodes and spleen through the interaction of chemokines CCL19 and CCL21 that are expressed in the T cell zone and CCR7, a chemokine receptor on naïve T cells. Dendritic cells (DCs), which also express CCR7, transport antigens from sites of infection to the T cell areas of the draining lymph node. Activation of a T cell occurs during interaction between a mature dendritic cell and a T cell with a receptor that recognizes the specific foreign peptide antigen and MHC molecule that presents the antigen on the dendritic cell surface (Fig. 5.1).

Dendritic cells reside in tissues where they express MHC class I but not MHC class II proteins. Once a pathogen is detected by its pattern recognition receptor (PRR), the DC ingests the pathogen and undergoes a maturation process. It expresses high amounts of both MHC class I and MHC class II proteins with antigen for presentation to T cells. The DC also expresses a lymph node homing receptor, CCR7, that facilitates its migration through afferent lymphatic vessels to the draining lymph node and then to the T cell zone. The activated DC also expresses co-stimulatory proteins that are important for T cell activation, including B7.1 (CD80) and B7.2 (CD86). Once the DC is in the T cell (paracortical) area of the lymph node, it interacts transiently with many different T cells until it encounters that particular T cell whose T cell receptor (TCR) and co-receptor (CD4 or CD8) binds peptide+MHC with a high enough affinity to transmit a signal into the T cell. This interaction of DC peptide-MHC with a naïve T cell TCR is termed signal 1.

In order to ensure that the T cell is only activated when a pathogen is present, a second signal is required. The co-stimulatory molecules, B7.1 (CD80) and B7.2 (CD86), on the mature DC bind to the

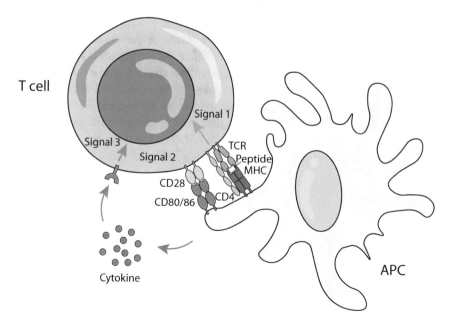

Fig. 5.1 Three signals are necessary to activate a naïve CD4 T cell. Signal 1, peptide plus MHC II; signal 2, costimulator; signal 3, cytokine. (©Ruddle 2020)

T cell surface protein CD28 receptor that then transmits signal 2 to the T cell. Signals 1 and 2 induce changes in the T cell, including an increase in cell surface adhesion molecules, that facilitate interactions between the T cell and the DC for several hours. At this point, the T cell is in a state of weak activation. For full activation and differentiation, a third signal is required. This occurs when a cytokine secreted by the DC binds to a cytokine receptor on the T cell. This process is called priming the T cell and constitutes signal 3 (Fig. 5.1).

Why are three signals necessary? Signal 1 through the T cell receptor provides specificity for a particular peptide from a particular pathogen so that the appropriate T cell proliferates. Signal 2 through the co-stimulatory proteins, B7.1 (CD80) and B7.2 (CD86), is the result of PAMP recognition by the DC through its pattern recognition receptor (PRR). This ensures that T cell activation occurs only when a pathogen is present. Cytokine signal 3 helps direct the nature of the T cell response so that its function is most appropriate for the type of invading pathogen. The cytokines made by the DC vary depending on which type of pathogen is present and the PRR that is activated. The naïve CD4 can differentiate into one of at least seven subtypes with different functions depending on the cytokines that are present in the milieu.

Once T cells are activated in the secondary lymphoid organs, they proliferate, differentiate, and produce effector molecules. This requires rewiring of cellular metabolism to meet the increased energy needs. The two main pathways to supply ATP are by glycolysis (breaking down glucose) and oxidative phosphorylation (OXPHOS) in the mitochondria. Naive and memory T cells rely on catabolic metabolism (energy-generating) whereas effector T cells engage in glycolysis and anabolic metabolism (energy-consuming). Building blocks for cell proliferation (lipids for membranes, proteins, nucleic acids) are produced by various anabolic processes. In addition, different metabolic pathways are activated for different kinds of effector responses. The fully activated effector T cells enter the circulation and migrate to the site of infection. This is accomplished by downregulating CCR7, upregulating S1P1 (the receptor for SIP in lymphatic vessels), and upregulating adhesion molecules and chemokine receptors that bind chemokines secreted by macrophages at the infection site. Effector T cells are short lived and die after the infection is cleared (Fig. 5.2). Some activated

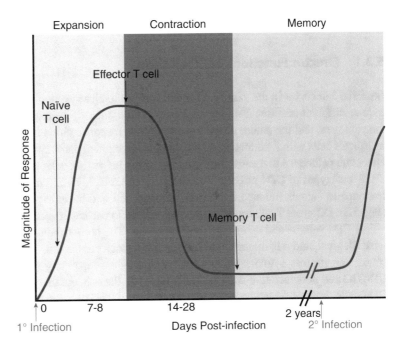

Fig. 5.2 Kinetics of a T cell response. Activated naïve T cells begin to proliferate and differentiate reaching a peak of effector cells between 7 and 10 days. These are short-lived cells, dying as the infection is cleared. Long-lived memory T cells remain that can be reactivated years later with the same pathogen. The response is more rapid and stronger than in the primary infection. (©Kavathas 2020)

T cells become memory T cells that are long lived. The next time the same pathogen is detected, they respond with a more rapid and vigorous response.

5.2.2   Activation by Superantigens

Superantigens are products of certain strains of *Staphylococcus aureus*, group A *Streptococcus*, or other microbes that are released extracellularly as toxins and act as nonspecific polyclonal T cell mitogens and cytokine inducers. Superantigens are not processed by antigen-presenting cells but, rather, are presented as intact proteins by macrophages to T cells. They simultaneously bind to MHC class II and the β chain of the TCR on CD4+ T cells. This crosslinking of the TCR and MHC class II mimics signal 1 and activates T cells; signals 2 and 3 are provided by the macrophage. A particular superantigen can activate 5–20% of an individual's total T cells, in contrast to the ability of a peptide+MHC complex to activate less than 0.01% of T cells. Superantigens induce massive production of cytokines, particularly TNF, IL-1, and IL-6. This cytokine storm can result in serious consequences with systemic toxicity, including shock and even death. *Staphylococcus aureus* toxic shock toxin (TSST-1) is a superantigen that induces fever, shock, and skin peeling. Human populations vary in their susceptibility to superantigens due to polymorphisms in MHC class II, which influences the binding of the superantigen. Treatment of superantigen-induced disease includes intravenous immunoglobulin (IVIg) and antibiotics.

5.3   T Cell Effector Functions

The pathway of differentiation that an activated naïve T cell takes is determined by the nature of the MHC molecule (class I or class II) presenting the peptide that is recognized by the T cell receptor, the concentration of antigen, and the identity of the cytokines in the immediate environment of the T cell when it recognizes its antigen. This microenvironment reflects the nature of the innate immune response at the site of infection and the site of priming.

5.3.1   Effector Functions of CD4 T Cells

Bacterial infections in the skin, viral infections in the airways, and helminth intestinal infections all require different adaptive immune responses. The tissue of origin of the activated DC, the nature of the pathogen, and the nature of the innate immune response guide the differentiation of CD4 T cells to effector cells with functions best suited to the infection at hand. Effector CD4 T cells do not directly attack the pathogens that cause infection but rather help other cells to achieve that goal.

Several types of CD4 effector T cells (Th1, Th2, Th17, Th22 Th9, Tfh, and Treg) differentiate in response to signals induced by various stromal cell and antigen-presenting cell-derived cytokines (Fig. 5.3). Different T cell transcription factors lead to particular sets of cytokines that define the individual CD4 subsets and determine their functions. The nomenclature of these effector cells is somewhat illogical, and it is important to keep in mind that a certain amount of plasticity exists so that one subset can express cytokines characteristic of another depending on the milieu. The CD4Th1 and CD4Th2 cell nomenclature was originally based on the concept that there were two different types of CD4 cells, both of which could "help" other cells. CD4Th1 cells that produce IL-2 and IFNγ were considered proinflammatory in their ability to activate other T cells and macrophages. CD4Th2 cells that produce IL-4 were originally considered as B cell helpers. In fact, it is clear that several additional

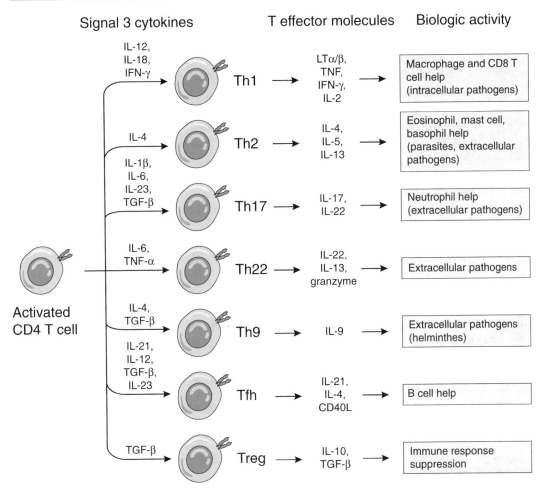

Fig. 5.3 Cytokine milieu (signal 3) determines CD4 T cell subset polarization. Signals 1 and 2 from the antigen-presenting cell activate the CD4⁺ T cell. Signal 3 polarizes the T cell to an effector cell subset that is defined by its cytokine profile. (©Ruddle 2020)

T cell subsets (Th1, Th17, Tfh) also help B cells. The logical step would have been to name the next functional type as Th3, but instead it was named Th17 because of its predominant production of the cytokines IL-17A and IL-17E. Th17 cells also produce IL-21 and IL-22. Later, it was realized that another T cell subset (Th22) produces even higher levels of IL-22, in addition to IL-13 and granzyme B. Th9 cells were named for their production of IL-9. Two other CD4 subsets were named for their functions. Tfh (follicular helper) cells help activate B cells in lymph node follicles; Treg (regulatory) cells dampen immune responses. After T cells have been "polarized" by DCs into various subsets (Th1, Th2, Th17, Th9, Th22, and Tregs), they move out of the lymph node to the site of infection. In contrast, Tfh cells downregulate CCR7 and upregulate CXCL13 which allows them to migrate to the CCR5-rich B cell follicular area of secondary lymphoid organs to help activate B cells. We now provide a more complete description of CD4⁺ T cell subsets to better appreciate the diverse role these cells play in the immune response.

Th1 cells help macrophages kill ingested bacteria, fungi, and viruses by producing the cytokine, interferon gamma (IFN-γ), which stimulates the formation of reactive oxygen species and nitric oxide in the phagolysosome within the macrophage. Infected macrophages present peptides from pathogen proteins on MHC-II molecules on their surface. The CD4 TCR binds to the specific peptide-MHC-II complex (signal 1). The CD4 T effector cell also expresses CD40 ligand that binds to it's receptor, CD40, on the macrophage (signal 2). This causes the CD4 cell to secrete IFN-γ that binds to another receptor on the macrophage and enhances formation of reactive oxygen species and nitric oxide. Neighboring macrophages can also bind IFN-γ as well. Th1 cells and macrophages produce TNFα that induces chemokines and adhesion molecules on blood endothelial cells, encouraging influx of additional inflammatory cells and complement-containing plasma through the blood vessels to the infected tissue. Th1 cells also secrete large quantities of IL-2 that enhances CD8 T cell proliferation and survival.

Th2 cells help eosinophils, basophils, mast cells, and B cells respond to and eliminate parasites and extracellular bacteria. The CD4 Th2 effector cells secrete the cytokines IL-4 and IL-13 that cause B cells to produce IgE antibody. IgE binds to eosinophils and mast cells by the Fc portion of the antibody. When the Fab portion of the antibody binds helminth (worm) antigen, these cells release their granules with broad-ranging effects that help eliminate helminths. Th2 cells also secrete IL-5 that recruit and activate eosinophils, mast cells, and basophils. Th2 cells are instrumental in allergic reactions.

Th17 cells help fight extracellular bacteria and fungi. Their cytokines IL-17 and IL-22 lead to the recruitment of neutrophils to eliminate the bacteria or fungus. They also promote production of antimicrobial peptides in the epithelial lining of the gastrointestinal tract and enhance the integrity of the epithelial barrier. Th17 cells contribute to pathogenesis of autoimmunity.

Th22 cells were originally confused with Th17 cells since both cell types produce the IL-22 cytokine. Recent studies strongly suggest that they are a distinct lineage with production of granzyme B and IL-13.

Th9 cells play a role in defense against helminths and tumors and have been implicated in the pathology of inflammatory bowel disease and allergic responses. They produce high levels of IL-9 and have been known to also produce IL-10 and IL-21.

Tfh cells migrate into the B cell follicle and produce Bcl6, IL-4, IL-21, and CD40L. They help activate naïve B cells in secondary lymphoid organs to differentiate, divide, mutate, and isotype switch to produce antibodies of different classes.

T reg cells recognize self tissue. They develop and are activated in the thymus as natural T regulatory cells (nTreg) or peripheral tissue as induced T regulatory (iTreg) cells. These cells produce IL-10 and IL-35 that control and limit the activities of other types of effector CD4$^+$ T cells and CD8$^+$ T cells. They function to dampen the activation of T cells to reduce tissue destruction and immunopathology. Treg cells are part of the peripheral tolerance sytem that inactivates T cells targeted against self tissue to help prevent autoimmunity.

5.3.2 Effector Functions of CD8 T Cells

Naïve CD8$^+$ T cells, like naïve CD4$^+$ T cells, are activated by three signals: (i) a T cell receptor signal after it recognizes and binds an antigen-MHC-I complex on an antigen-presenting cell, (ii) a costimulation signal when CD28 from an antigen-presenting cell binds to B7.1 or B7.2 on the T cell, and (iii) a cytokine receptor signal after the T cell binds cytokine released from an antigen-presenting cell. CD8$^+$ T cells primarily differentiate into CD8$^+$ cytotoxic T lymphocytes (CTL) that kill tissue cells infected by an intracellular pathogen such as a virus (Fig. 5.4). In general, they recognize "foreign" peptides that are synthesized by the target cell. CTLs move out of the secondary lymphoid organs to the site of the infection where they kill infected cells and their microbial contents.

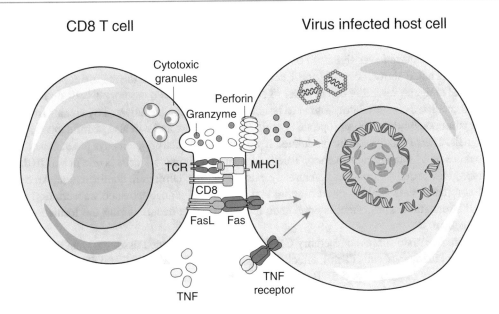

Fig. 5.4 Virus-specific cytolytic CD8+ cell induces apoptosis in virus-infected target cell. The CD8+ T cell recognizes a viral peptide on MHC class I on a host cell. It employs three different mechanisms to kill the target cell (FasL-Fas, TNF-TNFR1, cytotoxic granules). Perforin is released to form a pore through which caspase enters and induces apoptosis, apparent as DNA fragmentation. (©Ruddle 2020)

CTLs destroy infected cells with a variety of different molecules and induce either apoptosis or necroptosis. As noted in the chapter on innate immunity, apoptosis is an orderly process of programmed cell death that occurs in development and contributes to remodeling of tissues (e.g., digit formation) and is defined by characteristic changes including DNA fragmentation. Necroptosis is also a programmed cell death but occurs through different mechanisms and causes some inflammation, unlike apoptosis. CTLs initiate apoptosis when they express a cell surface molecule, Fas ligand (FasL), which triggers Fas protein on the target to direct that cell to undergo apoptosis. The Fas signal activates a series of proteolytic enzymes, including caspase 8. CTLs also contain cytotoxic granules containing granzymes and perforin. When the CTL recognizes its target, a change occurs in the microtubule-organizing center, and the granules move to a site of cell contact, allowing local and directed release of granule contents. Upon release, perforin undergoes a conformational change and is inserted into the membrane of the target cell, forming a pore. The granzymes enter the cell through the pore and induce apoptosis through activation of caspases. CTLs also express TNF and LTα which can kill by interacting with TNF receptors on the target cell and initiate apoptosis.

5.4   Memory

5.4.1   Introduction

The formation of long-lived memory T and B cells is a key feature of adaptive immunity. These antigen-experienced cells live for 25 years or more in constrast to the naïve T cell that can persist for 5–10 years. The ability of these cells to be more rapidly activated upon reencounter with a pathogen provides protection for decades against re-exposure to the same pathogen.

5.4.2 Memory T Cells

Memory T cells require fewer signals to be activated than naïve T cells and are activated more rapidly (1–2 days). As noted above, normally, the T cell needs three signals from the mature dendritic or other professional antigen-presenting cell in order to be activated. However, memory T cells do not require the CD28-mediated co-stimulatory signal to be activated. They can be activated by signals from the T cell receptor upon binding the appropriate peptide-MHC complex and will also be influenced by cytokine signals. Their function can be modulated if various co-stimulatory pathways are activated.

The more rapid activation of memory T cells compared with naïve T cells is due in part to the fact that those genes required for activation already exist in an open chromatin conformation. An open or poised chromatin state enables rapid binding and function of signal-activated transcription factors after cell stimulation. Thus, there is epigenetic remodeling that occurs during the formation of the memory cell.

There are five main subsets of memory CD4 and CD8 T cells named tissue-resident memory cells (Trm), central memory T cells (Tcm), effector memory T cells (Tem), peripheral memory (Tpm), and stem cell memory (Tscm) (Fig. 5.5). Both the Tcm and Tem cells are capable of producing the cytokine IL-2 for proliferation and effector cytokines after activation. However, Tcm cells exhibit lymphoid-homing properties and so are primarily found in lymphoid tissues, whereas Tem cells circulate in peripheral tissues and the blood. Tcm cells have a higher proliferative capacity compared with Tem cells; Tem cells generally produce higher levels of effector cytokines. Tscm is a relatively rare subtype. These cells are capable of self-renewal and proliferation but not effector function. Tissue

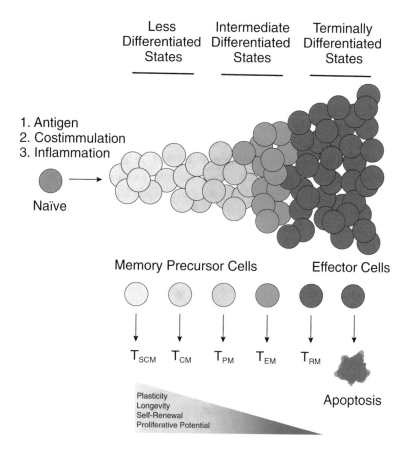

Fig. 5.5 Generation of CD8 effector and memory cells from precursor cells. Naïve CD8+ T cells are activated by a virus-infected cell (three signals). In a series of steps involving expansion and contraction, memory and effector cells ae generated from stem cell memory (Tscm) to central memory (Tcm), peripheral memory (Tpm), effector memory (Tem), and tissue-resident memory (Trm) cells. Finally, effector cells respond to virus-infected cells and can undergo apoptosis, although memory populations remain. Courtesy of Susan Kaech, PhD. Salk Institute. (©Ruddle 2020)

resident memory (Trm) cells are noncirculating cells located in the tissues poised to respond to pathogens that have previously infected that tissue such as Trm cells in the lung responding to lung respiratory viruses. Trm cells are found in multiple sites, including barrier sites such as the skin, intestine, reproductive tract, and lung, as well as in lymphoid sites. Functionally they have both proinflammatory and regulatory capabilities with low turnover. CD8 cells have one additional memory population which are end-stage cells that do not proliferate but can be cytotoxic. These are called T effector memory re-expressing CD45RA (Temra) cells. In the elderly almost half of the CD8 cells are T effector memory re-expressing CD45RA (Temra) cells.

5.5   B Cell Activation

5.5.1   Introduction

Humoral immunity is mediated by activated B cells that secrete antibodies and have functions not performed by cellular immunity. Antibodies are primarily directed against extracellular pathogens but also play a role in eliminating intracellular pathogens. For instance, neutralizing antibodies can bind to viruses and prevent them from infecting host cells. Humoral immunity is especially important in attacking microbes with polysaccharide and lipid capsules such as *Streptococcus pneumoniae* and *Neisseria meningitidis* because cellular immune mechanisms are less effective against such pathogens. Antibody induction is a primary focus of vaccine development.

Most B cells that recognize foreign protein antigen are located in B cell follicles of lymph nodes and the white pulp of the spleen. They are activated with the help of CD4$^+$ T cells (T cell-dependent B cells) (Fig. 5.6). T cell-dependent B cells show weak or no antibody responses without T cell help. T-dependent B cells require three signals to become fully activated. The activation process begins when the specific antigen binds two or more IgM receptors on the B cell surface (signal 1). Antigen may be free floating or presented to the B cells by follicular DCs (FDCs) or macrophages found in the follicles. The CD19 co-receptor associated with the BCR has a long cytoplasmic tail that anchors molecules important for BCR signaling, resulting in amplification of the signal. Some of the bound antigen+BCR is internalized in vesicles where the antigen is processed and presented on MHC class II for interaction with CD4 Tfh cells. The semi-activated B cells initially undergo limited clonal expansion and move to the periphery of the follicle because of decreased response to the chemokine CXCR5 receptor and increased expression of the CCR7 receptor. Simultaneously, CD4$^+$ T helper cells that have been activated by presentation of the same antigen by dendritic cells move toward the B cell follicles where they can interact with B cells in the parafollicular area. The CD4 Tfh cells bind to peptide-MHC-II presented by B cells. CD40L is expressed by the activated CD4 cells and binds to CD40 on the B cells (signal 2). The CD4$^+$ T cells secrete various types of cytokines depending on the type of microbial infection (bacteria, viruses, fingi, helminths) (signal 3). B cell activation is also facilitated by complement-induced activation of FDCs in lymph nodes. These FDCs can bind antibody–antigen–complement complexes, allowing them to present antigen to B cells and activate them to produce antibody.

After T cell cytokine secretion, T-dependent B cells undergo heavy chain isotype switching and become short-term plasmablasts (Fig. 5.6). The antibody isotype of the plasmablast that is created is most effective against the type of microbe that is causing infection. For example, a helminth infection will cause CD4$^+$ T cells to secrete IL-4, which in turn will cause the plasmablasts to switch to IgE antibody production. Long-lived antibody-secreting plasma cells develop and move to the circulation where they secrete antibody during acute infection. Some plasmablasts move to the bone marrow or mucosal tissue where they become plasma cells that produce antibody for many years. Memory B

T-dependent B cell activation:

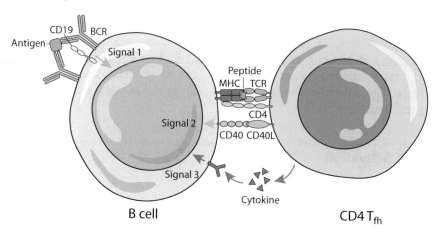

T-independent B cell activation:

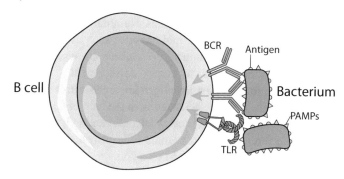

Fig. 5.6 B cell activation: T-dependent and T-independent. T-dependent B cell activation occurs for most B cells. Three signals are required. (i) Signal 1 occurs when the B cell receptor binds antigen. The co-receptor CD19 has a long cytoplasmic tail that binds adapter proteins to amplify signal transduction. The CD21 complement receptor may also contribute if a pathogen is opsonized by the complement protein C3d (ii). Signal 2 is transmitted by CD40 surface protein on the B cell upon interaction with a CD4 Tfh cell expressing CD40L. (iii) Cytokines secreted from the CD4 Tfh cell bind to cytokine receptors on the B cell which provide additional signals that influence the class of antibody the B cell will produce. For T-independent responses sufficient crosslinking of the receptor by binding pathogens with repeating structures and a signal from an innate receptor such as TLR receptors leads to B cell activation. (©Kavathas 2020)

cells are produced throughout the response. They do not produce antibody but will do so if reinfection with the same microbe occurs. These cells are activated by memory T cells.

Some B cells do not require T cell help for activation and are known as T-independent B cells. They recognize polysaccharides, lipids, and other nonprotein antigens. The repeating motifs in these molecules bind to multiple B cell receptors sending a strong signal for B cell activation. A second signal comes from another receptor such as a TLR innate receptor on the B cell that binds a ligand on the microbe (Fig. 5.6). The T-independent B-1 B cells are located in the marginal zone of the spleen, mucosal tissues, and peritoneum. They do not interact with T cells and undergo very little isotype switching so primarily express IgM. They produce "natural" antibodies that help protect from infections such as influenza.

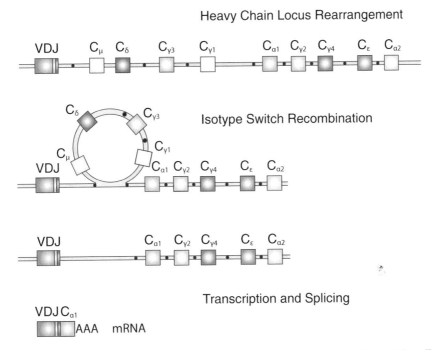

Fig. 5.7 B cell isotype switch. The heavy chain gene initially expressed by the B cell is of the IgM class. Further rearrangement can occur in the activated B cell in the presence of certain cytokines leading to looping out and cutting of the DNA so that the constant domain of another antibody isotype or class is moved close to the VDJ segments. In this example it is IgA. (©Kavathas 2020)

5.5.2 Isotype Switching

B cells (short-lived plasmablasts) initially secrete IgM antibody but as the infection continues, they begin to secrete different isotypes (IgA, IgG1, IgG2, IgG3, IgG4, or IgE). Each antibody isotype has specialized functional properties best suited for responding to different types of microorganisms. Isotype switching depends on cytokines secreted by CD4 Tfh cell-B cell interaction. The mechanics of isotype switching consist of DNA alteration in the B cell nucleus (Fig. 5.7). This occurs within germinal centers inside lymph nodes and spleen, areas where B cells proliferate at a high rate. The default antibody receptors on the surface of B cells and later secreted antibody are IgM and IgD antibody, although IgD is usually found in only small amounts in the serum. During early infection, IgM provides initial protection against invading pathogens. As the infection progresses, the B cells "adapt" and produce more effective antibody of a different isotype. Within the B cell nucleus, genes that encode the IgM heavy chain constant region of the antibody molecule are attached to a VDJ gene that encodes the antigen recognition portion of the antibody. After helper T cell interaction, a different heavy chain constant region segment that encodes for IgA, IgG, or IgE is substituted for the IgM heavy chain. T cell-independent B cells mainly become IgM-secreting plasma cells throughout the duration of infection.

5.5.3 Somatic Hypermutation and Affinity Maturation

As an infection progresses, there is prolonged and repeated exposure of B cells to protein antigen presented by FDCs in the germinal center of the lymph node and spleen. B cells proliferate at a high rate, and point mutations in the variable (V) region of the B cell genome occur with increasing

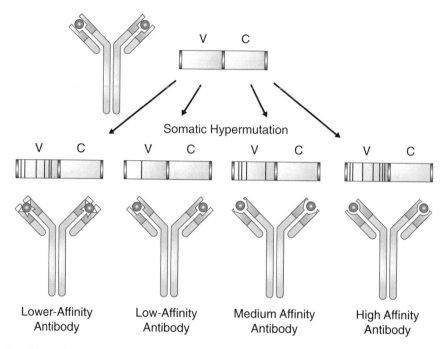

Fig. 5.8 B cell somatic hypermutation. The activation-induced cytidine deaminase (AID) gene is induced in activated B cells so that the rate of mutation in the heavy and light chain variable domains of the immunoglobulin genes is significantly increased. This leads to B cells producing antibody whose affinity is either unchanged (low), lower, medium, or high. Selection and survival of B cells with higher affinity antibody occur in a process called affinity maturation. (©Kavathas 2020)

frequency. Expression of activation-induced cytidine deaminase (AID) is responsible for the induction of mutations. The rate of mutation of dividing B cells is at a rate of about one base pair change per 10^3 base pairs per cell division which is 10^7-fold higher than the rate of other genes. This somatic hypermutation produces B cell clones whose antibody molecules bind with a wide variability in affinity to the antigen that initiated the response (Fig. 5.8). B cells that produce high-affinity antibody receptors interact strongly with FDCs and Tfh cells and survive, while B cells with lower antigen affinity die. The binding characteristics of antibody improve as the infection progresses, and as a result, antibody efficacy improves. This process is known as affinity maturation. After the pathogen has been eliminated, long-lived plasma cells and memory B cells are formed that can survive for years. If reinfection occurs at a later date, memory B cells are activated by memory T cells and multiply rapidly. They produce high-affinity IgA, IgG, or IgE antibody that helps prevent repeated infection or leads to a milder or asymptomatic infection. The different classes of antibody produced help eradicate microbes in multiple ways as described below (Fig. 5.9).

5.6   B Cell Effector Functions

5.6.1   Agglutination

Antibodies bind to the surfaces of microbial pathogens and can join two or more pathogens expressing the same antigen into an aggregate. This complex interferes with microbial function and allows clearance of multiple pathogens by phagocytes at one time rather than requiring multiple ingestion of individual pathogens.

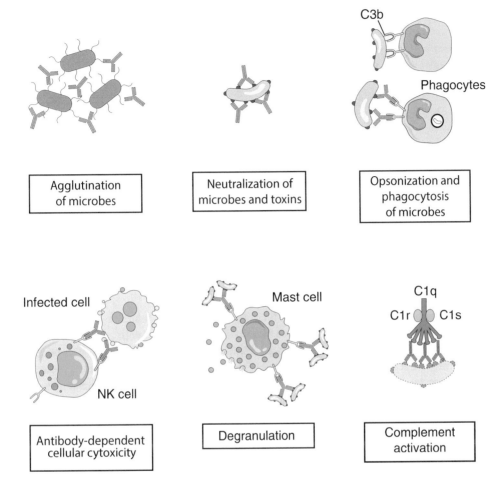

Fig. 5.9 Schematic of antibody effector functions. Antibodies function directly to agglutinate pathogens or neutralize microbes to prevent infection. They can also cooperate with components of the innate immune system in processes such as opsonization, ADCC with NK cells, mast cell degranulation, or complement activation. Antibodies that are attached to a pathogen surface that activate the complement system induce inflammation and cause lysis. (©Krause 2020)

5.6.2 Neutralization

Antibodies bind to microbes and prevent them from crossing epithelial barriers or binding to cell surfaces in order to enter cells. They also attach to microbial toxins and prevent them from binding to toxin receptors on healthy cells. Toxins cause many of the symptoms and complications of infection, and their blockage prevents pathological changes. This steric hindrance of microbes and their toxins is called neutralization.

5.6.3 Opsonization and Phagocytosis

Antibodies bind microbes with the antigen-binding portion of the molecule leaving exposed the Fc portion. Phagocytes (macrophages and neutrophils) have receptors on their surface for the Fc component of IgG1 and IgG3 isotypes. Attachment of the Fc portion of two or more antibodies with these receptors activates the phagocyte to ingest and kill the microbe. The coating of antibody on a microbial surface to facilitate phagocytosis is called opsonization and is especially important for microbes covered with polysaccharide-rich capsules such as *Streptococcus pneumoniae*. These microbes are not easily ingested by phagocytes but are readily ingested when antibody attaches to the polysaccharide capsule.

5.6.4 Antibody-Dependent Cellular Cytotoxicity (ADCC)

Antibody-dependent cellular cytotoxicity is the one antibody function that targets intracellular microbes. Cells infected with certain viruses or bacteria may express antigen on their surface membrane. Specific antibody can bind to these surface antigens through their antigen-binding sites. Natural killer cells have receptors for the Fc portion of the antibody molecule that is attached to infected cells. When the Fc receptor binds antibody, the NK cells become activated and release their granular contents, which destroy the infected cell and the infecting pathogen.

5.6.5 IgE and Eosinophil/Mast Cell Degranulation

IgE antibody is produced in response to parasitic infection, including helminths (worms) and protozoal parasites such as malaria. IgE antibodies bind to eosinophils, basophils, and mast cells via the Fc portion of the antibody. When two or more antibody molecules bind helminth antigen causing crosslinking of the antibodies on the surface of these cells, their granule contents are released and they kill the parasite. Most worms are too large to be phagocytized, and this mechanism has evolved to fight these infections. When mast cells coated with IgE antibody are activated they also produce cytokines that cause muscle contraction and production of mucus that help eliminate worms. Allergens such as pollen and cat dander also lead to IgE antibody production in people with those allergies. Such activity leads to hypersensitivity reactions such as asthma and hay fever. Mast cell and eosinophil degranulation in the lung elicit pathologic changes that cause respiratory difficulty in those who have asthma.

5.6.6 Complement Activation

Antibody of the IgM isotype and some IgG subset isotypes that are attached to microbial surfaces leave an exposed Fc portion that can bind to the C1 complement molecule. Once this attachment takes place, the complement cascade begins as described in Chap. 3. Antibody-induced complement activation was the first of three pathways of complement activation to be discovered and is termed the "classical" activation pathway. During acute infection, complement is first activated by either the alternative pathway or the mannose-binding lectin pathway because the components of these pathways are immediately available. Activation by the classical pathway is dependent on antibody that takes at least a few days to produce in a primary infection. The classical pathway is especially important if the other two do not function, as may occur with some encapsulated microbial infections.

Table 5.1 summarizes the different functions of the antibody isotypes (classes) as well as their properties.

Table 5.1 Different functions and properties of antibody isotypes

	IgM	IgG	IgE	IgA
Function	Complement activation	Neutralization, opsonization, ADCC; Complement activation	Mast cell sensitization and degranulation	Neutralization
Properties	Initial antibody	Transplacental transport	Helminth immunity Contributes to allergy	Mucosal immunity Transport into breast milk

5.7 Antibody Persistence and B Memory Cells

During a primary response when B cells are activated, some of the activated cells will develop into memory B cells and some into long-lived plasma cells. Plasma cells reside in the bone marrow and can make small amounts of antibody for years. Thus, when a pathogen infects a person who has been vaccinated, high-affinity antibody of the correct isotype is already present in the serum of the individual. The presence of memory B cells provides a rapid response (1–2 days) to reinfection. Somatic hypermutation is induced leading to the production and selection of cells with receptors that have even higher affinity. New plasma cells develop from these cells making high-affinity antibody. Thus, booster immunizations induce higher affinity antibodies than after primary immunization, and the amount of specific antibody is increased.

5.8 Regulating Immune Response

5.8.1 Introduction

There must be a balance during an immune response to restrict and eliminate a pathogen while maintaining host organ integrity and minimizing tissue damage. Every immune response has mechanisms to regulate the response, terminate it when a pathogen is cleared, and return to homeostasis. A number of mechanisms exist to dampen or end an immune response. These include (i) expression of inhibitory receptors on the surface of cells that send a negative signal upon ligand binding, (ii) effector T and B cells have a limited lifespan, (iii) T regulatory cells (described in Sect. 5.3) turn off immune responses (iv) negative feedback loops, and (v) T cells acquiring a state of "exhaustion." Both innate and adaptive immune cells express inhibitory receptors that are either always present or are induced at different times. This section will provide some examples of negative regulation to dampen or stop an immune response.

5.8.2 Negative Feedback Regulation

Upon ligand binding to certain PRRs in innate cells, the NF-κB signaling pathway is activated, which leads to the secretion of inflammatory cytokines and chemokines. This is a powerful response with a cost: tissue damage. To limit that damage, there is a negative feedback mechanism whereby a protein named A20, an ubiquitin-modifying enzyme, is induced after NF-κB signaling which limits its signaling. Interestingly, there are reduced levels of the A20 protein in bronchial epithelial cells of asthmatic patients; in mouse models of asthma, removing A20 worsens symptoms.

Another example of negative feedback regulation occurs after interaction of DCs with T cells in the lymph node when the DCs are presenting a peptide–MHC complex that engages the TCR on the T cell. Within hours of the interaction between the DCs and T cells, the T cells express a protein called

PROS1 (vitamin K-dependent plasma glycoprotein) that binds to phosphatidylserine (PtdSer) expressed at intermediate levels on the surface of activated T cells. The DCs express members of a family of receptor tyrosine kinases (RTK) that bind to PROS1 and send a negative signal into the DC leading to negative regulation of the immune response. These receptor tyrosine kinases (RTKs) TYRO3, AXL, and MERTK named TAM receptors are potent and indispensable inhibitors of inflammation and have a role in regulating many other types of immune responses such as CD4 Th2 immunity. Without Axl and Mertk, chronic inflammation and autoimmunity is enhanced in mice, and deletion of Tyro3 increases the risk of allergic responses.

5.8.3 Inhibitory Receptors (IRs)

There are many inhibitory receptors involved in regulating both innate and adaptive immunity. Two important inhibitory receptors on T cells are the cytotoxic T cell late activation antigen (CTLA-4) and the programmed death-1 protein (PD-1) (Fig. 5.10). The CTLA-4 cell surface protein is expressed

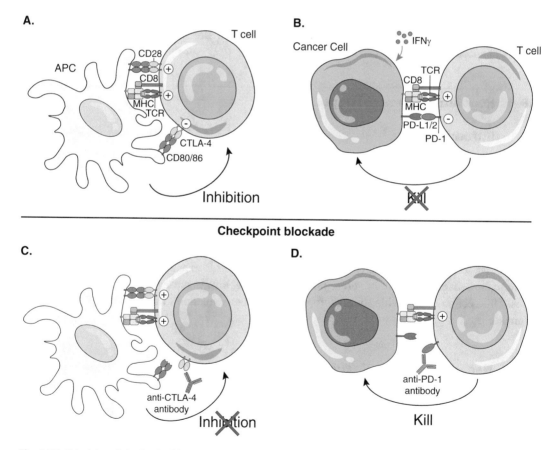

Fig. 5.10 Principles of checkpoint blockade therapy. Schematic of principle for interfering with T cell inhibitory receptor–ligand interactions that then modulate tumor immune response. (**a**) CTLA4 normally functions as an inhibitory receptor on activated T cells binding to the co-stimulatory proteins CD80/86 or B7.1/B7.2 on APCs. It competes for binding with the co-stimulatory protein CD28. (**b**) PD-1 also functions as an inhibitory receptor on T cells whose ligand, PD-L1 or PD-L2, is expressed on cells in the presence of IFNγ. (**c**, **d**) In checkpoint blockade immunotherapy, anti-CTLA-4, anti-PD-1, or anti-PD-L1 mAbs are used to block receptor–ligand interaction. This removes the "brakes" or inhibitory signals transmitted by these two receptors. (©Kavathas 2020)

around day 4 after T cell activation and binds to the co-stimulatory proteins B7.1 and B7.2 on mature antigen-presenting cells. In contrast to the CD28 protein which binds the same co-stimulatory ligands and sends an activating signal, CTLA-4 has a higher affinity for B7.1/B7.2 (CD80/86) than CD28, and it sends an inhibitory signal into the T cell limiting its activation. In addition, CD4 Tregs constitutively express CTLA-4.

The PD-1 protein on T cells binds to either ligand PD-L1 or PD-L2 induced on tissues in the presence of certain cytokines such IFN-γ. Therefore, when an immune response occurs in the tissues and PD-L1 or PD-L2 is expressed, the T cell receives a negative signal through the PD-1 receptor which limits its activity. Inhibiting the interactions between CTLA-4 and its ligand and/or PD-1 and its ligand is a new form of immunotherapy in cancer treatment described in Chap. 16. This therapy removes the "brakes" on T cells that enhances their ability to kill the tumor cells and is known as "checkpoint blockade immunotherapy" (Fig. 5.10). Blocking other inhibitory receptors such as TIGIT and TIM3 are also being explored for immunotherapy.

5.8.4 T Cell Exhaustion (Tex Cells)

Immune T cells can acquire a state of "exhaustion," whereby they are alive but have reduced function. This cell type (Tex) often develops during chronic infections such as that of the HIV virus infection or in certain cancers. When the immune system is unable to clear a pathogen, the antigen-specific T cells may acquire this phenotype. The exhausted cells (Tex) have functional defects, express multiple inhibitory receptors, and have an altered transcriptional epigenetic, metabolic, and differentiation program. The development of Tex cells minimizes damage due to the immune response, especially in the context of chronic infection and inflammation. Different subsets of Tex cells exist from progenitor to more terminally exhausted populations characterized by the presence or absence of inhibitory receptors such as PD-1 and TIM-3 and expression of certain transcription factors such as Eomes, Tcf1, and TOX. Their function can be rescued therapeutically through blockade of their inhibitory receptors.

5.8.5 Regulation of B Lymphocytes

After the amount of microbial antigen decreases during an infection, most of the remaining antigen is bound by IgG antibody that forms immune complexes. B cells express a low affinity receptor for IgG, the FcγII-A receptor (CD32A), which sends an inhibitory signal after receptor crosslinking with IgG. This contrasts with other Fc receptors that send activating signals. Another inhibitory receptor is CD22, which is expressed on mature B cells. It binds to sialic acid on transmembrane proteins, and its cytoplasmic domain is associated with the protein tyrosine phosphatase SHP-1. This phosphatase removes phosphate groups from signaling adaptor proteins and counteracts kinases that add phosphates to adaptors upon B cell receptor signaling.

5.9 Vaccination

The aim of vaccination is to induce a protective adaptive immune response that prevents disease. This is achieved by immunizing individuals with a form of the pathogen, or a part of the pathogen, so that when the vaccinated individuals subsequently reencounter the pathogen, they make a rapid secondary immune response that eliminates infection before disease develops.

5.9.1 Types of Vaccines

For many years the two major approaches to develop antigens for vaccine development were either to inactivate the pathogen (such as a virus) by heat or chemicals or to develop a weakened live form of the pathogen. The former product was called a killed vaccine and the latter an attenuated vaccine. Each type of vaccine has certain advantages and disadvantages. In the case of a killed vaccine, it was important that antigens eliciting a protective immune response maintained their immunogenicity after pathogen inactivation. Although it was difficult to develop an attenuated virus that was both immunogenic and did not cause disease, both types of vaccines are in use today, including killed vaccines such as the pertussis vaccine and attenuated live virus vaccines such as those for measles, mumps, rubella, and yellow fever. Some vaccines, such as influenza and polio are available in both killed and attenuated forms.

With the advent of recombinant DNA technology in 1975, it became possible to isolate single genes from different microorganisms and to create subunit vaccines. A gene from a pathogen can be inserted into bacteria, yeast, or cell lines (e.g., insect or mammalian cells) for protein production. Large quantities of the protein can be produced and purified for a vaccine. One example is the vaccine against human papilloma virus. The major capsid protein L1 can be produced in yeast and assembles into a capsid which is purified for the vaccine. Another example is the vaccine against tetanus. The *Clostridium tetani* bacteria secrete a toxin that is harmful. The vaccine contains an inactivated toxin (toxoid), in order to generate protective antibodies against the toxin which neutralizes it.

In order for a subunit vaccine to be effective, it is necessary to add a substance that will activate a pattern recognition receptor. The antigen-presenting cells must receive a signal from a pattern recognition receptor (PRR) binding a ligand (PAMP) in order to undergo changes so that it is capable of activating a T cell. Therefore, a substance is added to a vaccine to trick the immune system into thinking a pathogen is present, which is called an adjuvant. *Adjuvant* is a word that means "helper." In some cases, the adjuvant consists of inactivated bacteria to stimulate the innate immune system. For instance, DTP is a widely administered vaccine that provides protection against three bacterial diseases, diphtheria, tetanus, and pertussis (whooping cough), the latter caused by the bacterium *B. pertussis*. It is called a combination vaccine and consists of the two protein toxoids for diphtheria and tetanus, as well as inactivated *B. pertussis* bacteria. The inactivated bacteria provide both antigen and a PAMP that is recognized by dendritic cells and activates them to initiate an adaptive immune response.

Another type of vaccine is called a *conjugate vaccine* for the development of high-affinity antibodies against polysaccharides on the surface of bacteria which generally are weak antigens. A strong antigen is linked (conjugated) to the purified polysaccharide, and this is used for immunization. The strong antigen activates CD4 Tfh cells, which help activate B cells that bind to the polysaccharide portion of the conjugate. An example of a conjugate vaccine is the *Haemophilus influenzae* type b (hiB) vaccine.

The ability to rapidly sequence the genomes of pathogens at a reasonable cost has allowed the development of vaccines that were not previously possible. For instance, *N. meningitidis* of serogroup B was sequenced, and genes were identified. Three genes encoded antigenic targets that were used to develop Bexsero, the vaccine against *N. meningitidis* B that was approved in Europe in 2013. In addition, genes from a pathogenic microbe can be added to a nonpathogenic microbe to serve as a carrier for immunization.

There are three ways in which vaccines are protective against infectious pathogens:

1. *Prophylactic*—this is the most common form of vaccination. They are preventive vaccines to protect the host prior to exposure to the pathogen. They often induce neutralizing antibodies.

2. *Therapeutic*—these are vaccines designed to treat individuals already infected with the pathogen (common for chronic viral infections).
3. *Herd immunity*—individuals in a population may be protected from the pathogen without vaccination because the frequency of vaccinated individuals is so high that spread of infection and risk of exposure drops to such a significant degree that they are, in essence, protected. This is particularly important for individuals with compromised immune systems who cannot be vaccinated. For a highly infectious microorganism that is airborne such as measles, it is estimated that at least 94% of the population needs to be immunized to achieve effective herd immunity.

In order for a vaccine to be effective, it must be safe with minimal side effects and protective against the live pathogen when encountered naturally. An ideal vaccine also is inexpensive, biologically stable for shipping and storage, and easy to administer. It needs to provide sustained and long-lived immunity. For example, smallpox and yellow fever vaccines have demonstrated protection for more than 50 years in humans. In some cases, a booster vaccination is recommended since immunity can wane. An example is the vaccine against *Varicella zoster* (causing chicken pox) that is recommended for children to prevent chicken pox and in previously infected older adults to prevent shingles. Shingles occurs when the virus, which is dormant in nerve cells, is reactivated in people as they age. Another issue with the elderly is that their immune system has diminished, a condition termed *immunosenescence*. Both adaptive and innate immunosenescence contribute to impaired vaccine responses among the elderly.

5.9.2 Summary of Types of Vaccines

Live attenuated virus vaccine The virus has mutations that impair its ability to cause disease but can induce an immune response and best mimics the natural infection. Generally, these are effective vaccines. An example is the vaccine for chicken pox.

Heat-killed/formalin-fixed vaccine Pathogens can be killed and injected. Sometimes relevant antigens are destroyed in the process, but this approach works well in some cases. An example is the hepatitis B vaccine.

Conjugate vaccine These vaccines link a highly immunogenic antigen with a weakly antigenic bacterial antigen, such as polysaccharide, in order to generate CD4 Tfh cell help to B cells with a receptor binding the polysaccharide.

Recombinant protein subunit vaccine A gene is isolated that encodes an immunogenic protein from a microorganism, which is grown in large quantities in another species, and the protein used for immunization. The immunogenic protein can be given with an adjuvant to activate dendritic cells through PRRs. Alternatively, the gene encoding the protein can be inserted into the genome of a nonpathogenic microorganism that is used for immunization and provides the PAMP.

DNA vaccine The vaccine consists of DNA which encodes an antigen(s) against which an immune response is sought. The DNA is taken up by host cells, transcribed, and then translated into protein.

Related microorganism vaccine Vaccination against the virus causing smallpox was performed using the related, nonpathogenic viruses, such as the vaccinia virus which causes cowpox. Sufficient sharing of antigens made this vaccine highly effective for preventing smallpox for more than 50 years.

Despite great advances in the field of vaccine research, effective vaccines are still not available for HIV, malaria, and tuberculosis (TB). One challenge is that some viruses have very high mutation rates so they are continually changing. This is the reason that a new influenza vaccine is developed every year. With persistence, human ingenuity, global cooperation, and support of biomedical research, further progress will be made.

5.9.3 Immunoassays to Monitor Pathogen Exposure and Vaccine Efficacy

The specificity of the adaptive immune system makes it possible to determine whether an individual has been exposed to a pathogen and whether a vaccine resulted in an immune response. The commonly used methods involve analysis of the blood for the presence of antigen-specific antibody or memory T lymphocytes in the blood. A wide variety of antibody tests are available such as chemiluminescence immunoassays (CLIA, flash of light is signal), enzyme-linked immunoassays (ELISA, change of substrate to a color by an enzyme), immunoblot/Western blot (recombinant or native proteins applied to a filter paper), agglutination, or lateral flow immunochromatography. For some tests, the strength of the immune response is evaluated by the extent that the serum or plasma can be serially diluted. The last positive reaction is termed the *titer* of antibody. For other tests a specified volume of sample is diluted in buffer and tested. The result may be given as a qualitative positive, negative, or indeterminate.

For detecting exposure to some pathogens such as *Mycobacterium tuberculosis* or *Cytomegalovirus*, T cell responses are evaluated by stimulating T cells with a mixture of peptides corresponding to proteins from the microbe and assaying for cytokine release such as IFN-γ. Quantiferon-TB Gold and ELISpot assays are examples of two assays. In the latter assay the number of T cells on a filter paper making the cytokine of interest can be counted.

Websites www.who.int World Health Organization

www.cdc.gov Centers for Disease Control and Prevention (CDC)

References

1. Allman D, Wilmore JR, Gaudette BT. The continuing story of T-cell independent antibodies. Immunol Rev. 2019;288(1):128–35.
2. Angajala A, Lim S, Phillips JB, Kim JH, Yates C, You Z, et al. Diverse roles of mitochondria in immune responses: novel insights into immuno-metabolism. Front Immunol. 2018;9:1605.
3. Bengsch B, Ohtani T, Khan O, Setty M, Manne S, O'Brien S, et al. Epigenomic-guided mass cytometry profiling reveals disease-specific features of exhausted CD8 T cells. Immunity. 2018;48(5):1029–45 e5.
4. Cinquanta L, Fontana DE, Bizzaro N. Chemiluminescent immunoassay technology: what does it change in autoantibody detection? Auto Immun Highlights. 2017;8(1):9.
5. Cooper MD. The early history of B cells. Nat Rev Immunol. 2015;15(3):191–7.
6. de Kouchkovsky DA, Ghosh S, Rothlin CV. Negative regulation of type 2 immunity. Trends Immunol. 2017;38(3):154–67.

7. Forthal DN. Functions of antibodies. Microbiol Spectr. 2014;2(4):1–17.
8. Geltink RIK, Kyle RL, Pearce EL. Unraveling the complex interplay between T cell metabolism and function. Annu Rev Immunol. 2018;36:461–88.
9. Kumar BV, Connors TJ, Farber DL. Human T cell development, localization, and function throughout life. Immunity. 2018;48(2):202–13.
10. LeBien TW, Tedder TF. B lymphocytes: how they develop and function. Blood. 2008;112(5):1570–80.
11. McLane LM, Abdel-Hakeem MS, Wherry EJ. CD8 T cell exhaustion during chronic viral infection and cancer. Annu Rev Immunol. 2019;37:457–95.
12. Mosmann TR, Cherwinski H, Bond MW, Giedlin MA, Coffman RL. Two types of murine helper T cell clone. I. Definition according to profiles of lymphokine activities and secreted proteins. J Immunol. 1986;136(7):2348–57.
13. Neurath MF, Kaplan MH. Th9 cells in immunity and immunopathological diseases. Semin Immunopathol. 2017;39(1):1–4.
14. Plank MW, Kaiko GE, Maltby S, Weaver J, Tay HL, Shen W, et al. Th22 cells form a distinct Th lineage from Th17 cells in vitro with unique transcriptional properties and Tbet-dependent Th1 plasticity. J Immunol. 2017;198(5):2182–90.
15. Rubin SJS, Bloom MS, Robinson WH. B cell checkpoints in autoimmune rheumatic diseases. Nat Rev Rheumatol. 2019;15(5):303–15.
16. Sharma P, Wagner K, Wolchok JD, Allison JP. Novel cancer immunotherapy agents with survival benefit: recent successes and next steps. Nat Rev Cancer. 2011;11(11):805–12.
17. Thakar J, Mohanty S, West AP, Joshi SR, Ueda I, Wilson J, et al. Aging-dependent alterations in gene expression and a mitochondrial signature of responsiveness to human influenza vaccination. Aging (Albany NY). 2015;7(1):38–52.
18. Treanor B. B-cell receptor: from resting state to activate. Immunology. 2012;136(1):21–7.

Disorders of the Immune System

6

Paula B. Kavathas, Peter J. Krause, and Nancy H. Ruddle

6.1   Introduction

Thus far the emphasis in this text has been on a description of the beneficial functions of the immune system, primarily in its response to infection. We have described the organs, cells, and effector molecules of the innate and adaptive systems and indicated the ways in which they coordinate and cooperate to clear the body of pathogens. However, there are monogenic diseases in which the immune system does not function to the optimal benefit of the individual. These disorders of the immune system include immunodeficiencies affecting the innate and/or adaptive immune system. On the other hand, the immune response may be inappropriately activated in allergic disease to innocuous substances or in autoimmunity when the adaptive immune system acts against the host. Still another disorder of the immune system occurs when, through genetic mutation, the innate immune system becomes aberrantly activated in the absence of antigen and induces autoinflammation. We describe principles and a few select diseases as illustrations.

6.2   Immunodeficiency

Genetic variants in coding or noncoding genomic regions can result in inborn errors of immunity/primary immunodeficiency diseases (PID). There are more than 350 inborn errors of immunity that have been identified as of 2017, and the number is growing with increasing access to next-generation sequencing. Approximately 1.7% of the ~21,000 genes in the human genome have been implicated in these monogenic disorders. Approximately 1/1200 live births in the US have this type of disorder.

P. B. Kavathas (✉)
Departments of Laboratory Medicine and Immunobiology, Yale School of Medicine,
New Haven, CT, USA
e-mail: paula.kavathas@yale.edu

P. J. Krause
Department of Epidemiology of Microbial Diseases, Yale School of Public Health and Departments
of Medicine and Pediatrics, Yale School of Medicine, New Haven, CT, USA

N. H. Ruddle
Department of Epidemiology of Microbial Diseases, Yale School of Public Health, New Haven, CT, USA

© Springer Nature Switzerland AG 2019
P. J. Krause et al. (eds.), *Immunoepidemiology*, https://doi.org/10.1007/978-3-030-25553-4_6

In contrast IgA deficiency which is the most common PID occurs in about 1/300 to 1/500 people. Disease-causing genetic lesions can be single nucleotide variants, insertions or deletions, or chromosomal changes such as translocations. Initially, the disorders were identified as susceptibility to infection accompanied by antibody deficiencies, phagocyte dysfunction, or complement deficiencies. It is now recognized that immunodeficiency can also lead to immune dysregulation that can manifest as autoimmunity, lymphoproliferation, or autoinflammation. Therefore, rather than calling these disorders PID or primary immunodeficiencies, some propose the broader description of inborn errors of immunity. Nine major categories of these disorders described by the International Union of Immunological Societies are listed in the Textbox.

Textbox: Major Categories of Immune Deficiencies

Immunodeficiencies affecting both cellular and humoral immunity
Combined immunodeficiencies with associated or syndromic features
Predominantly antibody deficiencies
Diseases of immune dysregulation
Congenital defects of phagocyte number, function, or both
Defects in intrinsic and innate immunity
Autoinflammatory disorders

The first genetic immunodeficiency, Bruton's agammaglobulinemia, was discovered in 1952 as a failure to produce antibody. Infants had recurrent infections with pyrogenic bacteria. Intravenous immunoglobulin replacement therapy was used for treatment. It was not until 1993, however, that the causative gene defect was identified as *Bruton tyrosine kinase (BTK)*. The BTK protein is important for signal transduction through the pre-B cell receptor so that B cells that lack this protein do not develop beyond the pre-B cell stage. Another well-known immunodeficiency is severe combined immunodeficiency (SCID) that involves defects in both T and B lymphocytes. Children with SCID present with serious infections and can also fall ill from some vaccines containing live attenuated viruses. An X-linked form presents in males due to mutation in the gene encoding the common gamma chain (γ_c) which is a shared receptor subunit for multiple important cytokine receptors (including IL-2, IL-4, IL-7, IL-9, IL-15, and IL-21). The gene is located on the X chromosome; males have only one copy of the X chromosome in contrast to females who have two copies of the X chromosome and the potential for an unmutated gene. Untreated children with SCID generally do not survive beyond the second year of life. SCID was made famous in the 1970s and 1980s by a young boy with X-linked SCID who lived for 12 years in a plastic germ-free bubble and was known as the "bubble boy." Most states now include newborn screening for SCID. Bone marrow transplantation early in life is standard treatment.

An example of a genetic defect affecting T regulatory cells is "CTLA-4 haploinsufficiency with autoimmune infiltration" (CHAI) disease. As we learned earlier, CTLA-4 is an inhibitory receptor competing with the costimulatory protein CD28 for shared ligands B7.1 and B7.2 (CD80 and CD86) on activated T cells. In addition, it is constitutively expressed on regulatory T cells and in certain contexts is crucial for proper CD4 Treg suppressive function. In this disease one copy of the CTLA-4 gene is defective, so that the amount of CTLA-4 protein is reduced. This causes severe immune dysregulation disrupting B and T cell homeostasis. Patients have extensive and destructive lymphocytic infiltrates in multiple nonlymphoid organs.

Understanding the genetic basis for these primary immunodeficiency disorders is essential for their diagnosis, prognosis, genetic counseling, and the development of precision therapeutics, particularly as these disorders are characterized by a high degree of phenotypic heterogeneity. When an individual with a suspected inborn error of immunity is identified, determining the genetic basis can be a challenge. The DNA sequence of the affected individual is compared with unaffected family members and databases of human genome sequences so that common variants in the population can be excluded. If individuals with the same genetic variant and immune phenotype from different families are identified, this strongly supports the hypothesis that the identified genetic variant is causing the immune defect. These candidate variants for rare inborn errors of immunity are usually validated with biochemical and molecular analysis. For some genes, mutations can lead to normally expressed proteins that show increased (hypermorphic) or decreased (hypomorphic) activity compared with the wild-type protein. There can also be incomplete penetrance, whereby not everyone with a specific gene mutation becomes ill, suggesting other genetic, epigenetic, or environmental factors impact disease susceptibility. For instance, if the gene defect makes an individual susceptible to certain viral pathogens, it will not be evident until exposure to the specific pathogen causes severe disease.

Determining mechanisms for inborn errors of immunity is important not only for helping the patients therapeutically but also for providing fundamental insight into how the immune system works in humans. For instance, there are patients who lack neutrophils or IgA, and the role of neutrophils or IgA in immunity can be determined based on the patient's susceptibility to various pathogens. Two types of autoimmune diseases led to the discovery of two important genes called AIRE and FOXP3. In autoimmune polyglandular syndrome type I (APS1; also known as APECED), there is a mutation in the AIRE (autoimmune regulatory) gene that encodes a transcriptional regulator expressed in the thymus. AIRE was thus identified as important for negative selection of autoreactive T cells during their development as described in Chap. 4. In another autoimmune disease called IPEX syndrome (immunodysregulation, polyendocrinopathy enteropathy, X-linked), a mutation in the transcription factor FoxP3 impairs CD4 T regulatory cell development and function, which established the critical role of FoxP3 for CD4 Tregs.

Immunodeficiencies can also result from nongenetic causes and are called secondary or acquired immunodeficiencies. Causes include malnutrition, infection by the human immunodeficiency virus, or chemotherapy for cancer treatment. A classic example of the effect of malnutrition on immune function involves vitamin A deficiency. Dr. Alfred Sommer was studying vitamin A deficiency and its impact on blindness. He noticed in his data that children with even the mildest xerophthalmia were dying much more frequently than children with normal eyes in developing countries because of infectious disease. Supplementation with low-dose vitamin A restored immune function and reduced these deaths. By 1993 global efforts to prevent vitamin A deficiency were launched to prevent blindness and death from infectious disease. Vaccines are often ineffective in individuals with primary or secondary immunodeficiencies. In addition, the elderly experience *immunosenescence* reducing vaccine efficacy.

6.3   Hypersensitivity and Allergy

Hypersensitivity is a pathological immune response to antigens that normally pose little or no threat. Hypersensitivity has traditionally been classified into four disease types based on the immunologic mechanism causing the reaction: type I, immediate hypersensitivity (IgE-mediated allergic disease); type II, antibody-mediated disease; type III, immune complex disease; and type IV, delayed hypersensitivity (lymphocyte-mediated disease) (Fig. 6.1).

Fig. 6.1 Allergy skin testing. A small area of swelling with surrounding redness known as a wheal and flare is typical of a positive allergy skin test. (Used with permission of Mayo Foundation for Medical Education and Research. All rights reserved)

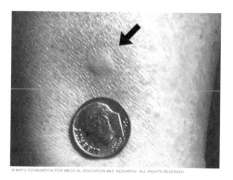

Immediate hypersensitivity or allergic disease is mediated by induction of CD4 Th2 immunity and the production of IgE antibodies directed against certain antigens (allergens) that can be infectious or noninfectious. The reason that this occurs is not well understood. People with allergies react to specific allergens delivered through specific routes that cause the production of CD4 Th2 lymphocytes and B cell secretion of IgE antibody (Fig. 6.2). The Fc portion of IgE antibody binds to mast cells, basophils, and activated eosinophils by an FcεR1 receptor on these cells so that their cell surfaces become coated with IgE. Each time a person with allergies is exposed to a particular allergen, more IgE is produced, and more allergen binds to mast cell and eosinophil-bound IgE. When allergin binds to enough IgE on mast cells and eosinophils, there is a cellular release of granules, cytokines, and lipid mediators such as histamine that lead to numerous deleterious physiological changes. Cytokines released include IL-4, IL-5, IL-13, and GM-CSF. Immediate hypersensitivity may occur within minutes of allergen exposure and may cause anaphylaxis, asthma attacks, food allergies, or hay fever. Asthma is a major health burden affecting about 350 million people worldwide. Anaphylaxis is a serious allergic response that often involves swelling, hives, lowered blood pressure, or shock. Anaphylactic shock can be fatal. Anaphylaxis typically involves more than one organ system, while other allergic reactions generally are more localized. Anaphylactic symptoms usually start within 5–30 minutes of coming into contact with an allergen to which an individual is allergic. Occasionally, it may take more than an hour to notice anaphylactic symptoms. A few anaphylaxis triggers that can cause death include bee stings, peanuts, and penicillin. Common allergens include house dust mites, pollen, pet dander, and mold. The array of allergic clinical syndromes depends on the location and number of mast cells, eosinophils, and their mediators.

Asthma occurs primarily in people who have a genetic tendency to develop allergic disease, although some asthma patients have a minimal allergic family background. Asthma is not a single disease as individuals can have mild to very severe disease phenotypes, sometimes arising in childhood and later in life. The mechanisms for these different forms are still being determined. Asthmatic patients experience acute and chronic pulmonary inflammation. Risk factors besides allergy include obesity, early viral infections, smoking, diet, and indoor and outdoor allergens. Asthma attacks can be triggered by allergens, respiratory infections such as rhinovirus infections, exercise, cold air, air pollution, and stress. Initial attacks usually are mild because only a small number of IgE molecules are bound to mast cells and eosinophils. More IgE molecules are bound with repeated exposure to the allergen. For asthmatics, allergen binding to multiple IgE molecules causes mast cell and eosinophil activation in lung tissue. They release a number of vasoactive substances that lead to constriction of the small airways in the lung. In later stages of an asthma attack, fluid and neutrophils collect in airway lumens, which are more refractory to therapy than earlier in the course when bronchodilators may be sufficient to end an attack. Patients experience wheezing, coughing, and difficulty breathing

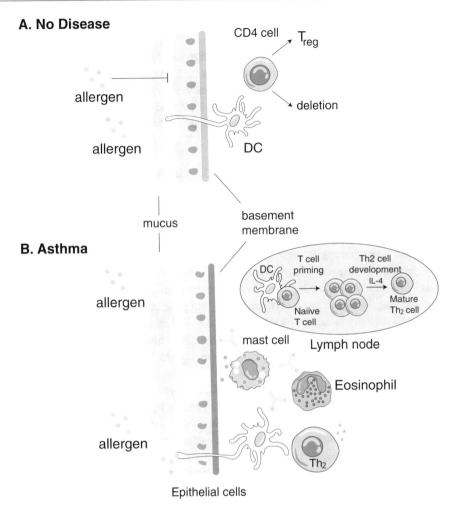

Fig. 6.2 Asthma/allergy. Airway responsiveness to inhaled allergens in a person with asthma and person without asthma. (**a**) For a person without asthma, the epithelia cell and mucus layer are intact, limiting the amount of inhaled allergen that is picked up by dendritic cells. Allergens that are brought to the lymph node do not induce an inflammatory response. (**b**) For a person with asthma, the disease process begins when an allergen enters the lung and is picked up by pulmonary dendritic cells and presented to T cells in lymph nodes. T cells differentiate into CD4 Th2 cells that then help B cells to produce IgE antibody. IgE binds to Fcε receptors on activated eosinophils and mast cells. When allergen binds to the IgE antibody leading to crosslinking, the mast cells are activated. Granules, cytokines, and inflammatory mediators are released from these cells that have a wide range of physiologic effects, including airway smooth muscle constriction and neutrophil infiltration of the airways, epithelial damage, and breathing difficulty. These effects lead to persistent inflammation and airway remodeling, unless the allergen exposure is removed. (©Krause 2020)

and, in the most severe form of the disease, death by asphyxiation. Asthma is treated with bronchodilators to counteract airway constriction, steroids to suppress inflammation, and drugs that inhibit mast cell degranulation. Desensitization therapy or allergen immunotherapy (allergy shots) is a long-term treatment for many people with allergic rhinitis, allergic asthma, conjunctivitis, or stinging insect allergy. Immunotherapy involves exposing people to larger and larger amounts of allergen to attempt to induce or restore tolerance to the allergen. Recently, monoclonal antibody therapy directed against IgE, IL-4, IL-5, and IL-13 has had some success.

Type II hypersensitivity is caused by IgM or IgG antibody directed against fixed self-tissue. It may be due to a response to foreign antigen that damages healthy tissue in the area where microbes are being destroyed (innocent bystander damage) or foreign antigen that binds to self-tissue, such as occurs with drug hypersensitivity reactions, or molecular mimicry when microbial antigens have a similar molecular structure as self-tissue. An example of the latter is rheumatic fever where antibody against *Streptococcus pyogenes* also attacks the heart, joint, and brain tissue. In certain autoimmune diseases, antibody directed against self leads to autoantibody-mediated cellular destruction. Examples of such autoimmune disease include autoimmune hemolytic anemia such as Rh disease, Goodpasture's syndrome, Graves' disease, and myasthenia gravis.

Type III hypersensitivity occurs when two or more IgG antibody molecules attach to soluble antigen during a bloodstream infection and form immune complexes. Immune complexes deposit on the endothelial lining of blood vessels. The Fc portion of antibody molecules in the complex bind to neutrophils and complement that cause inflammation of the vascular endothelium. Vasculitis is usually generalized because immune complexes occur throughout the vascular system. Circulating mononuclear cells and neutrophils clear immune complexes by binding to them with both Fc and complement receptors. They are phagocytosed and destroyed in phagolysosomes. The ability of phagocytic cells to clear immune complexes is overwhelmed in immune complex disease. Examples include Farmer's lung, systemic lupus erythematosus, and poststreptococcal glomerulonephritis.

Type IV hypersensitivity is caused by activated T cells that recruit an inflammatory infiltrate. This type of hypersensitivity is described as delated-type hypersensitivity when T cells react to a foreign antigen such as a bacterium or virus. The TB skin test to identify individuals infected with *Mycobacterium tuberculosis* is based on the delayed hypersensitivity reaction. After tuberculin protein is injected intradermally, skin swelling and erythema occur and are maximal after 48–72 h when the skin reaction is interpreted as positive or negative. Type IV hypersensitivity also includes contact sensitivity when T cells react to a self-antigen that is modified by an external agent, such as poison ivy or nickel. The poison ivy plant contains a protein called urushiol that can be absorbed into the dermis. Urushiol breaks down into metabolites that are picked up by dendritic cells, which present this antigen to T cells in the draining lymph node. T cells that are activated by these metabolites proliferate and move to the skin site where they release cytokines that activate local macrophages resulting in skin blisters and itching. Mechanisms causing type IV hypersensitivity include CD4+ lymphocyte release of cytokines such as IL-17 and TNF, which attract neutrophils and macrophages that release cytokines, proteolytic enzymes, and toxic oxygen species. These damage local tissue or cause CD8+ cytotoxic T lymphocyte destruction of healthy tissue.

6.4   Autoimmunity

Autoimmunity occurs when T cells and/or B cells recognize self as foreign and attack self-tissue, causing pathology. Autoimmune diseases can involve individual cells (the beta cells in the pancreas in type I diabetes), organs (the joints in rheumatoid arthritis), or the entire body (nucleic acid protein complexes in systemic lupus erythematosus). The pathologic mechanisms can be due to inflammatory T cells (Th1 or Th17), and/ or antibodies and/ or antigen-antibody complexes. Autoimmunity is the result of a complicated series of interactions that can be said, in a somewhat simplistic way, to be influenced by gender, genes, and geography. In all situations, loss of tolerance to self is the important characteristic.

6.4.1 Mechanisms of Peripheral Tolerance

Multiple mechanisms exist to protect the individual from an attack on self. In an earlier chapter we learned about the mechanisms of central tolerance that eliminate self-reactive T cells in the thymus and self-reactive B cells in bone marrow. However, some cells with the potential for autoreactivity can escape into the periphery. Once a T cell leaves the thymus and begins to circulate throughout the body, additional mechanisms, broadly categorized as peripheral tolerance, come into play. T regulatory cells can regulate autoreactive T or B cells through secretion of inhibitory cytokines. Some T regs develop in the thymus and are called "natural" T regs, whereas others can be induced in the periphery. Anergy is another form of peripheral tolerance. T cells that only receive a signal through their T cell receptor, but no costimulatory signal, either die or are no longer able to be activated.

Another form of peripheral tolerance is ignorance. In this situation, the T cell lacks access to the self-antigen. This can be due to the fact the antigen is inaccessible to the T cell because it is hidden inside a cell or is in an organ which lacks T cell access. The eye, the brain, and the testis are examples of such "privileged sites" that are normally protected from T cell circulation. If the privileged site is breached by physical or pathogen-induced damage, the cellular contents become accessible to the immune system. Antigens can leak to the draining lymph node and activate those T cells that have not been eliminated in the thymus. If the T cell has a TCR that recognizes peptide+MHC, it is activated, and can migrate to the affected organ, and damage can occur. One example of a pathology associated with a physical breach is sympathetic ophthalmia. In this case a blow to the eye releases antigens into the circulation, T cells become activated and then proceed to damage the other eye by an immune attack.

6.4.2 Gender, Genes, and Geography

As noted above, autoimmune diseases are multifactorial, and the "three Gs" (gender, genes, and geography) all contribute. In many, but not all autoimmune diseases, females are more susceptible than males. This is true for multiple sclerosis (MS), a disease of the central nervous system, and systemic lupus erythematosus. On the other hand, males are as likely as females to develop type I diabetes. Genetics plays a major role in autoimmunity, and the particular genes that influence propensity for disease vary with the autoimmune disease. The MHC has been strongly implicated in some autoimmune diseases, but other genes are also in play. In the case of MS, the chance in the USA of developing the disease is 0.1%. This rises to 2.5–5% with first-degree relatives of an affected individual. However, an identical twin of an individual with MS has only a 25% chance of developing the disease, indicating a 75% chance of *not* developing the disease even with identical genome. This indicates that the environment plays a role. Epidemiologic studies indicate that proximity to the equator can be protective against the development of MS. Another example of environmental influence on autoimmunity is viral infections that triggers the first manifestation of Type 1 diabetes. This has given rise to the hypothesis that exposure to particular microorganisms might trigger an autoimmune disease, perhaps through the phenomenon of "molecular mimicry" whereby a T cell population activated by a pathogen might expand and cross-react with a self-antigen. Another hypothesis is that a "cytokine storm" induced by a systemic infection might provide signal 3 for a small, primed but not activated population of T cells, to differentiate into an effector population. The role of the microbiome has recently come under intense scrutiny, indicating that both the external and internal environments may influence the propensity to develop an autoimmune disease (Fig. 6.3).

Fig. 6.3 Several factors contribute to autoimmune diseases. A rough approximation of the influence of genetics, sex, and the environment on autoimmune disease. This varies widely between different diseases. (©Ruddle 2020)

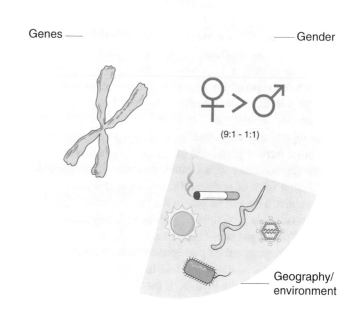

6.5 Autoinflammatory Diseases

6.5.1 Definition

Autoinflammatory diseases are inherited disorders characterized by activation of the innate immune system in the apparent absence of infection. They are usually characterized by an absence of auto-antibodies or autoreactive T cells, thus distinguishing them from autoimmunity. The symptoms of these diseases are frequently systemic, usually with recurrent fevers of unknown origin and involvement of multiple different organs and tissues, and frequently with ulcers affecting the skin and mouth and amyloid deposits in the kidney. These conditions usually have a genetic component, which is triggered by poorly understood environmental factors, in the absence of a defined microbial component.

6.5.2 History

Several disorders of periodic fevers such as familial Mediterranean fever (FMF) and familial Hibernian fever (FHF) that include inflammation in multiple organs, such as the skin, heart, lungs, and kidneys, appeared to be sporadic and not due to a known viral or bacterial infection. The basis of these fevers was a mystery until a series of family studies revealed that they were due to defects in innate immune signaling. In the case of FMF, mutations in MEVF (the gene that encodes pyrin, a key component of the inflammasome) result in unchecked activation of IL-1β. The term "autoinflammation" was first used in a publication describing an autosomal dominant defect in the TNF receptor I as the cause of FHF. The original definition of autoinflammation due to familial fevers has been expanded to encompass many syndromes that include defects in the genes encoding the type I interferon and complement pathways and even some protein-processing enzymes. The original definitions of monogenic autoin-flammatory diseases now include polygenic diseases and even some diseases characterized by sterile skin and joint inflammation that are not accompanied by fevers.

6.5.3   Mechanisms and Classifications

6.5.3.1 Monogenic Autoinflammatory Diseases

There are at least six types of monogenic inflammatory diseases. They include pyrin activation, IL-1 activation TNF receptor mutations, mutations in regulators of the NF-kB pathway, interferon activation, and complement activation. Mutations in MEVF, the gene coding for pyrin, were the first to be associated with an autoinflammatory disease. Familial Mediterranean fever (FMF) is generally inherited as a monogenic autosomal recessive. There are now at least 80 known mutations of MEVF associated with FMV. Elucidation of the function of pyrin through studies of FMV have revealed that it contributes to an inflammasome that is independent of the well-known NLRP3 inflammasome whose function is to recognize toxins of invading pathogens or host proteins modified by invading pathogens. The persistence of mutations in MEVF in the heterozygous state in certain populations has suggested that it may provide a survival advantage by conferring resistance to such pathogens as *Mycobacterium tuberculosis* and *Yersinia pestis*.

Mutations in several different genes involved in the production or constitutive activation of IL-1, ranging from an inactive IL-1 receptor antagonist to activation of NLRP1 or NLRP3 inflammasomes, have been identified as contributing to autoinflammatory diseases. In many cases, gain-of-function mutations lead to activated inflammasomes, activated caspase-1, production of IL-1β and IL-18, and activation of NF-κb.

TNFRI mutations result in an autosomal dominant fever syndrome whose etiology was identified in members of a large Scottish-Irish pedigree. The TNFR1-associated periodic syndromes (TRAPS) are characterized by unchecked activation of the NF-κB signaling pathway and sustained production of inflammatory cytokines, such as TNF and IL-1. TRAPS were originally thought to be due to increased signaling through TNFR1 but more recently have been postulated to be due to a defect in receptor shedding or protein misfolding and retention in the endoplasmic reticulum.

Mutations in genes regulating NF-κb activation have now been linked to several autoinflammatory diseases. Blau syndrome and early-onset sarcoidosis are due to mutations in NOD2, a pattern recognition receptor. Constitutive activation of NOD2 results in activation of NF-κb and release of inflammatory cytokines. Other disorders of TNF- and IL-1-induced NF-κb signaling are due to defects in genes controlling negative regulators of the NF-κB pathway, manifested as inflammation, arthritis, and fever.

Type I interferon (IFN) is a product of the innate system that can be induced after viral infection. Several pattern recognition receptors (PRRs) recognize viral RNA, DNA, or RNA/DNA hybrids resulting in release of type I interferon, its interaction with the IFN receptor, and then activation of IFN response genes, leading to inflammation. Interferonopathies are associated with inappropriate activation of this pathway and mutation of sensing molecules and high levels of type I interferon. The diseases include Aicardi-Goutières syndrome, which is characterized by calcifications in the brain, encephalopathy, leukocytosis, and puffy skin (chilblains) and are associated with mutations in either TREX1, a DNA sensor or one of the RNA-DNA hybrid sensors, RNASEH2A, RNASEH2B, or RNASEHC. The neurologic pathology results in mental impairment. Other diseases are associated with high levels of interferon, and no obvious viral infection may also be due to defects in interferon production or signaling.

Several autoinflammatory conditions are caused by mutations of genes that normally regulate proteins in the complement pathway, resulting in constitutive activation. Atypical hemolytic uremic syndrome is due to loss-of-function mutations in complement factor H. Its loss allows unrestricted activation of C3bBb in the alternative pathway. Paroxysmal nocturnal hemoglobinuria (PNH) is due to mutations in the gene encoding PIGA, an enzyme that is required for anchoring two complement inhibitory proteins, CD55 and CD59, that regulate the membrane attack complex, again leading to unchecked complement activity and tissue damage.

6.5.3.2 Polygenic Autoinflammatory Diseases

An additional group of diseases that do not appear to be monogenic are considered as autoinflammatory. They are characterized by inflammation of unexplained origin with no apparent association with a microbial infection and no apparent antibody or T cell activation. A few of these fascinating syndromes are noted below.

Behçet's disease was originally considered to be an autoimmune disease because of its association with HLA-B51 and hyperreactivity to streptococcal antigens but is now considered as an adult-onset autoinflammatory disease with high levels of IL-1β. Behçet's disease is characterized by a series of apparently unrelated symptoms, such as canker sores, eye inflammation, and skin rashes. A monogenic form of the disease that closely resembles the classic form has been described in six families. All are afflicted with a mutation in a NF-κB negative regulator gene.

Several other diseases fall under the category of autoinflammation. Still's disease, a systemic juvenile idiopathic arthritis, is associated with fever and skin rash and/or swollen lymph nodes, hepatomegaly, or splenomegaly. The disease is characterized by activated macrophages and high levels of IL-18. The absence of an association with a particular HLA is one feature that distinguishes it from other forms of juvenile arthritis. Adult-onset Still's disease is associated with inflammasome activation and high levels of IL-1β. Some types of inflammatory bowel diseases including Crohn's disease and ulcerative colitis involve chronic inflammation of the gastrointestinal tract with additional symptoms involving several organs, including the skin, eyes, bones, kidneys, and lungs. Schnitzler's syndrome is a rare disease with rash, fever, increased neutrophils, and amyloid deposits. It is considered an autoinflammatory disease because of recurrent fevers of unknown etiology and high levels of IL-1β and IL-18. Sweet's syndrome, also known as acute febrile neutrophilic dermatosis, is characterized by fever and red papules on the skin with infiltrates of neutrophils.

6.5.4 Treatment

The original treatment of autoinflammatory disorders was colchicine, which destabilizes microtubules among other actions. Now that the mechanisms of many of the monogenic autoinflammatory disorders are known, specific therapies can be employed, including treatment with cytokine inhibitors. Anti-IL-1 and anti-TNF therapies have been useful in some of the monogenic and polygenic autoinflammatory diseases. JAK inhibitors are sometimes useful for treatment of the interferonopathies.

6.5.5 Further Areas of Research

Phenotypic heterogeneity is an issue in even the monogenic autoinflammatory disorders. That is, individuals with the same mutation exhibit different clinical manifestations with involvement of the gut, skin, and/or gastrointestinal system. Furthermore, an individual may have different symptoms at different times. What cells are contributing to pathogenesis? Monocytes? Innate lymphoid cells? What is the trigger? Recent studies suggest there may be a role for the microbiome. Another unresolved issue is the occasional overlap with autoimmune symptoms, immunodeficiency, and defects with hyper- or hypoproduction of immunoglobulins. A recently articulated concept that chronic inflammation can contribute to type II diabetes, gout, and atherosclerosis is called "inflammaging."

Website *Infevers* http://infevers.umai-montpellier.fr, a database of hereditary auto-inflammatory disorder mutations

References

1. Ciccarelli F, De Martinis M, Ginaldi L. An update on autoinflammatory diseases. Curr Med Chem. 2014;21(3):261–9.
2. Fischer A, Provot J, Jais JP, Alcais A, Mahlaoui N, members of the CFPIDsg. Autoimmune and inflammatory manifestations occur frequently in patients with primary immunodeficiencies. J Allergy Clin Immunol. 2017;140(5):1388–93 e8.
3. Gauthier M, Ray A, Wenzel SE. Evolving concepts of asthma. Am J Respir Crit Care Med. 2015;192(6):660–8.
4. Kalish RS, Wood JA, LaPorte A. Processing of urushiol (poison ivy) hapten by both endogenous and exogenous pathways for presentation to T cells in vitro. J Clin Invest. 1994;93(5):2039–47.
5. Lenardo M, Lo B, Lucas CL. Genomics of immune diseases and new therapies. Annu Rev Immunol. 2016;34:121–49.
6. Manthiram K, Zhou Q, Aksentijevich I, Kastner DL. The monogenic autoinflammatory diseases define new pathways in human innate immunity and inflammation. Nat Immunol. 2017;18(8):832–42.
7. McCusker C, Upton J, Warrington R. Primary immunodeficiency. Allergy Asthma Clin Immunol. 2018;14(Suppl 2):61.
8. McDermott MF, Aksentijevich I, Galon J, McDermott EM, Ogunkolade BW, Centola M, et al. Germline mutations in the extracellular domains of the 55 kDa TNF receptor, TNFR1, define a family of dominantly inherited autoinflammatory syndromes. Cell. 1999;97(1):133–44.
9. Moghaddas F, Masters SL. The classification, genetic diagnosis and modelling of monogenic autoinflammatory disorders. Clin Sci (Lond). 2018;132(17):1901–24.
10. Picard C, Bobby Gaspar H, Al-Herz W, Bousfiha A, Casanova JL, Chatila T, et al. International Union of Immunological Societies: 2017 Primary Immunodeficiency Diseases Committee Report on Inborn Errors of Immunity. J Clin Immunol. 2018;38(1):96–128.
11. Raje N, Dinakar C. Overview of immunodeficiency disorders. Immunol Allergy Clin N Am. 2015;35(4):599–623.
12. Ray A, Raundhal M, Oriss TB, Ray P, Wenzel SE. Current concepts of severe asthma. J Clin Invest. 2016;126(7):2394–403.
13. Sommer A. Vitamin A, infectious disease, and childhood mortality: a 2 solution? J Infect Dis. 1993;167(5):1003–7.
14. Uzzaman AC, Cho SH. Classification of hyersensitivity reactions. In: Greenberger PA, Grammer LC, editors. Allergy asthma proceedings. 33 Suppl 1: OceanSide Publications, Inc; 2012. Providence, Rhode Island, USA. p. S96–S9.
15. Zharkova O, Celhar T, Cravens PD, Satterthwaite AB, Fairhurst AM, Davis LS. Pathways leading to an immunological disease: systemic lupus erythematosus. Rheumatology (Oxford). 2017;56(suppl_1):i55–66.

IMMUNOEPIDEMIOLOGY BASICS: IMMUNOLOGY OF POPULATIONS

Immunoepidemiology of Selected Components of the Innate and Adaptive Immune Systems

7

Nancy H. Ruddle and Paula B. Kavathas

7.1   Introduction

Immunoepidemiology is the study of immune variation within populations. In this chapter, we will provide examples of genetic variation or polymorphisms in selected components of the immune system. We have chosen components that represent the innate system, the adaptive system, and those that bridge both. We have also chosen components representative of recognition molecules as well as antigen nonspecific and specific effector functions.

DNA polymorphisms are differences in gene sequences that can give rise to changes in gene regulation (generally in enhancers or promoters), gene function (in exon sequences), or simple intronic sequence changes with no apparent effect on function. The latter are nonetheless useful in identifying populations. Polymorphisms can be single-nucleotide polymorphisms (SNPs), microsatellite repeats, and minisatellite or variable-number tandem repeats. These polymorphisms may be detected as restriction fragment polymorphisms (RFLP) or by a variety of newer methods (TaqMan, mass array, single base extension). Targeted genome sequencing with high-density methods used for genome-wide association studies (GWAS) is also used. The vast majority of GWAS hits are in the noncoding regions. As sequencing of the genome becomes ever more accessible and inexpensive, additional polymorphisms will be detected. Whatever the method, it is clear that the detection of polymorphisms is already available and will continue to be a key tool in understanding the variation of the immune system in human populations and in advancing personalized medicine. Often, polymorphisms act as disease modifiers, but in some cases are simply correlated with a specific disease. While here we introduce the concept of polymorphisms of selected components of the immune system, in later chapters, it will be apparent how immune system polymorphisms contribute to resistance or susceptibility to particular diseases.

N. H. Ruddle (✉)
Department of Epidemiology of Microbial Diseases, Yale School of Public Health, New Haven, CT, USA
e-mail: nancy.ruddle@yale.edu

P. B. Kavathas
Departments of Laboratory Medicine and Immunobiology, Yale School of Medicine,
Yale University, New Haven, CT, USA
e-mail: paula.kavathas@yale.edu

© Springer Nature Switzerland AG 2019
P. J. Krause et al. (eds.), *Immunoepidemiology*, https://doi.org/10.1007/978-3-030-25553-4_7

7.2   Innate Immunity: Polymorphisms of Pattern Recognition Receptors

Pattern recognition receptors (PRR) have been co-evolving with pathogens. While the ligands for PRR are generally invariant structures on pathogens, some pathogens can alter their ligand such that binding is no longer as strong or even nonexistent. In this scenario, the host can become vulnerable and the pathogen can be lethal. Individuals in a population with a rare variant PRR capable of binding to the altered pathogen ligand would recognize the pathogen, mount a response, and have a selective advantage. Over generations, this would potentially increase the frequency of the variant PRR. Polymorphisms in signaling adaptor proteins downstream of a particular PRR that affect the response from that PRR can also impact immune response to a pathogen.

An interesting case study identified genetic variants in the *PRR IFIH1* gene also known as MDA5, which recognizes RNA viruses [1]. Viral respiratory tract infections are the most common childhood illnesses worldwide, with almost 100% of children being infected during the early years of life. Often, they are mild and self-limiting, but approximately 3% of individuals have more severe disease. These infections account for 21% of childhood mortality worldwide. A genetic sequencing study was performed on children who required intensive care support even though they were previously healthy and did not have any additional major risk factors such as immunosuppression or preterm birth. Interestingly, defects in the innate recognition of RNA viruses by the MDA5 PRR variant prevented an efficient antiviral IFN response in the hospitalized patients. Thus, alterations in a PRR affected susceptibility to a certain class of microbes.

Of the 10 human toll-like receptors (TLRs) discussed in Chap. 3, a range of roughly 2–12 SNPs has been reported for each receptor [2]. The frequency of these variants can vary depending on the ethnic group. Specific SNPs were reported to be risk factors for disease susceptibility, septic shock, or cancer. For instance, the TLR-4 receptor has approximately 10 genetic variants with the highest frequency in the extracellular LRR domain that binds the ligand. Two genetic variants, Asp299Gly (rs4986790) and Thr399Ile (rs4986791), were associated with hyporesponsiveness to the ligand LPS found in gram-negative bacteria. The Asp299Gly (rs4986790) variant was associated with the risk of severe sepsis after burn injury and increased mortality in systemic inflammatory response syndrome (SIRS) patients. The Asp299Gly (rs4986790) variant was a risk factor for the development of chronic periodontitis in humans. This is an inflammatory disease affecting the connective tissue surrounding the teeth that leads to tooth loss. In contrast, the two variants were reported to have a protective association with Legionnaire's disease and leprosy.

Polymorphisms in the NLR family member NOD-2 have been reported. The highest genetic risk for developing Crohn's disease, an inflammatory bowel disease (IBD), is due to SNPs in the NOD2 gene. Crohn's disease is an inflammatory disorder in the GI tract leading to the breakdown of the intestinal barrier and an aberrant inflammatory response to the intestinal microbiota. NOD2 detects muramyl dipeptide found in the peptidoglycans of most bacteria. The NOD2 receptor is located in the cytoplasm of cells detecting intracellular bacteria or bacterial ligands taken up by cells and delivered into the cytosol. Homozygosity at three different single-nucleotide polymorphisms in NOD2 had a greater odds ratio compared with heterozygotes (20–40 vs. 2–4) [3] of developing Crohn's disease. The three NOD2 mutations affected the ligand-binding domain of NOD2 and resulted in diminished signaling. This may impair the detection and control of intestinal microbiota, pathogens, or both. Additional NOD2 polymorphisms are associated with autoinflammatory conditions (Blau syndrome) resulting in augmented signaling.

7.3 Complement

An extensive literature exists regarding the polymorphisms of the complement system which includes roughly 50 different proteins. These include activators (mannose-binding lectin), pathway components, and inhibitors. One polymorphism that is of particular interest is in Factor H, a negative regulator of the alternative complement pathway. Factor H inhibits C3 convertase (Chap. 3) that cleaves C3 to C3a and C3b and thus inhibits complement effector functions. Adult onset or age-related macular degeneration (AMD) is a major cause of severe vision loss. A coding variant in Factor H, resulting in Y402H (rs1061170), is associated with this condition in Caucasian populations [4–6]. Predicting the likelihood of disease can be used for early detection and potential therapeutic intervention. An excellent review article describing this and several SNPs in other complement genes describes in detail their worldwide distribution [7].

7.4 Innate and Adaptive Immunity: Cytokines, Chemokines, and their Receptors

7.4.1 Introduction

The biological activities of cytokines, chemokines, and their receptors have been well described in previous chapters. Their production by macrophages and stromal cells suggests their role in the innate system in immediate responses to invading pathogens. These include the proinflammatory molecules, TNF, IL-1, IFN-α, and IL-6. On the other hand, cytokines such as TNF, IL-4, and IFN-γ are produced by T and B cells as part of the adaptive system. As noted in previous chapters, the cytokines play key signaling roles in inflammation and adaptive effector functions. The chemokines are crucial molecules in guiding cell trafficking. Thus, it is natural to assume that polymorphisms in cytokines would play major roles in disease, and they do.

7.4.2 Cytokine Gene Polymorphisms in Human Disease

7.4.2.1 General Comments

Several examples exist in which polymorphisms of cytokines, chemokines, or their receptors play direct roles in disease. Polymorphisms in the TNF receptor and IL-1 are the direct causes of autoinflammatory diseases. Mutations in the γ-chain that are common to the receptors of IL-2, IL-4, IL-7, IL-9, IL-15, and IL-21 result in severe immunodeficiency. CCR5 and CXCR4 chemokine receptors act as co-receptors for HIV, and thus their polymorphisms are associated with susceptibility to viral infection, disease progression, and response to antiretroviral therapies (see Chap. 10).

On the other hand, many of the polymorphisms are associated with multifactorial diseases where cytokines act as disease modifiers. There are many analyses of the effects of SNPs, GWAS, or individual cytokine sequence polymorphisms on particular diseases. A particularly accessible, early analysis [8] provides data associating particular polymorphisms in several different cytokines with cancer, coronary artery disease, and autoimmune and inflammatory diseases, in addition to occupational and environmental diseases such as silicosis and farmer's lung. Data from these studies and others were compiled in an online database in 1999 and supplemented several times [9–12]. The publications from these websites delineate cytokine polymorphisms associated with particular diseases during the period up to 2005. A more recent review [13] concentrates on Alzheimer's disease and polymorphisms in a limited group of cytokine genes (IL-1, IL-6, TNF-α, and transforming growth factor-β).

Another large and more recent database is presented by Kveler et al. [14]. These authors have built a global immune-centric view of diseases that can predict cytokine–disease associations. They present an online site (http://www.immunexpresso.org) that can be queried regarding cytokine–disease associations.

7.4.2.2 Cytokine Polymorphisms Associated with Diseases

We note a few examples of immunoepidemiological studies of cytokine polymorphisms and diseases that are based on studies of individual human populations. Promoter region polymorphisms in the gene for migration inhibitory factor (MIF) were studied with regard to severe malarial anemia in Kenyan children [15]. The authors studied - 794 $CATT_{5-8}$ repeat polymorphisms and found that the there was an association with more severe disease in those individuals that had seven or eight CATT repeats, whereas MIF - 794 $CATT_6$ was associated with protection. Furthermore, individuals with long repeats tended to have lower MIF serum levels, suggesting that this marker might reflect functions resulting in reduced inflammation and thus lower the chance of developing severe anemia and death.

More than 600 SNPs have been identified in the TNF-α gene and potential disease association. For example, four TNF promoter SNPs were studied in an Iranian population with regard to the severity of hepatitis B infection. Those with −308 G (rs1800629), −857 C, and −863 A were significantly more likely to suffer from chronic hepatitis B infection [16]. Several promoter polymorphisms have been associated with the levels of the cytokine. In a study of age-related macular degeneration (AMD) in a Russian population, no association was found with either one of the two of the SNPs, −863 and −238 (rs361525). However, there was a higher frequency of *TNF-α* -308 AA and *TNF-α* -308 GA (rs1800629) in AMD patients than controls. The issue is somewhat less straightforward in that certain combinations of SNPs of the three studied polymorphisms were more frequently associated with AMD [17]. Given the importance of TNF-α in inflammation affecting multiple tissues, it is perhaps not surprising that there would be so many polymorphisms.

7.5   Presentation and Recognition of Self and Foreign Antigens: MHC and KIR Polymorphisms

7.5.1   MHC

The major histocompatibility complex (MHC), termed human leukocyte antigen (HLA) complex in humans located on chromosome 6, contains the most polymorphic genes in the entire human genome, namely those encoding the cell surface proteins MHC class I and II that were discussed in Chap. 4. These proteins function as antigen-presenting molecules and are important for disease susceptibility/resistance, transplantation, and autoimmunity. An Immuno Polymorphism Database (IPD) was established in 2003 to provide a centralized system for the study of polymorphisms in the genes of the immune system. The IPD-IMGT/HLA (International ImMunoGeneTics) database provides the sequences of the human MHC proteins. It contains a locus-specific database for all the different alleles for each HLA gene. Initially, the sequences were determined using protein sequencing; later they were determined by DNA sequencing of exomes or whole genomes. Information regarding the ethnic origin of the sequences in the database is available, as well as frequencies of alleles in different ethnic groups. As of December, 2018, there were 14,800 MHC class I alleles and 5288 MHC class II alleles. The number of different MHC class I proteins were 4638 (HLA-A), 5590 (HLA-B), and 4374 (HLA-C). For MHC class II, the most polymorphic genes were DRB (1908 proteins), DQB1 (878), and DPB1 (728). This section will discuss the significance of MHC polymorphism for infectious disease susceptibility, and in Chap. 8, for autoimmunity.

The high level of diversity of MHC genes is the result of both balancing and directional selection [18, 19]. The latter occurs when a mutation increases reproductive fitness and provides a selective advantage within an environment such as pathogen-driven selection. Several findings support directional selection. First, the polymorphism is not randomly found at all amino acids of the MHC or HLA protein, but is primarily at those amino acids located in the groove, that is, that part of the protein involved in peptide presentation to T cells. The analysis of nucleotide substitution patterns shows that the rate of amino acid replacement substitutions is higher than that of synonymous substitutions (a nucleotide change that does not result in amino acid substitution) in regions of the gene that encode the peptide-binding groove, while the opposite occurs in the regions of the gene that do not encode the groove. This argues for positive natural selection, a process that drives advantageous variants to high frequencies due to the enhanced survival of individuals carrying those variants. For example, viruses generally express a limited number of proteins (e.g., HPV virus expresses 9–10 proteins). If an individual does not express an MHC protein that can present a foreign viral peptide to a cytotoxic T cell, then cells infected with that intracellular virus will not be recognized and killed. The individual could succumb to a lethal virus such as the small pox-causing variola virus.

The advantage of different individuals within a population expressing different MHC types is that some members of a population may be able to present a peptide that elicits a T cell response to a particular pathogen and survive, even if others succumb. On the other hand, other members of the population could express different MHC proteins and respond well to a different pathogen. Thus, MHC allele diversity or polymorphism in the population increases the probability that some members of a population will survive infection by a lethal pathogen. The fact that MHC allele frequency differs in the populations in different geographical locations supports directional selection as pathogen exposure would not be the same. There are many examples throughout the history of lethal pathogens such as malaria and the bubonic plague during the middle ages in Europe that have had a selective force impacting human genetics.

The impact of diversity in the MHC type of members of the population is illustrated by examining HIV infection and progression to AIDS. Some HIV-infected individuals with certain HLA types do not progress to AIDS [20]. Individuals expressing the HLA proteins HLA-B57, HLA-B27, and HLA-B14 are able to present viral peptides from the conserved regions of the viral genome in the groove of those HLA proteins on the surface of infected cells. Viral mutations in those conserved viral sequences are not viable or have reduced fitness. Therefore, the virus cannot "escape" detection by CD8 cytotoxic T cells by mutating those peptide sequences that are presented to T cells. Individuals who express the above-noted HLA proteins are called "elite controllers." Given the high rate of mutation by the HIV virus, viral escape from cytotoxic CD8 T cell killing is a major problem in host defense against HIV.

It is not surprising that the frequencies of MHC alleles for different ethnic groups vary as people are exposed to the same or different pathogens depending on where they live. Endemic pathogens exert evolutionary pressures that drive higher or lower rates of certain MHC alleles in a population. A large case-control study of children in West Africa where malaria is prevalent showed that HLA-Bw53 and the HLA class II haplotype DRB1*1302–DQB1*0501 were independently associated with protection from severe malaria [21]. These MHC types were common in West Africans where malaria is endemic but rare in other racial groups.

Another driver of MHC polymorphism is balancing selection. In this case, heterozygous individuals have a selective advantage as they can potentially present peptides to T cells from multiple MHC proteins. This can result in several alleles being maintained in a population at intermediate frequencies. The HIV epidemic provided evidence for the advantages of both certain HLA alleles (example above) as well as for balancing selection. The rate of progression to AIDS in HLA heterozygous individuals is relatively slower compared with the HLA homozygous people. In addition, certain HLA alleles encoded by MHC class I and/or class II genes can be found together in individuals more frequently than expected based on their frequencies within the population. This linkage disequilibrium is thought to represent the advantage of having certain combinations of HLA proteins that can together present peptides.

Migration of people from different isolated geographical areas into cities adds to the diversity of HLA types within those cities and impacts *tissue transplantation* for kidney, bone marrow, and other organs. Approximately 0.5–0.1% of CD4 and CD8 T cells are able to cross-react and bind to foreign HLA antigens on a graft. These T cells will respond to the foreign HLA antigens expressed on the graft and lead to rejection. Thus, HLA typing is performed for donors of both organs and bone marrow in an effort to select potential donors based on HLA/MHC matching with the host.

In addition to the direct selection of HLA alleles, there can be multilocus interactions called epistasis whereby the effect of one gene is dependent on that of another. HLA proteins interact with the killer cell immunoglobulin-like receptors (KIRs) described in the following section. Both are very polymorphic systems. The combination of high frequencies of ligands and receptors or, at the other extreme, the combination of low frequencies is associated with autoimmunity and susceptibility to infection, respectively [19]. The combination also influences reproduction as described in the following sections.

7.5.2   NK Cell KIR Polymorphisms

Natural killer cells are a subpopulation of lymphocytes important both for innate response to virally infected and tumor cells as well as in the establishment of the placenta during reproduction. These cells were first characterized in the 1970s by their ability to kill tumor cells lacking self-MHC class I expression without prior sensitization. This was known as detection of "missing self " described in Chap. 3. NK cells do not harm normal healthy cells expressing MHC class I, but do attack cells compromised by infection, malignancy, or other forms of stress. Inhibitory receptors that bind MHC class I proteins are the key determinants of NK activity. In humans, there are two types of NK cell receptors that detect MHC class I: CD94/NKG2A and KIR. As NK cells are developing, they have a variegated expression pattern of these receptors. If the ligands for these receptors are expressed on host cells, it affects NK cells during their development so that they will have increased responsiveness to activation and sensitivity to "missing self." This is referred to as NK cell education.

The contribution of the NK cell CD94/NKG2A inhibitory receptor to NK education depends on the expression of its ligand, the HLA-E protein. The nonclassical MHC class I protein HLA-E is nonpolymorphic. However, its expression on the cell surface varies among people. This is because HLA-E has a peptide-binding groove, like classical MHC class I proteins, that must bind a nonamer peptide with methionine at position 2 to fold properly. This peptide is created when the leader sequences of HLA-A, HLA-B, and HLA-C (−22 to −14) proteins are cleaved after synthesis. While the leader sequences of HLA-A and HLA-C have the correct nonamer peptide, only some HLA-B-type leader sequences have methionine at position 2. The others have threonine. In that case, the peptide does not bind to HLA-E, and thus the protein does not fold properly and is not expressed on the cell surface. Because HLA-B proteins are more highly expressed than HLA-A and HLA-C, the HLA-B type of the individual has a major effect on HLA-E expression. Individuals who are HLA-B M/M homozygotes express much higher HLA-E levels relative to T/T homozygotes. Thus, NK cells with CD94/NKG2A are more educated in M/M individuals and have an increased ability to mediate the missing-self response.

The other set of receptors detecting HLA proteins are called killer cell immunoglobulin-like receptors (KIRs). They are the second most polymorphic gene family in the human genome after

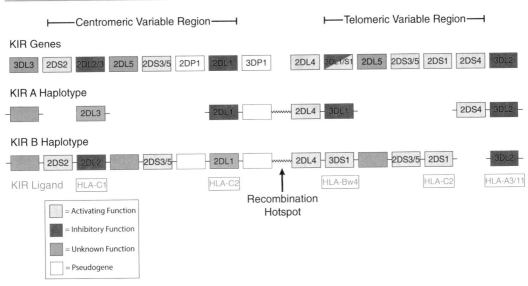

Fig. 7.1 *Human KIR locus.* Of the 15 KIR genes located on chromosome 19, the common A and B haplotypes have a subset of genes encoding activating receptors (green), inhibitory receptors (red), pseudogenes (white), or have unknown function (gray). The receptor nomenclature reflects the number of immunoglobulin-like domains (two or three) and the length of their cytoplasmic tail with short tails found in activating receptors and long tails in inhibitory receptors. The KIR B haplotype has a greater gene content diversity and can have either the 2DS3 or 2DS5 gene (slashed line). Rarer haplotypes include a shorter variant of the A haplotype with the genes deleted or a longer B haplotype with a duplication. The HLA ligands for KIR receptors are indicated. A difference is that the A haplotype gene 3DL1 binds HLA class I proteins with the Bw4 epitope, whereas the B haplotype gene 3DS1 binds HLA-F. The lighter shade indicates weaker ligand binding by the receptor. A repetitive sequence between the centromeric and telomeric regions creates a recombination hotspot. (Adapted from Parham and Guethlein [22]) (©Kavathas 2020)

HLA. The IPD-KIR database, located in the Immuno Polymorphism Databases (IPD), provides a centralized repository of human KIR receptor sequences. KIRs only exist in humans and great apes, an indication of their rapid evolution. The number of genes can vary depending on the two haplotypes an individual inherits from their mother and father. The two main haplotypes called A and B have different numbers of KIR genes out of the 15 possible genes, including some pseudogenes (Fig. 7.1). Both haplotypes include genes encoding inhibitory or activating receptors. However, the A haplotype has more genes encoding inhibitory receptors relative to activating receptors, and the B haplotype has a greater proportion of activating receptors. KIRs recognize the HLA epitopes HLA-A3/11, Bw4, C1, or C2. All HLA-C proteins express either C1 or C2. Some HLA-A or B proteins have the Bw4 epitope, and the A3/11 epitope is present on a subset of HLA-A proteins. Therefore, individuals can have from one to four KIR receptor ligands. Polymorphisms within the KIR genes lead to receptors with different affinities for their ligands, differences in expression levels, and differences in the strength of the inhibitory signal. Thus, the contribution of KIR receptors to NK education for "missing self" will depend on the pattern of KIR receptor expression on the NK cells and an individual's HLA type. Because the pattern of expression of these receptors on NK cells is variegated, if an individual has all four KIR ligands, they will possess a range of NK cells educated by KIRs.

Thus, NK education during development is determined by an individual's KIR genes, their HLA class I type, and their HLA-E expression levels. If the developing NK cell expresses KIR inhibitory receptors and/or the CD94/NKG2A inhibitory receptor and there is strong ligand binding, the NK cell will develop so as to be sensitive to the loss of self-MHC class I on host cells. NK cell education is dominated by CD94/NKG2A if there is good HLA-E expression and only one KIR ligand present.

Interestingly, there are HLA-B and HLA-C haplotype groups with certain HLA-C alleles in linkage disequilibrium with certain HLA-B polymorphisms: one biased to providing ligands that educate CD94/NKG2A+ NK cells and the other biased to providing ligands that educate KIR+ NK cells [22]. Thus, NK cells can potentially express a spectrum of receptors binding to HLA from none to weak to strong. If the NK cell's inhibitory receptor(s) for HLA strongly bind ligand, the cell exerts a vigorous response to the loss of HLA on damaged or infected target cells. NK cells that either do not bind or weakly bind HLA proteins are less "educated" but are beneficial for fighting pathogens that do not modulate HLA levels [23]. They work well in ADCC or proinflammatory microenvironments. Thus, NK education determines the threshold for NK reactivity, with the strength of NK education inversely correlated with the requirement for additional signals from activating receptors. This has important ramifications regarding the response to infectious agents and to tumors that have lost HLA class I expression.

Another impact of the combination of KIR and HLA proteins an individual expresses is on *reproduction*. Successful pregnancy is fostered by specialized *uterine NK cells* (uNK). These cells are the predominant cell types in the decidua (maternal tissue interfacing with the placenta) playing an important role in the development of the placenta and formation of the spiral arteries that bring maternal blood to the fetus [24]. Fetal trophoblast cells invade maternal tissues for remodeling. This process must be balanced, as extensive invasion is associated with high birthweight and high-risk delivery, whereas poor invasion is associated with pre-eclampsia, low birthweight, and recurrent miscarriage. The NK cells do not kill the trophoblast cells but instead assist them in tissue remodeling.

Some combinations of KIR receptors on the NK cells and HLA types of the mother and fetus are associated with poor invasion of the decidua for a first pregnancy [23]. Mothers homozygous for the KIR A haplotype have an increased rate of miscarriage, pre-eclampsia, and babies of low birth when the mothers also carry an HLA-C1 allele and the fetus has an HLA-C2 allele inherited from the father. The trophoblast cells express HLA-C and HLA-E but not HLA-A and HLA-B. The cognate CD94/NKG2A and KIR2D receptors which are overexpressed on the uNK cells encounter C1/C2 heterozygous fetal cells. The KIR A haplotype has inhibitory receptors for C1 and C2 but lacks the activating receptor KIR2DS1 that could bind to HLA-C2 of paternal origin. In this case, the educated NK cells are presumably insufficiently activated to promote tissue remodeling. The uNK education and the HLA type of the fetus which favors maternal NK responsiveness over inhibition would promote successful placentation and spiral artery formation.

7.6   T Cell Receptor Polymorphisms

T cell receptors (TCR) are cell surface molecules that consist of two chains: either αβ or γδ. The receptors' variable domains are generated in a manner similar to that of immunoglobulins (Chap. 4). For TCRαβ, each α chain is encoded by a variable (TRAV), a joining, and a constant gene (VJC). There are 70–80 Vα segments and 61 Jα segments. Similarly, each β chain is encoded by a variable (TRBV), a diversity, a joining, and a constant gene (VDJC). There are 52 Vβ1 sequences, 2 Dβ sequences, 13 Jβ sequences, and 2 Cβ sequences (Figs. 7.2 and 7.3). Further variability is generated by the random insertion of nucleotides during somatic recombination of VJ or VDJ gene segments. The combination of the two alpha and beta variable domains is the recognition moiety of the receptor that interacts with the peptide presented by HLA Class I or II. The constant domains are the regions that cluster with the associated CD3 molecules to transmit signals to the nucleus after the engagement of the receptor with the antigen. In this section, we consider polymorphisms in human TCRs as detected through the analysis of SNPs, GWAS studies, and functional polymorphisms in antigen-specific TCRs. The majority of the polymorphisms that have been identified are in the α-and β-chains, since they comprise the

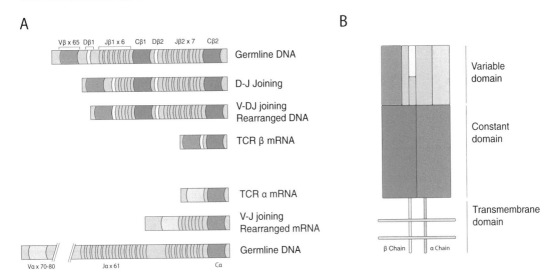

Fig. 7.2 *Somatic recombination to generate the αβ-T cell receptor (TCR).* The VDJ recombination mechanism used for creating B cell receptor diversity is used for creating T cell receptor diversity. Instead of the light and heavy chains found in the B cell receptor, the T cell receptor is composed of alpha (α) and beta (β) chains, or in a subset of T cells, gamma (γ), and delta (δ) chains. Panel A shows the transition from the germline DNA with many possible V D J segments for the beta chain and VJ segments for the alpha chain to a single VJ or VDJ sequence in TCR mRNA of the α and β chains, respectively. This occurs through somatic recombination in a T lymphocyte during development. Panel B shows the TCR that is created from the TCR mRNA and how each protein component of the TCR has been encoded from a specific V, D, or J gene segment. The variable region is responsible for antigen recognition while the constant region is embedded in the T cell surface. (Adapted from DeSimone et al. ref [8] Chap.4) (©Krause 2020)

majority of TCRs. The International Immunogenetics database (IMGT) noted earlier for HLA, KIR, and immunoglobulin also includes data on the TCRs of multiple species, although we concentrate on the identified human polymorphisms.

Multiple SNP allelic polymorphisms have been described in *TCRA* and *TCRB* genes, with some resulting in amino acid changes. In one of the earliest and most comprehensive studies, Subrahmanyan et al. [25] analyzed sequence variation in the *TCRBV* locus in 10 individuals in each of four populations (African American, Chinese, Mexican, and Northern European.). They evaluated 63 V region genes and found 279 SNPs that were located throughout the sequence of each TCRBV segment representing the promoter, exons, an intron, and even the recombination signal sequence. A large number (111) of polymorphic sites were found in a single population: 86 in the African American population, 13 in the Chinese population, 6 in the Mexican population, and 6 in the Northern European population. Later studies evaluated the same four populations with regard to the *TCRA/D* locus SNP [26] and sequence [27] polymorphisms. Again, a large number (284) of SNPS were identified that encompassed all parts of the genes (promoters, exons, and introns). An average of five SNPs per V gene was identified (ranging from 0 to 15). As in the previous study on *TCRB* polymorphisms, there was significant variation among the populations, where 79 of the 284 variants were found in a single population. The largest number were found in the African American population.

There have been numerous attempts to correlate TCR polymorphisms with disease. An early study on germline polymorphisms evaluated the relationship of TCR polymorphisms to the autoimmune disease, systemic lupus erythematosus (SLE). An association was found between a particular TCRα RFLP and the disease in Mexican and American individuals [24, 28, 29]. Despite the capacity for an enormous amount of heterogeneity in TCRs, it has actually been possible in a few instances to define

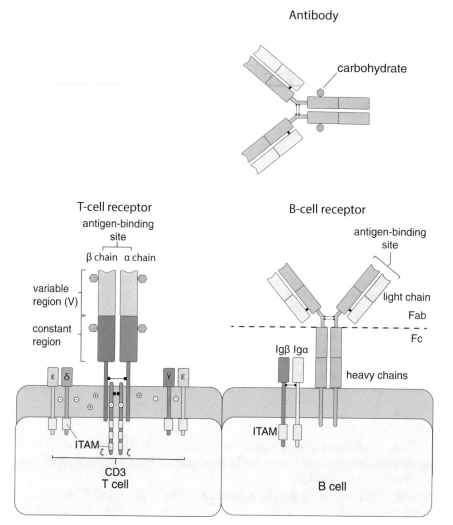

Fig. 7.3 *Structure of the B cell and T cell receptors.* Lymphocyte antigen receptors consist of the *T cell receptor* (TCR) on the T cell surface, the *B cell receptor* (BCR) on the B cell surface, and the *secreted antibody molecule.* The antibody lacks the transmembrane domain of the BCR. The antibody can be cleaved by papain, and the reduction of the disulfide bonds in the hinge region results in (i) two fragment antigen-binding (Fab) components and (ii) one fragment crystallizable (Fc) component (the effector moiety of the antibody molecule). The TCR contains α and β chains that recognize antigen, but signals are transmitted by the associated CD3 complex of proteins (εδ, γε, and ζ ζ). Interaction between proteins is in part mediated by positive and negative charges within the transmembrane domains. Immunoreceptor tyrosine-based activation motifs (ITAMS) are motifs in the cytoplasmic tail that interact with adaptor proteins for signal transduction. The Igα and Igβ chains interacting with the BCR contain ITAM motifs as do CD3 proteins (©Krause 2020)

certain *public specificities,* that is, the V gene usage is prevalent across a human population that is associated with reactivity to a particular pathogen. These have included HIV and Epstein–Barr virus. In a study of reactivity to Gag293, a determinant of HIV, Benati et al. [28] compared TCR usage of a population of HIV controllers to a group of patients who were on antiretroviral therapy (HAART group). The controllers had a highly skewed TCR repertoire to Gag293 with a preferential usage of TRAV24 and TRBV2 variable gene segments compared to the HAART group, even though there was considerable clonotypic diversity in the T cells of the controllers. These data indicate preferential usage of a "public" specificity in a group of individuals who appear to be mounting a defensive immunological response to the virus.

Another example of preferential usage of a public specificity was reported by Gras et al. [30] who studied the T cell reactivity of 27 healthy Caucasian individuals against an epitope of an Epstein–Barr virus protein. They noted the predominant use of *TRBV9*01* as a public TCR, that is, used by many individuals. The authors noted that the common allelic variant TRBV9∗02, which differs by a single amino acid, was never used. These studies suggested that it will be possible to predict TCR usage based on epitope characteristics. Recent advances in bioinformatics and the analysis of repertoire usage in populations of individuals [31] and in individual cells in an individual during aging [32] provide great promise for the further understanding regarding functional polymorphisms. Repertoire analysis, and reactivity to individual pathogens will have implications for vaccine development and disease susceptibility.

7.7 Immunoglobulin Polymorphisms

Immunoglobulin polymorphisms are beginning to be appreciated with increased genomic sequencing. Antibody molecules consist of two heavy and two light chains (Fig. 7.3) that are generated through the process of somatic recombination (Chap. 4). There are currently more than 420 identified polymorphisms in Ig genes for the heavy and light chain genes. This gene diversity arises from single-nucleotide polymorphisms (SNPs) and copy number variation (CNV), which include insertions, duplications, and deletions [33–35]. These data emerged from the 1000 Genomes Project [35, 36], a multicenter project designed to examine human genetic variation. Immunoglobulin diversity exists between people of a given population as well as among human ethnic groups. This variation may result in differences in the development of B cell receptors, B cell memory, and antibody function [33].

There is evidence to suggest that the Ig germline polymorphisms have functional implications for mounting an antibody response against an antigen important for a particular disease, in this case influenza virus infection. Interesting data were reported for the IG heavy chain variable gene cluster (IGVH) gene *IGHV1–69*. The immunoglobulin heavy chain V region genes are organized into subgroups. The IGHV1 subgroup has several members including the *IGHV1–69* gene [37]. The hemagglutinin (HA) major capsid protein of influenza has a stem region that is relatively invariant. It was determined that there was predominant usage of the *IGHV1–69* alleles with a critical phenylalanine at position 54 (F54) (SNP rs5589101) in the CDR2 loop for broadly neutralizing antibodies against the stem region of HA. Alleles of *IGHV1–69* that substitute an alanine (A54) or leucine (L54) at the same position 54 in the heavy-chain protein showed dramatically decreased binding affinities of antibodies against influenza [33, 34]. Africans and Europeans had the highest percentage of F/F alleles, and South Asians have the lowest percentage (Fig. 7.4). Although no studies compared the incidence or severity of influenza infection in these study populations, the *IGHV1–69* alleles were shown to confer differences in antigen binding, clonal expansion, affinity maturation, and class switching [33]. These differences suggest that the study populations may vary in the quality of their antibody responses to influenza and influenza vaccination [35, 38]. The absence of an F/F antibody alone does not necessarily mean a poorer outcome from influenza as other genes are available that may produce alternative and equally effective antibodies.

The gene usage of a second *IGVH1–69* SNP (rs1184524) with multiple alleles was also analyzed in the 1000 Genomes Project. The ability of an antibody to bind the *Staphylococcus aureus* NEAr iron transporter 2 (NEAT2) domain was assessed. Better neutralizing Abs were found when individuals had glycine at position 50 (G50) than if they had alleles encoding arginine at position 50 (R50).

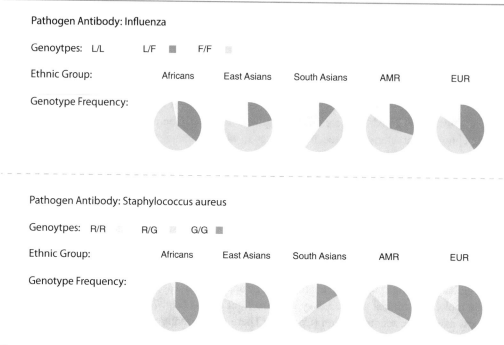

Fig. 7.4 *Impacts of IG germline polymorphism on antibody repertoire/structural diversity.* Two single-nucleotide polymorphisms (SNPs) in the highly variable *IGHV1–69* gene (in B cell germline) have been shown to encode functional residues critical for neutralizing antibodies against the influenza virus hemagglutinin stem region (F54 and L54 amino acid-associated alleles; SNP rs55891010) and the "NEAT2" domain of *Staphylococcus aureus* (R50 and G50 alleles; SNP rs11845244). The frequency of these SNPs differs between five human ethnic groups (Africans, East Asians, South Asians, Central/South Americans, and Europeans). In the top panel, the F allele encodes the functional critical phenylalanine residue for influenza antibody, while in the bottom panel, the G allele encodes the functional critical phenylalanine residue for the *Staphylococcus aureus* antibody. The figure demonstrates different genetic prevalence for antibody formation among several populations in different parts of the world. (Figure 7.4 originally copyright obtained from Elsevier (Roopa Lingayath) 5/2719/ from Watson et al The Individual and Population Genetics of Antibody Immunity, *Trends Immunology* Volume 38, Issue 7, July 2017, Pages 459–470. Original source: The 1000 Genomes Project Consortium. A global reference for human genetic variation. *Nature* 526: 68-74, 2015.) Creative Common

Antibodies that had glycine at position 50 had the higher affinity. As with the antibody directed against influenza, the distribution of the *IGVH1–69* alleles for the *Staphylococcus aureus* antibody differed among the five geographically dispersed populations, with the Africans and Europeans having the highest frequency of G/G alleles (Fig. 7.4). With better understanding of Ig germline polymorphisms and biased antibody responses to specific epitopes, it may be possible to understand the immunogenetic potential of an individual's baseline naïve repertoire.

The Fc component of an antibody is also polymorphic and varies in its structural and functional characteristics among immunoglobulin classes and in its distribution among human subpopulations [39, 40]. An intact antibody Fc region and its target receptors are required for several antibody-mediated immune responses, including the clearance of immune complexes by phagocytes. Immune complexes contribute to the pathogenesis of several autoimmune diseases, including systemic lupus erythematosus (SLE). SLE has been associated with certain Fc receptor variants located on neutrophils and monocytes that do not effectively bind and remove immune complexes [41, 42]. Certain Fc receptor variants are less able to facilitate neutrophil phagocytosis than others and may thereby inhibit the resolution of infection. Interestingly, immune cells with lower affinity Fc receptors respond less well to monoclonal antibody therapy [41], as noted in Chap. 16.

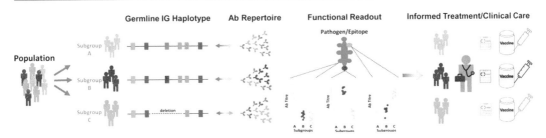

Fig. 7.5 *A paradigm for integrating genotypic information into the study of the Ab-mediated response in disease and clinical phenotypes.* In the proposed paradigm, a population cohort is partitioned into subgroups based on functional genotypes/haplotypes that are directly associated with subgroup-specific signatures in the expressed repertoire and other relevant phenotypes (e.g., Ab titer; clinical outcome) associated with the Ab response to a given antigen/epitope. This partitioning can be used to inform tailored clinical care and treatment (e.g., vaccination regime). (Used with permission from Watson et al. [35])

A framework for carrying out future studies to integrate genotypic information on antibody polymorphisms with antibody responses to infection and vaccination was suggested by Watson et al. based on several studies of the *IGHV1–69* SNPs [35] (Fig. 7.5). The sequential steps in this algorithm are as follows: (i) identify different germline antibody genotypes/haplotypes (alleles) in a population and partition the population into subgroups based on their inferred type of antibody response, (ii) characterize the antibody repertoire of these different subgroups, (iii) characterize the epitopes on the microbe that each antibody is reacting against, and (iv) analyze the antibody titer to each epitope for each subpopulation and the clinical outcome from infection. This information can then be used to tailor the vaccine type (e.g., subunit vs. inactivated organism) and clinical care during a pathogen outbreak for each patient subpopulation.

References

1. Asgari S, Schlapbach LJ, Anchisi S, Hammer C, Bartha I, Junier T, et al. Severe viral respiratory infections in children with IFIH1 loss-of-function mutations. Proc Natl Acad Sci U S A. 2017;114(31):8342–7.
2. Noreen M, Arshad M. Association of TLR1, TLR2, TLR4, TLR6, and TIRAP polymorphisms with disease susceptibility. Immunol Res. 2015;62(2):234–52.
3. Zhang H, Zeng Z, Mukherjee A, Shen B. Molecular diagnosis and classification of inflammatory bowel disease. Expert Rev Mol Diagn. 2018;18(10):867–86.
4. Edwards AO, Ritter R 3rd, Abel KJ, Manning A, Panhuysen C, Farrer LA. Complement factor H polymorphism and age-related macular degeneration. Science. 2005;308(5720):421–4.
5. Haines JL, Hauser MA, Schmidt S, Scott WK, Olson LM, Gallins P, et al. Complement factor H variant increases the risk of age-related macular degeneration. Science. 2005;308(5720):419–21.
6. Klein RJ, Zeiss C, Chew EY, Tsai JY, Sackler RS, Haynes C, et al. Complement factor H polymorphism in age-related macular degeneration. Science. 2005;308(5720):385–9.
7. Ermini L, Wilson IJ, Goodship TH, Sheerin NS. Complement polymorphisms: geographical distribution and relevance to disease. Immunobiology. 2012;217(2):265–71.
8. Yucesoy B, Kashon ML, Luster MI. Cytokine polymorphisms in chronic inflammatory diseases with reference to occupational diseases. Curr Mol Med. 2003;3(1):39–48.
9. Bidwell J, Keen L, Gallagher G, Kimberly R, Huizinga T, McDermott MF, et al. Cytokine gene polymorphism in human disease: on-line databases. Genes Immun. 1999;1(1):3–19.
10. Bidwell J, Keen L, Gallagher G, Kimberly R, Huizinga T, McDermott MF, et al. Cytokine gene polymorphism in human disease: on-line databases, supplement 1. Genes Immun. 2001;2(2):61–70.
11. Haukim N, Bidwell JL, Smith AJ, Keen LJ, Gallagher G, Kimberly R, et al. Cytokine gene polymorphism in human disease: on-line databases, supplement 2. Genes Immun. 2002;3(6):313–30.
12. Hollegaard MV, Bidwell JL. Cytokine gene polymorphism in human disease: on-line databases, Supplement 3. Genes Immun. 2006;7(4):269–76.

13. Su F, Bai F, Zhang Z. Inflammatory cytokines and Alzheimer's disease: a review from the perspective of genetic polymorphisms. Neurosci Bull. 2016;32(5):469–80.

14. Kveler K, Starosvetsky E, Ziv-Kenet A, Kalugny Y, Gorelik Y, Shalev-Malul G, et al. Immune-centric network of cytokines and cells in disease context identified by computational mining of PubMed. Nat Biotechnol. 2018; 36(7):651–9.

15. Awandare GA, Martinson JJ, Were T, Ouma C, Davenport GC, Ong'echa JM, et al. MIF (macrophage migration inhibitory factor) promoter polymorphisms and susceptibility to severe malarial anemia. J Infect Dis. 2009; 200(4):629–37.

16. Heidari Z, Moudi B, Mahmoudzadeh Sagheb H, Moudi M. Association of TNF-alpha gene polymorphisms with production of protein and susceptibility to chronic hepatitis B infection in the south east Iranian population. Hepat Mon. 2016;16(11):e41984.

17. Chernykh V, Shevchenko A, Konenkov V, Prokofiev V, Eremina A, Trunov A. TNF-α gene polymorphisms: association with age-related macular degeneration in Russian population. Int J Ophthalmol. 2019;12(1):25–9.

18. Cagliani R, Sironi M. Pathogen-driven selection in the human genome. Int J Evol Biol. 2013;2013:204240.

19. Meyer D, VR CA, Bitarello BD, DY CB, Nunes K. A genomic perspective on HLA evolution. Immunogenetics. 2018;70(1):5–27.

20. McMichael AJ, Jones EY. Genetics. First-class control of HIV-1. Science. 2010;330(6010):1488–90.

21. Hill AV, Allsopp CE, Kwiatkowski D, Anstey NM, Twumasi P, Rowe PA, et al. Common west African HLA antigens are associated with protection from severe malaria. Nature. 1991;352(6336):595–600.

22. Parham P, Guethlein LA. Genetics of natural killer cells in human health, disease, and survival. Annu Rev Immunol. 2018;36:519–48.

23. Boudreau JE, Hsu KC. Natural killer cell education in human health and disease. Curr Opin Immunol. 2018;50: 102–11.

24. Mor G, Abrahams VM. Immunology of pregnancy. In: Resnick R, Lockwood CJ, Moore TR, Greene ME, Copel JA, Silver RM, editors. Creasy and Resnik's maternal-fetal medicine: principles and practice: Elsevier Health Sciences; 2018. p. 128–41.

25. Subrahmanyan L, Eberle MA, Clark AG, Kruglyak L, Nickerson DA. Sequence variation and linkage disequilibrium in the human T-cell receptor beta (TCRB) locus. Am J Hum Genet. 2001;69(2):381–95.

26. Mackelprang R, Carlson CS, Subrahmanyan L, Livingston RJ, Eberle MA, Nickerson DA. Sequence variation in the human T-cell receptor loci. Immunol Rev. 2002;190:26–39.

27. Mackelprang R, Livingston RJ, Eberle MA, Carlson CS, Yi Q, Akey JM, et al. Sequence diversity, natural selection and linkage disequilibrium in the human T cell receptor alpha/delta locus. Hum Genet. 2006;119(3):255–66.

28. Benati D, Galperin M, Lambotte O, Gras S, Lim A, Mukhopadhyay M, et al. Public T cell receptors confer high-avidity CD4 responses to HIV controllers. J Clin Invest. 2016;126(6):2093–108.

29. Tebib JG, Alcocer-Varela J, Alarcon-Segovia D, Schur PH. Association between a T cell receptor restriction fragment length polymorphism and systemic lupus erythematosus. J Clin Invest 1990;86(6):1961–67.

30. Gras S, Chen Z, Miles JJ, Liu YC, Bell MJ, Sullivan LC, et al. Allelic polymorphism in the T cell receptor and its impact on immune responses. J Exp Med. 2010;207(7):1555–67.

31. Dash P, Fiore-Gartland AJ, Hertz T, Wang GC, Sharma S, Souquette A, et al. Quantifiable predictive features define epitope-specific T cell receptor repertoires. Nature. 2017;547(7661):89–93.

32. Lu Y, Biancotto A, Cheung F, Remmers E, Shah N, McCoy JP, et al. Systematic analysis of cell-to-cell expression variation of T lymphocytes in a human cohort identifies aging and genetic associations. Immunity. 2016;45(5): 1162–75.

33. Avnir Y, Watson CT, Glanville J, Peterson EC, Tallarico AS, Bennett AS, et al. IGHV1-69 polymorphism modulates anti-influenza antibody repertoires, correlates with IGHV utilization shifts and varies by ethnicity. Sci Rep. 2016;6:20842.

34. Pappas L, Foglierini M, Piccoli L, Kallewaard NL, Turrini F, Silacci C, et al. Rapid development of broadly influenza neutralizing antibodies through redundant mutations. Nature. 2014;516(7531):418–22.

35. Watson CT, Glanville J, Marasco WA. The individual and population genetics of antibody immunity. Trends Immunol. 2017;38(7):459–70.

36. Genomes Project C, Auton A, Brooks LD, Durbin RM, Garrison EP, Kang HM, et al. A global reference for human genetic variation. Nature. 2015;526(7571):68–74.

37. Watson CT, Breden F. The immunoglobulin heavy chain locus: genetic variation, missing data, and implications for human disease. Genes Immun. 2012;13(5):363–73.

38. Wheatley AK, Whittle JR, Lingwood D, Kanekiyo M, Yassine HM, Ma SS, et al. H5N1 vaccine-elicited memory B cells are genetically constrained by the IGHV locus in the recognition of a neutralizing epitope in the hemagglutinin stem. J Immunol. 2015;195(2):602–10.

39. Ahmed AA, Giddens J, Pincetic A, Lomino JV, Ravetch JV, Wang LX, et al. Structural characterization of anti-inflammatory immunoglobulin G Fc proteins. J Mol Biol. 2014;426(18):3166–79.

40. Bournazos S, Chow SK, Abboud N, Casadevall A, Ravetch JV. Human IgG Fc domain engineering enhances anti-toxin neutralizing antibody activity. J Clin Invest. 2014;124(2):725–9.
41. Kaifu T, Nakamura A. Polymorphisms of immunoglobulin receptors and the effects on clinical outcome in cancer immunotherapy and other immune diseases: a general review. Int Immunol. 2017;29(7):319–25.
42. Tsang ASMW, Nagelkerke SQ, Bultink IE, Geissler J, Tanck MW, Tacke CE, et al. Fc-gamma receptor polymorphisms differentially influence susceptibility to systemic lupus erythematosus and lupus nephritis. Rheumatology (Oxford). 2016;55(5):939–48.

Immunoepidemiology of Immune Dysfunction

Eric Meffre, Peter J. Krause, and Nancy H. Ruddle

8.1   Introduction

In Chap. 6, we introduced the concept of dysfunction in the immune system. Here, we delve more deeply into some of these topics from the perspective of advances that have been made in our understanding of immune dysfunction by evaluating the immunoepidemiology of immune deficiency and immune hyperresponsiveness/hypersensitivity. Hypersensitivity reactions have traditionally been classified mechanistically as (I) immediate hypersensitivity (allergic diseases, usually mediated by IgE antibody), (II) antibody-mediated, (III) immune complex, and (IV) lymphocyte-mediated reactions. In this chapter, we shall approach immune dysfunction with a more clinical focus and discuss the immunoepidemiological aspects of immunodeficiency, allergy, and autoimmunity. Immunoepidemiology is the study of the diversity of immune responses in populations and the factors influencing this diversity. A subset of the general population develops immunodeficiency, allergy, or autoimmunity, and within each of these subpopulations is an array of immune dysfunction. Previous studies of these groups have provided a clearer picture of how the immune system works, how it can malfunction, the risk factors for the development of immune dysfunction, and how we may diagnose and treat those afflicted with these conditions.

E. Meffre
Departments of Immunobiology and Internal Medicine, Yale School of Medicine,
New Haven, CT, USA
e-mail: eric.meffre@yale.edu

P. J. Krause
Department of Epidemiology of Microbial Diseases, Yale School of Public Health and Departments of Medicine and Pediatrics, Yale School of Medicine, New Haven, CT, USA
e-mail: peter.krause@yale.edu

N. H. Ruddle (✉)
Department of Epidemiology of Microbial Diseases, Yale School of Public Health, New Haven, CT, USA
e-mail: nancy.ruddle@yale.edu

© Springer Nature Switzerland AG 2019
P. J. Krause et al. (eds.), *Immunoepidemiology*, https://doi.org/10.1007/978-3-030-25553-4_8

8.2 Lessons from Patients with Primary Immunodeficiencies Resulting from Specific Gene Mutations

8.2.1 Definition of Primary Immunodeficiencies

Primary immunodeficiencies are a heterogeneous group of syndromes resulting from gene mutations affecting the function of the immune system [1]. Primary immunodeficiencies were first evidenced by impairments of the adaptive immune system and characterized by early onset infectious events in young infants who failed to thrive due to their inability to produce either T cells or B cells or both in severe combined immunodeficiency diseases (SCID). It became clear that most of these syndromes were monogenic and caused in most cases by recessive deleterious mutations in a single gene on either the autosomal (chromosomes 1–22) or the X chromosome. In the case of autosomal genes, recessive deleterious mutations cripple both alleles and therefore prevent the production of a functional molecule, whereas a single recessive X-linked gene mutation is sufficient to induce a phenotype in males because they only carry a single X chromosome. Of note, many genes encoding molecules that mediate important roles in the immune system (*BTK, TNFSF5/CD40L, FOXP3, WAS, SH2D1A*) are located on the X chromosome, and their mutations induce X-linked syndromes affecting young boys, whereas carrier mothers are mostly asymptomatic due to the presence of a second X chromosome harboring a functional gene.

In addition to the susceptibility to various infectious microorganisms, patients with primary immunodeficiencies often develop paradoxical autoimmune manifestations with autoantibody production, while they fail to secrete high-affinity antigen-specific protective antibodies and mount ineffective responses to vaccines. The origins of autoimmune complications in these patients will be discussed.

8.2.2 Novel Concepts in Primary Immunodeficiencies

8.2.2.1 Gene Mutations May Display Incomplete Penetrance

While the initial reports of primary immunodeficiency diseases followed a Mendelian inheritance, meaning that all individuals with deleterious mutated alleles were affected, more recent studies showed that gene mutations associated with primary immunodeficiencies may have an incomplete penetrance. For instance, some individuals carrying heterozygous mutations in either *CTLA4* or *TNFRSF13B* gene that encodes cytotoxic T-lymphocyte-associated protein 4 (CTLA-4 aka CD152) and transmembrane activator and CAML interactor (TACI), respectively, were not affected, whereas other carriers from the same family suffer from immunodeficiency, suggesting that either other gene modifiers or environmental factors influence disease development [2].

8.2.2.2 Gene Mutations May Induce Various Phenotypes and Syndromes

In addition, different mutations in the same gene may differentially affect immune cell development and responses, resulting in various syndromes. For instance, mutations in recombination-activating genes 1 (RAG1) and RAG2, the enzymes that catalyze V(D)J recombination are associated with a broad spectrum of clinical and immunological manifestations. RAG mutations, resulting in either SCID or Omenn syndromes, induce lower enzymatic activity compared to those in patients with less severe diseases characterized by defective antibody production and autoimmunity [3].

8.2.2.3 Early Diagnosis of Primary Immunodeficiency Diseases

The diagnosis of primary immunodeficiency diseases often relies on the recurrence or multiplicity of infectious episodes that are not immediately noticed by physicians and may delay the provision of appropriate therapeutic approaches. The previous occurrence of primary immunodeficiency diseases in some families may obviously alert physicians who may otherwise be unaware of such diagnosis. While global increasing awareness of primary immunodeficiency diseases favors their diagnosis, newborn screening for life-threatening primary immunodeficiencies such as SCID is now performed in many states of the United States and allows the early identification of these patients before any symptoms occur. This screening consists of assessing the presence of T cells in neonate's blood by detecting T-cell receptor excision circles (TREC) generated during the recombination of the T-cell receptor genes by PCR [4]. A failure to detect TREC reveals the absence of T cells that warrants further blood investigations in these newborns and potentially leads to the diagnosis of SCID and the rapid initiation of therapeutic approaches such as bone marrow transplantation or gene therapy (see Sect. 8.2.7).

8.2.2.4 Gene Mutations May Manifest Phenotype Later in Life and Confer Restricted Susceptibility to Specific Pathogens

The first primary immunodeficiency diseases that were characterized were identified in young patients who were subject to a broad spectrum of infections. It has now been shown that gene defects can induce immune dysregulation later in life, can sometimes be associated with a primary immunodeficiency diagnosis in adulthood, and can induce deficiency to a limited array of pathogens. The immune susceptibility of more recently characterized primary immunodeficiencies can even be restricted to specific types of pathogens and sometimes to a single one such as herpes simplex virus (HSV), which causes encephalitis in patients deficient in TLR3, UNC93B1, TRIF, TRAF3, TBK1, or IRF3. These are key molecules of the TLR3 pathway essential for mediating the immune response against HSV [5]. Mendelian susceptibility to mycobacterial diseases is associated with inborn errors of IFN-γ immunity. X-linked lymphoproliferative disease (XLP) caused by mutations in the X-linked *SH2D1A* gene encoding SAP is another example of restricted susceptibility to a single pathogen, that is, Epstein–Barr virus.

8.2.3 Gene Mutations Affecting Early Lymphoid Development and Severe Combined Immunodeficiency Diseases (SCID)

SCID are life-threatening syndromes caused by gene mutations impairing the development of the adaptive immune system and more specifically T cells. A famous patient inspired the expression "Bubble Boy" in reference to the fact that he was forced to live in a sterile environment to prevent infections. SCID is subdivided into T–B, in which patients display near complete absence of T and B cells in circulating blood, and T–B+ SCID, in which patients lack T cells but possess B cells. Both groups of SCID include forms with or without NK cells.

8.2.3.1 T–B–NK- and NK+ SCID and Omenn Syndrome

T–B–NK–SCID may result from mutations in the autosomal *adenosine deaminase* (*ADA*) gene that encodes an enzyme that transforms toxic purine metabolites; as a consequence, ADA loss of function results in the apoptosis and death of early lymphoid precursors. Mutations abrogating RAG activity in T–B–NK + SCID patients prevent the recombination of immunoglobulin and T-cell receptor (TCR) gene segments, thereby impairing the production of B-cell receptors (BCR) and TCRs necessary for

B and T cell development, respectively, whereas NK cells can develop. Of note, *RAG* mutations that allow the formation of a few T cells may result in Omenn syndrome, which is characterized not only by high susceptibility to fungal, bacterial, and viral infections as in SCID patients but also severe autoimmune manifestations combined with erythroderma, eosinophilia, and allergies [3]. Circulating B cells are rarely detected in the blood of Omenn syndrome patients, but some are produced, as evidenced by their elevated serum IgE concentrations. Mutations in other molecules involved in V(D)J recombination such as Artemis encoded by the *DNA cross-link repair 1C* (*DCLRE1C*) gene and the DNA-dependent protein kinase (DNA-PK) encoded by the *PRKDC* gene may also result in either T–B–NK+ SCID or the Omenn syndrome.

8.2.3.2 T–B+ SCID

Some gene mutations may only affect the development of T cells with or without NK cell involvement and without altering B cell development in T–B + NK+/− SCID patients. Mutations in X-linked *common gamma chain* (*IL2RG*) gene and autosomal mutations in *IL7RA* or *Janus kinase 3* (*JAK3*), which encodes JAK3 that binds the common gamma (γc) chain, prevent the assembly and signaling of the IL-7 receptor, thereby revealing the essential role of interleukin-7 (IL-7) for T cell development [6]. Since the γc chain is also part of the IL-2, IL-4, IL-9, IL-15, and IL-21 receptors and since IL-15 is necessary for NK cell development and survival, γc chain-deficient SCID patients lack both T and NK cells. Rare forms of T–B + NK+ SCID are associated with mutations in *CD3D* and *CD3E* genes that encode CD3δ and CD3ε, the two key components of the CD3 complex that associate with the TCR and mediate its signaling.

8.2.3.3 Bare Lymphocyte Syndromes (BLS)

BLS type I and type II are characterized by the absence of either major histocompatibility complex (MHC) class I or class II molecules, respectively, the latter being induced by mutations in the transcription factors regulating MHC class II expression. BLS I and BLS II result in severe immunodeficiency in the absence of proper CD8+ or CD4+ T cell development, respectively.

8.2.4 Mutations Affecting T Cell Selection and Function

Gene mutations may specifically alter the selection of T cells in the thymus and interfere with the production or the function of regulatory T cells (Tregs) that play an essential role in maintaining tolerance.

8.2.4.1 Autoimmune Polyendocrinopathy–Candidiasis–Ectodermal Dystrophy (APECED) Syndrome

Mutations in immune regulator (AIRE) result in APECED syndrome also named autoimmune polyglandular syndrome type 1 (APS-1), which is characterized by defective central T cell tolerance, autoimmunity targeting the parathyroid and adrenal glands, the production of many autoantibodies targeting tissue-specific antigens and cytokines, and fungal infections such as chronic mucocutaneous candidiasis. AIRE mediates the ectopic expression of peripheral tissue antigens (PTAs) in medullary thymic epithelial cells (mTECs), thereby ensuring immunological tolerance by regulating the selection of the TCR repertoire through the deletion of autoreactive thymocytes and directing the autoreactive clones into the Treg lineage [7]. Hence, the absence of functional AIRE allows some autoreactive T cells to enter the conventional T cell compartments instead of becoming Tregs, which likely favors the development of autoimmune conditions.

8.2.4.2 Immune Dysregulation, Polyendocrinopathy, Enteropathy, X-Linked (IPEX) Syndrome

IPEX syndrome caused by mutations in the X-linked *forkhead box protein 3* (*FOXP3*) gene demonstrates the key role played by Tregs in maintaining tolerance [8]. Indeed, mutations in FOXP3, a transcription factor critical for Treg function, result in a severe autoimmune disorder mostly targeting endocrine glands and the production of various autoantibodies in IPEX patients. This syndrome is very severe, and affected newborns may already manifest some autoimmune condition such as type 1 diabetes.

Mutations in genes encoding CD25/IL-2Rα, CTLA-4, and LRBA molecules important for Treg survival or function also induce autoimmune conditions that may resemble IPEX syndrome, although milder phenotypes have been reported in individuals with heterozygous *CTLA4* gene mutations who may only display autoimmune disease of the thyroid alone or even no clinical manifestation [2].

8.2.4.3 Wiskott–Aldrich Syndrome (WAS)

Mutations in the X-linked *WAS* gene induce eczema, thrombocytopenia, and immunodeficiency, as initially described by Drs. Wiskott and Aldrich. Abnormal WAS protein induces cytoskeleton rearrangement defects resulting in small platelets and low platelet counts, a failure to form an immunological synapse after TCR activation, altered antibody production, nonsuppressive Tregs linked to autoimmune manifestations, and susceptibility to develop lymphoma. The assessment of gene therapy for Wiskott–Aldrich patients revealed promising outcomes and may be considered as the therapeutic approach for this syndrome. Milder mutations of the *WAS* gene may induce less severe disorders such as X-linked thrombocytopenia (XLT) or X-linked congenital neutropenia (XLN).

8.2.5   Gene Mutations Specifically Affecting Antibody Production

Dr. Ogden C. Bruton described for the first time in 1952 a young boy susceptible to recurrent pneumococcal infections who lacked gamma globulins in his serum, revealing that he could not produce immunoglobulins [9]. Bruton also postulated that supplementation with serum gamma globulins isolated from healthy individuals might be beneficial to these patients, and this is currently the standard of care for many patients with primary immunodeficiencies. It was only decades later that mutations in the X-linked *Bruton tyrosine kinase* (*BTK*) gene were demonstrated to result in the virtual absence of B cells in the blood of male patients with X-linked agammaglobulinemia (XLA) syndrome. Autosomal gene mutation may also result in either impaired B cell development and agammaglobulinemia or normal B cell development but defective antibody responses and are presented in the paragraphs below.

8.2.5.1 Defects in Early B Cell Development and Agammaglobulinemia

Mutations in several genes have been reported in humans that specifically block or inhibit the production of B cells and result in the lack of immunoglobulins in patients' sera. Known mutations impact B cell development primarily at the pre-B cell stage in the bone marrow.

These patients with agammaglobulinemia harbored recessive deletions or critical base pair substitutions in the immunoglobulin mu constant region gene, in *IGLL5* gene encoding one of the components of the surrogate light chain that binds IgM in the absence of conventional light chains to form the pre-B cell receptor (Pre-BCR), or in *CD79A* or *CD79B* genes that produce CD79A/Igα and CD79B/Igβ, respectively, and form the IgM signaling complex. All these mutations prevent the expression of pre-BCR that is essential for pre-B cell proliferation, survival, and differentiation into B cells [6].

Alternatively, mutations in the X-linked *BTK* gene, encoding a tyrosine kinase-mediating pre-BCR and BCR signaling, are responsible for XLA syndrome, also characterized by severely impaired B cell and antibody production. Of note, Btk mutation in mice induces a much milder phenotype due to redundancy with another tyrosine kinase, Tec, that permits BCR signaling.

Mutations in the *BLNK* gene, which encodes the B-cell linker/SLP-65 adaptor protein that binds CD79A and BTK, also lead to a block of B cell development at the pre-B cell stage in the bone marrow.

8.2.5.2 Gene Mutations Altering Antibody Production but Not Early B Cell Development

Hyper IgM (HIGM) Syndromes

A group of patients suffer from specific impairments in antibody production, especially IgG and IgA, whereas naive B cell production appears unaffected. These defects in class switch recombination (CSR), also illustrated by severely decreased numbers of circulating isotype-switched memory B cells, are often associated with elevated IgM concentrations in the serum of HIGM syndrome patients and recurrent bacterial infections.

The genetic basis of HIGM is diverse and may be caused by defects in the CD40L/CD40 pathway essential for B cell activation, germinal center (GC) formation, and the induction of class switch recombination (CSR) [6]. The majority of HIGM cases result from mutations in the X-linked *CD154 (CD40 ligand)* gene. CD40L is expressed by T cells and plays an essential role in activating B cells. Recessive *CD40* gene mutations result in an autosomal rare form of the disease, with B cell intrinsic defects clinically indistinguishable from HIGM due to defective CD40L. Indeed, both CD40-L and CD40-deficient patients lack GCs and fail to produce isotype-switched antibody responses against pathogens. Altered CD40 signaling in the absence of functional nuclear factor-κB essential modulator (NEMO/IKKγ) also induces a form of HIGM associated with anhydrotic ectodermal dysplasia, a key feature of this syndrome.

HIGM may also result from mutations in genes encoding enzymes involved in CSR and somatic hypermutations (SHM). Activation-induced cytidine deaminase (AID) is the enzyme induced in GC B cells that catalyzes CSR and SHM [6]. Mutations in the *AICDA* gene that encodes AID cause an autosomal recessive form of HIGM characterized by the presence of enlarged GCs and the absence of CSR and SHM in both mice and humans.

Another CSR deficiency has been correlated with mutations in the *uracil–DNA glycosylase (UNG)* gene that encodes an enzyme that excises from DNA uracils resulting from enzymatic deamination of cytosines by AID. As a consequence, UNG-deficient patients have impaired CSR but functional SHM processes, although with a skewed pattern.

In contrast to AID deficiency, lack of UNG does not induce hyperplastic GC responses or the emergence of autoreactive naive B cells. Since the production of high-affinity mutated antibodies downregulates GC reactions likely by eliminating specific antigens on follicular dendritic cells (FDCs), a failure to induce SHM and generate high-affinity specific antibodies in AID-deficient patients may therefore result in sustained antigen expression on FDCs in GCs, leading to prolonged B and T cell activation and proliferation, increased production of T follicular helper cells (Tfh), and cytokines, such as IL-4, IL-10, and IL-21 [10]. These cytokines interfere with Treg-suppressive function and may contribute to the accumulation of autoreactive naïve B cells in the blood of AID-deficient patients that could be activated by Tfh cells and systemic cytokines that support not only autoantibody secretion but potentially the development of autoimmune manifestations frequently reported associated with AID deficiency. In addition, some HIGM patients have normal *CD40L, CD40, NEMO, AICDA,* or *UNG* genes, suggesting that mutations in other unknown genes may induce additional forms of HIGM.

Common Variable Immunodeficiency Disease (CVID)

CVID includes a heterogeneous group of antibody deficiency disorders characterized by decreased serum IgG combined with decreased IgM and/or IgA concentrations, low isotype-switched B-cell frequencies, and poor ability to produce specific antibody titers after vaccination [11]. CVID mostly occurs sporadically, suggesting the prevalence of recessive inheritance. However, 5–20% of patients may present some family history, which suggests an autosomal dominant transmission as evidenced for heterozygous mutations in *CTLA4*, *NFKB1*, *NFKB2*, and *IKZF1* genes.

The identification of monogenic forms of CVID is in constant progression due to next-generation sequencing technologies. Gene mutations inducing a CVID-like phenotype affect either the ability of T cells to activate B cells or intrinsically prevent B cell activation, survival, or their development into antibody-secreting plasma cells. For instance, defective inducible T cell costimulator (ICOS) expression due to biallelic recessive *ICOS* mutations in T cells abrogates their differentiation into Tfh cells necessary for the development of GC B cells and antibody secretion. Similarly, the inability to produce IL-21 due to homozygous recessive *IL21* gene mutations also impairs GC B cell development. IL-21 receptor deficiency induces a phenotype similar to the absence of functional IL-21. Heterozygous *CTLA4* gene mutations inducing CTLA-4 haploinsufficiency that alters the downregulation of T cell activation and Treg function [2] or homozygous *LRBA* gene mutations that prevent LRBA-dependent rescue of CTLA-4 degradation in endosomes, both induce defective antibody production frequently combined with autoimmune manifestations that may be severe, especially in LRBA-deficient patients.

Gene mutations affecting B cell survival and activation also result in defective antibody secretion. BAFF receptor deficiency induces a severe loss in peripheral B cells, thereby illustrating the important role for BAFF for naïve B cell survival. Heterozygous gene mutations in TNFRSF13B encoding TACI, another TNF receptor family member that also binds BAFF or APRIL, interferes with plasma cell survival and therefore with antibody production. In addition, TACI mutations also diminish TLR-mediated B cell activation because TACI binds and amplifies the signaling of TLR7 and TLR9 [12]. Biallelic recessive mutations in genes encoding the components of the CD19/CD81/CD21 BCR co-receptor lead to defective BCR signaling and an impairment of B cell activation and antibody production. Mutations in other genes involved in B cell activation such as *CD20, NFKB1, NFKB2*, and *IKZF1* encoding Ikaros DNA-binding molecules also result in CVID-like phenotypes. Some of these patients carry only a heterozygous gene mutation that exerts either a dominant negative effect on the unmutated allele or haploinsufficiency. Paradoxically, about 20% of CVID patients also develop autoimmune complications, especially autoimmune cytopenias mediated by autoantibodies targeting erythrocytes and inducing autoimmune hemolytic anemia, or platelets resulting in immune thrombocytopenia, or both in Evans syndrome. Similar to AID-deficient patients, CVID patients with autoimmune cytopenias exhibit hyperplastic GC, associated with severely decreased SHM frequencies and an IgA deficiency-associated inability to contain gut microbiota that may result in the production of antibodies cross-reactive with self-antigens [13]. Finally, some patients may specifically suffer from IgA deficiency; the etiology of this syndrome is not well understood.

8.2.6 Lymphoproliferative Syndromes

These syndromes result from defects in lymphocyte cytotoxicity. Two main pathways are involved: FAS/FASL interactions that induce caspase activation and cell death or the perforin-dependent secretory pathway that depends on the exocytosis of cytolytic granules.

8.2.6.1 Autoimmune Lymphoproliferative Syndrome (ALPS)

ALPS are characterized by the abnormal survival of lymphocytes, polyclonal T and B cell expansion, and the accumulation of unusual TCRαβ$^+$CD4$^-$CD8$^-$ double-negative mature T cells [14]. Autoimmunity in ALPS patients is associated with the emergence of anti-red blood cell autoantibodies. ALPS are often caused by mutations in the *TNFRSF6* gene encoding CD95/FAS, which is a membrane receptor inducing caspase activation and cell death by apoptosis. Other rare mutations in *TNFSF6/CD95L/FAS ligand* or *Caspase 10* (*CASP10*) genes may also result in ALPS.

8.2.6.2 Hemophagocytic Lymphohistiocytosis (HLH) Syndrome

HLH syndrome is characterized by fever and splenomegaly resulting from the phagocytosis of red blood cells, platelets, and other cells by macrophages in the absence of autoimmune manifestations [15]. In addition, cytotoxic T cells and NK cells are unable to eliminate their targets, which result in CD8$^+$ and CD4$^+$ T cell activation and expansion after antigenic challenges and organ damage that may be fatal. HLH syndromes can be caused by mutations in the perforin gene and failure to form pores in the membranes of target cells necessary to their killing. Alternatively, HLH may result from mutations in genes encoding molecules that control the exocytosis of secretory cytolytic granules. Hence, defects in either RAB27 or lysosomal trafficking regulator (LYST) by preventing the release of cytolytic molecules contained in granules result in Griscelli syndrome and Chediak–Higashi syndrome, respectively.

X-linked lymphoproliferative (XLP) syndrome is another form of HLH induced by Epstein–Barr virus (EBV)-induced mononucleosis in male patients carrying a mutation in their X-linked *SH2D1A* gene encoding SAP (signaling lymphocytic activation molecule/SLAM-associated protein) that mediates specific cytotoxic T-cell and NK functions.

8.2.7 Treatment Strategies for Patients with Primary Immunodeficiencies

Treatment strategies differ greatly among patients with primary immunodeficiencies due to the heterogeneity of these diseases. Intravenous immunoglobulin replacement therapy (IVIg) is the commonly used regimen to prevent recurrent infections in many primary immunodeficiency patients with defects in immunoglobulin secretion and diminish infectious episodes associated with this condition. However, IVIg needs to be provided on a regular basis throughout life and does not correct the origins of primary immunodeficiencies.

More severe and potentially life-threatening conditions such as SCID or IPEX syndrome may require bone marrow transplantation, which represents a curative option for these patients. Donor stem cells allow the development of a functional immune system in transplanted patients. Since transplantation of stem cells have shown a better efficacy in young infants below 1 year of age, newborn screening for SCID performed in many states of the USA improve the outcomes of bone marrow transplantation in these patients.

However, despite the early diagnosis of SCID, HLA-matched bone marrow donors may not be available for transplantation. Gene therapy may now be considered as an alternative therapeutic option for some patients with primary immunodeficiencies and currently consists in delivering a novel functional gene that compensates for the mutated endogenous gene using either a retroviral or lentiviral delivery strategy in the patient's own stem cells in vitro before reimplantation [16]. This strategy has shown efficacy for ADA SCID patients and more recently in WAS patients, whereas retroviral-driven expression of γc chain in IL2RG-deficient SCID patients allowed the production of T cells but led subsequently in 5 out of 20 patients to an uncontrolled clonal T cell proliferation due to deregulated oncogene expression caused by the retroviral integration in the patient's genome. Novel gene therapy approaches are currently being developed and aim at repairing the gene mutation in situ through targeted genome editing mediated by CRISPR/Cas9 nuclease. This improved gene therapy strategy may therefore erase previous gene defects and allow the normal expression of a functional gene in the patient's own cells [17].

In conclusion, hundreds of mutated genes have now been reported to be associated with the development of primary immunodeficiencies and induce many and various defects of the immune system in humans. The study of primary immunodeficiency patients identifies molecules and pathways involved in cellular or humoral immune responses toward specific pathogens or in mediating T and B cell tolerance in humans.

8.3 Allergy

8.3.1 Introduction

Allergies are aberrant responses to the types of foreign antigens called allergens. Most allergens are noninfectious and cause no symptoms in nonallergic persons. People with allergies typically respond with a Th2 cell response and the formation of IgE antibody against particular antigens. Allergic diseases are common, especially in developed countries, and are increasing. In this section, we shall focus on food allergies because they are among the most common allergic reactions, are increasing in frequency, and have attracted much recent scientific and public interest. Food allergies are sometimes confused with food intolerance because symptoms of both are often similar, but food intolerance is nonimmune-mediated. It can be triggered by carbohydrates (e.g., lactose intolerance), fat intolerance (e.g., gall bladder disease), caffeine, food additives, and other food products.

8.3.2 Food Allergy Classification

Food allergies are among the most common hypersensitivity reactions. They are increasing in frequency and have attracted much recent scientific and public interest. They have been defined as "'an adverse health effect arising from a specific immune response that occurs reproducibly on exposure to a given food" [18–23]. It is important to distinguish food allergy from food intolerance. Both can cause similar gastrointestinal symptoms, but food allergy is driven by aberrant immune responses and can cause severe systemic and gastrointestinal symptoms, while food intolerance is not caused by immune dysfunction and generally does not produce systemic symptoms [19, 22]. There is no universally recognized classification of food allergy, but it can be broadly classified as IgE-mediated (immediate) and non-IgE-mediated (delayed response) mechanisms [19, 20, 22] (Fig. 8.1). The former is caused by IgE antibody and the latter are caused either by cell-mediated or by multiple immunoglobulin subtype mechanisms. Examples of IgE-related disorders include life-threatening shock due to peanut or shellfish allergy, while non-IgE-mediated conditions include celiac disease and food protein-induced enterocolitis syndrome [19, 20, 22]. Most recent scientific work on food allergies has focused on IgE-mediated reactions. Another classification of food allergy consisting of five subtypes of the classic food allergy phenotype has been proposed: (1) persistent, (2) transient, (3) food-dependent exercise-induced allergy (FDEIA), (4) nonsteroidal anti-inflammatory drug (NSAID)- or aspirin-induced allergy, and (5) alcohol-dependent allergy [18]. Transient phenotype means that a person who develops a food allergy as a child "outgrows" their allergy over time, whereas a person with persistent phenotype does not. For example, more than 80% of children with egg, soy, wheat, or milk allergies lose their allergy over time. Investigation of hypotheses regarding the mechanisms of these two phenotypes is ongoing. The other categories describe cofactors that will elicit an allergic

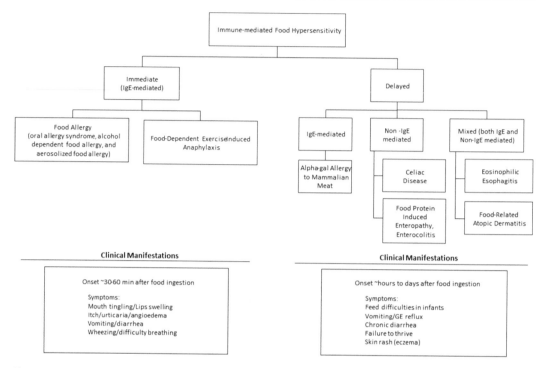

Fig. 8.1 A schematic classification and clinical characteristics of food hypersensitivity (IgE-mediated, non-IgE-mediated, and mixed [IgE-mediated and non-IgE-mediated]). (Adapted from Lin [22]). (©Krause 2020)

response to food when the food allergen is ingested around the same time as the cofactor exposure (exercise, nonsteroidal anti-inflammatory drugs [NSAID], aspirin, or alcohol).

8.3.3 Epidemiology and Immunoepidemiology of Food Allergies

An estimated 15 million people in the USA have food allergies [21]. The prevalence of food allergies has increased over the past 25 years. An array of studies has found that 4–8% of children younger than 5 years and 1–3% of adults report food allergies. Even higher estimates have been noted based on self-reporting methodologies without laboratory confirmation. In sum, the overall prevalence of food allergies in the US population is somewhere between 1–2% and 10% [18–27]. The wide range of prevalence estimates is due to the variability in definitions, methodologies, and population characteristics of these studies. A small subset of people with food allergies suffers life-threatening symptoms with an estimated 150 fatalities a year in the USA [23].

Food allergies often begin in childhood, but some food allergies, especially those due to shellfish and tree nuts, begin de novo in adulthood [19, 28]. Although more than 170 foods have been documented to cause allergy, almost all (~90%) are caused by eight food items [19, 20, 22, 23, 25, 28]. *Cow's milk* is the most common cause of food allergy in children with an estimated prevalence of 3.5% (95% CI, 2.9%–4.1%) from self-report studies and 0.6–0.9% from studies with confirmation by laboratory or food challenge [25]. Milk allergy usually develops in the first year of life, and in most cases resolves by age 6. *Eggs* are the second most common cause of food allergy in children, also developing in the first year of life and often resolving by age 6. *Peanut* allergy can develop at any time in life and usually is permanent. Severe reactions are more common with peanuts than other foods. Peanut allergy appears to be increasing in frequency. *Tree nut* allergy can first present during either childhood or adulthood. Allergy to *fish and shellfish* tend to develop in adulthood. Allergy to *soy and wheat* are the least common of the top eight food allergies but are more common than food allergies to meat, fruits, or vegetables.

Risk factors for food allergy include *genetic causes* that explain an increase in food allergies among those who have a family history of atopy. They also include *race* (a person's physical characteristics, such as skin, hair, or eye color) and *ethnicity* (cultural factors, such as nationality, ancestry, and language). There is a higher overall incidence of allergy to food in non-Hispanic blacks and Asians compared with Caucasians but a decrease in allergy to peanuts in Asians compared with Caucasians. Another risk factor is *gender*, with an increased risk of food allergy in males. *Other allergies* are also risk factors, as those with allergic dermatitis and physician-diagnosed asthma have an increased risk of food allergy. Finally, certain environmental factors increase the risk of food allergies. For example, there is an increased risk in US children born to immigrant parents, a decreased risk in children with more food diversity in infancy, and a decreased risk of food allergy in children with older siblings and pets in the home [20, 21, 28]. The decreased risk of food allergy among children who are exposed to a wider microbiome (as listed in the environment category) is consistent with the hygiene hypothesis. This hypothesis posits that early exposure to a wide array of microbes and especially helminths decreases the development of allergy and possibly food allergy [29].

8.3.4 Clinical Manifestations of Food Allergies

Food allergy symptoms usually develop within a few minutes to 2 hours after eating the offending food. There is great diversity in the clinical presentation of food allergy from mild local oropharyngeal reactions to life-threatening anaphylaxis. Multiple organ systems can be affected including skin (erythema, swelling, itch), gastrointestinal tract (vomiting, diarrhea), lungs (wheezing, difficulty breathing), and heart/vascular system (shock, cardiac arrest). The most common food allergy signs and symptoms include hives; itching or eczema; tingling or itching in the mouth; swelling of the lips, face, tongue, and throat or other parts of the body; wheezing, nasal congestion, or trouble breathing; abdominal pain, diarrhea, nausea, or vomiting; and dizziness, lightheadedness, or fainting. A life-threatening anaphylactic response is characterized by a swollen throat that impairs breathing, constriction and tightening of the airways, shock with a severe drop in blood pressure, a rapid pulse, and dizziness, lightheadedness, or loss of consciousness. Overall, peanuts are the most common food allergens causing fatal or near-fatal anaphylaxis, while shellfish are the most common triggers in adults.

8.3.5 Mechanism of IgE-Induced Food Allergy Symptoms

The mechanism of IgE-induced food allergy symptoms can be extrapolated from studies of how other antigens (allergens) cause allergic symptoms [28–30]. Allergens are presented to T lymphocytes by antigen-presenting cells in the presence of cytokines that polarize them to Th2 cells. The T cells produce cytokines (IL-4, 5, 13) that activate B cells to switch to IgE-producing plasma cells. The secreted IgE binds to IgE Fc receptors on mast cells, eosinophils, and basophils. Repeated allergen exposure increases the amount of allergen-induced IgE binding. Once a threshold is exceeded, allergen binding to multiple IgE molecules on mast cells, eosinophils, or basophils causes a rapid granule release, synthesis, and secretion of lipid mediators and vasoactive amines, and synthesis and secretion of cytokines. These have numerous downstream effects that cause the rapid onset of hives and/or gastrointestinal pain, diarrhea, hypotension, and death in some severe cases. It takes very little allergen to trigger the rapid onset of serious reactions. For example, as little as 0.1 mg of peanut protein can cause severe symptoms within minutes to an hour [22].

8.3.6 Example of an IgE-Mediated Food Allergy: The Alpha Gal Story

Meat allergy associated with tick bite is a recently recognized food allergy that is increasing in frequency and geographical range [28, 31]. The first report of red meat allergy associated with tick bite was published in 2009 in Australian residents who developed urticaria, anaphylaxis, and gastrointestinal upset 2–6 hours after eating red meat, including beef, pork, and lamb. A similar reaction was subsequently noted in US residents, primarily those living in the southeastern USA. Immediate hypersensitivity reactions were noted shortly after eating red meat and within a few weeks or months of exposure to Lone Star tick bites [31]. The cause for this association was determined in a somewhat circuitous fashion. Urticarial and anaphylaxis reactions had been reported in a few patients receiving cetuximab (a monoclonal antibody used to treat cancer) and more so in the residents of the Southeast than the Northeast. Patients experiencing these reactions were found to have high serum concentrations of IgE antibodies directed against the mammalian oligosaccharide, galactose alpha-1, 3-galactose (alpha-gal). Additional studies showed that alpha gal IgE antibodies were more common in people living in the southeastern USA (>20% seroprevalence) than in the northeast (<1% seroprevalence) [31]. Investigation of potential causative factors revealed that high levels of alpha gal were found in red meat, cetuximab solution, and in larval and adult Lone Star tick saliva. It is now thought that many people develop anti-alpha gal IgM and IgG antibodies after ingestion of red meat without allergic symptoms. In contrast, people who are exposed to alpha gal through a different route (intravenously with cetuximab or intradermally through Lone Star tick bites) develop IgE antibody to alpha gal. IgE antibodies lead to allergic responses. The Lone Star tick is expanding northward. As an increasing number of people become exposed to these ticks, the incidence of red meat allergy is expected to increase. The European tick, *Ixodes ricinus,* also transmits alpha gal in its saliva, and several reports have been published of red meat allergy in Europe. The alpha gal/red meat allergy story demonstrates that cross-reactivity between disparate sources of allergen can have significant clinical consequences, that the mode of exposure can determine whether allergy-inducing IgE antibodies are formed, and that both genetic and environmental factors can act in concert to define the subpopulations of allergic individuals.

8.3.7 Diagnosis, Treatment, and Prevention

The diagnosis of food allergy is often difficult, as it may be dangerous to challenge an allergic person with the suspected food item. A medical history can be suggestive of food allergy, but laboratory testing for IgE antibodies and skin prick or intradermal testing are usually necessary to confirm the diagnosis [19, 21, 22, 25]. As noted above, food allergies that develop in childhood may resolve by adulthood. It is recommended that physicians follow patients at least yearly to document the loss of allergy and slowly reintroduce the food that caused allergic symptoms [19]. Desensitization works in a subset of food allergy patients. Some patients with peanut allergy have responded to the reintroduction of gradually increasing amounts of peanut protein [19]. Early introduction of peanuts in the first year of life in many children considerably reduces the risk of peanut allergy. For those with persistent allergy, avoidance of the allergy-inducing food and carrying an epi pen are recommended. One recent promising approach has been the administration of the anti-IgE medication omalizumab to these patients during peanut desensitization [32]. Patients receiving omalizumab over as little as 8 weeks were able to tolerate higher doses of peanut allergen compared with the control subjects, and the desensitization was sustained after omalizumab was discontinued.

8.4 Autoimmunity

8.4.1 Introduction

In Chap. 6, we introduced the concept of autoimmune diseases—those conditions where the immune system turns against the body and attacks host tissues, employing the full armamentarium of cells and substances that would normally be enlisted in the fight against pathogens. As noted above, autoimmune diseases can be directed against a particular cell such as the insulin-producing β cell in Type I diabetes (T1D), an organ, such as the joints in rheumatoid arthritis (RA), or the contents of all cells, as in systemic lupus erythematosus (SLE). The autoimmune diseases are complex and multifactorial with both genetic and acquired considerations—summarized as "genes, gender, and geography," with an influence of lifestyle. There are racial differences in autoimmune diseases, with Blacks and Asians disproportionally affected by SLE, and Blacks, but not Asians, disproportionally affected by multiple sclerosis (MS) [33]. Most autoimmune diseases have a genetic component. This is apparent in family studies where the chance of a sibling manifesting an autoimmune disease is higher than the overall population, and the chances of an identical twin are even higher, *but rarely 100%*. This indicates that other factors must be considered, and this is where the environment (geography) comes into play. Although there are many animal models of autoimmune diseases that have provided insight into possible mechanisms and modifying factors, in this chapter, we emphasize those human epidemiological studies that have enlightened the field.

8.4.2 Genes

8.4.2.1 Introduction

As noted above, there is an increased chance of a sibling of an affected individual exhibiting an autoimmune disease. In the case of MS, the risk is 7% for a sibling, but even higher (23%) for a monozygotic twin [34]. Thus, there is clearly a genetic component to autoimmunity. Even when a particular gene is identified as a risk factor, further risk may be due to combinations of genes and/or the function of a gene at another locus that serves to modify function (epistasis). The identification of individual genes as risk factors for autoimmunity first began with family studies and then progressed to studies of populations, then to large data studies with GWAS, and now has advanced to high throughput genetic sequencing.

8.4.2.2 Major Histocompatibility Complex (MHC)

By far, the highest risk factor for autoimmune disease is found within the genes of the major histocompatibility complex (MHC) (Fig. 8.2 as described in Chap. 4). Most of these associations are positive, that is, the presence of a particular allele is associated with a particular disease, although there are also protective alleles [35]. All three members of the TNF family of cytokines that map within the locus have been implicated in autoimmune diseases. The earliest and most dramatic association of MHC with autoimmunity was that of HLA B∗27 with ankylosing spondylitis, an autoimmune condition involving inflammation of the spinal cord [36]. In the original description, 35 of 40

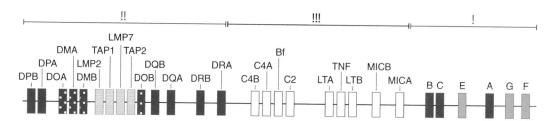

Fig. 8.2 Map of the human major histocompatibility complex, HLA. The MHC region, called HLA in humans, is located on chromosome 6p spanning about 4 kb. The genes encoding the MHC class I genes (HLA-A, HLA-B, and HLA-C) and nonclassical MHC class I genes (HLA-E, HLA-F, and HLA-G) are closely linked (region I). The MHC class II genes (HLA-DR, HLA-DQ, and HLA-DP) are linked to the genes for the peptide transporter (TAP), the proteasome components (LMP), and the DO and DM genes involved in peptide loading of MHC II. Other immune-related genes are clustered in region II including complement proteins (C4A, C4B, Bf), cytokines (TNF, LTα, LTβ), and stress-induced proteins (MICB, MICA) (©Kavathas, 2020)

(88%) of patients expressed an allele of this gene, whereas only 72 of 406 controls (8%) did. This early observation has been confirmed in multiple studies in multiple populations, generally indicating an odds ratio of 39, although this gene is in epistasis with endoplasmic reticulum aminopeptidase 1 (ERAP1), which trims the peptides in the endoplasmic reticulum for binding to MHC class I molecules [37]. Additional MHC haplotypes are associated with predisposition to other autoimmune diseases, although the odds ratios are not quite as high. The extensive list of these associations is reviewed in [38]. Many of the genes in the MHC are in linkage disequilibrium with other genes, making interpretations difficult regarding the mechanisms of disease. The obvious mechanism would be a propensity to present particular tissue-restricted self antigens. However, recent advances have revealed a variety of ways in which MHC alleles contribute to the various diseases, as summarized in [39]. For example, HLA-DR15, a risk factor for MS, has been shown to allow myelin basic protein peptide-specific T cells to escape thymic selection. HLA-A*02:01, a risk for T1D, has a low affinity for an insulin peptide and also allows autoreactive T cells to escape selection. Other alleles regulate HLA expression and influence HLA stability.

The Class III region of the MHC contains many genes associated with the immune system, including some complement genes and those of the "immediate" TNF family (TNF-α, LT-α, and LT-β). Polymorphisms in both TNF-α and LT-α have been associated with several autoimmune diseases [40, 41], and complement genes, C4 and C2, have been linked to SLE [42]. However, it is difficult to separate these polymorphisms from those of the class I and II genes as they are in linkage disequilibrium. It is clear that these cytokines contribute to the pathology of many autoimmune diseases. Furthermore, genes of the TNF signaling pathway through NF-κB have been implicated in MS [43]. Therapy to inhibit the TNF pathway gene activity has been remarkably effective in some autoimmune diseases (see Chap. 16).

8.4.2.3 PTPN22

Lymphoid protein tyrosine phosphatase (nonreceptor-type 22 (Lyp), encoded by *PTPN22*) is a signaling molecule expressed on many cells of the innate and adaptive immune system. A variant (PTPN22R620T) has been identified as a risk factor in at least 17 different autoimmune diseases including rheumatoid arthritis, T1D, Graves's disease, and SLE, with odds ratios ranging from 1.16 to 1.98. On the other hand, at least four diseases, including celiac disease, MS, psoriasis, and ulcerative colitis (UC), are *not* affected by this variant, and there is a *decreased* risk associated with Behçet disease and Crohn's disease (CD) (reviewed in [44]). Lyp is expressed by many cell types (myeloid, T, and B), and the exact function that contributes to immune dysregulation and a risk factor for some autoimmune diseases is under investigation. It has been identified as a negative regulator of TCR signaling, but binding partners in addition to TCR have been identified.

8.4.2.4 Genome-Wide Association Studies

Tremendous advances have been made in the identification of genes associated with autoimmunity through genome-wide association studies (GWAS). In these studies, DNA from two groups of people are studied—those with a particular (autoimmune) disease and those without. DNA is then analyzed for the increased presence of particular single-nucleotide polymorphisms (SNP) in the affected group. In an early study of MS, 110 SNPs were identified that were strongly associated with the disease; two were within the IL-2 receptor alpha gene (*IL2RA*), one in *IL7RA*, and multiple SNPs in the HLA-DRA locus [45]. Since that time, over 233 susceptibility genes for MS have been identified by this technique. The same technique has been used to identify susceptibility genes for RA and Crohn's disease, and it has begun to be possible to identify the pathways, particularly in the immune system, that underlie the mechanisms of these diseases. However, the field has realized that although the "era of GWAS is not over" [46, 47], it behooves researchers to move beyond the identification of the segments of DNA, many of which are noncoding variants, to chromatin structure and structure–function mapping (Todd, 2018). A recent publication using the approach of exome sequencing has identified four rare coding variants associated with MS that were not detected by GWAS [43].

8.4.3   Gender

Many autoimmune diseases have a pronounced sex bias in prevalence with a preponderance of females, including multiple sclerosis (MS) (3:1), systemic lupus erythematosus (SLE), and Sjögren's syndrome (SS) (both 9:1), while T1D has an almost equal ratio of males to females. On the other hand, several studies indicate an increased prevalence of ankylosing spondylitis in males (summarized in [48]). In addition to differences in the incidence of disease, there are also differences between the sexes in severity and mortality. In general, clinical symptoms and cognitive disability of MS are more severe in males than females [48]. A registry-based study of over 14,000 patients revealed that male primary progressive MS patients became disabled more rapidly than females [49]. Clinical symptoms have also been reported to be more severe in male SLE patients, but higher mortality was seen in female SLE patients (summarized in [48]).

The biological reasons for gender differences in autoimmune diseases must be considered in light of the different and complex pathogenic mechanisms in the various diseases and differences in the various gene products that contribute to them. The multiple explanations for discrepancies between the sexes have included differences in biological factors and social and cultural exposures.

8.4.3.1 Biological Explanations

Sex Hormones

The most obvious difference between males and females that could contribute to sex prevalence in autoimmunity is sex hormones. Many autoimmune diseases that have a predominant female ratio, such as SLE, MS, and RA, occur after puberty. T1D, which does not exhibit a skewed sex ratio, has a mean onset before puberty. Strikingly, SLE with a ratio of 9:1 in adults, though rare in children, has a 1:1 ratio before puberty (summarized in [50]). In general, female hormones tend to suppress Th1 and Th17 responses, whereas male hormones tend to suppress B cell responses. Since women tend to produce higher antibody titers to vaccines, one would expect females to be skewed toward antibody-mediated diseases like SLE, and that is the case. However, that would not explain the preponderance of female victims of MS and Sjögren's syndrome (SS), diseases which, though characterized by antibody production, clearly have T cell-mediated pathogenic mechanisms.

Endogenous estrogens include estrogen, estradiol, and estriol. The estrogens have multiple effects on the cells of the immune system. In general, they are immunosuppressive for T cells and enhance the activity of B cells. Estriol is produced only during pregnancy and is especially high in the third trimester, a time when there is a reduced relapse rate in MS and RA (see below). Estriol has been evaluated in a phase 2b clinical trial in combination with a widely used agent copaxone (glatiramer acetate). The trial was designed for women with relapsing remitting MS (RRMS), a particularly difficult group to treat. The study met its primary end point with 70% relapse reduction [51] and additional effects that included slowing of gray matter atrophy on magnetic resonance imaging [52]. Progesterone, another female sex hormone, is produced at high levels by the placenta, although it is also produced at low levels by males. Studies suggest that this hormone may suppress B cell differentiation and that it may affect post-translational glycosylation of immunoglobulins [50].

Testosterone, a hormone associated with masculine characteristics, is a known inhibitor of antibody and thus is likely a protective factor in SLE. Furthermore, males with MS and low testosterone levels fared poorly with regard to disability and cognitive decline [48]. A recent study demonstrated that testosterone inhibits BAFF, a B cell survival factor, and thus could explain lower antibody responses in males [53]. Clinical studies with testosterone patches in both SLE and MS have had only modest success. There have been multiple studies on the activities of sex hormones in vitro and in vivo in mouse models of autoimmunity. These studies cannot fully explain the reasons for the gender skewing in some autoimmune diseases. They suggest that hormones can influence disease development in individuals who are already genetically and geographically prone to the disease.

Pregnancy

Severity of MS clinical symptoms decreases during pregnancy. This was initially confirmed by an observational study of the disability scores and relapse rates of 254 women with MS in 269 pregnancies in 12 European countries [54]. The relapse rate was reduced during pregnancy and was reduced by 72% in the third trimester. However, disturbingly, severity and frequency of relapses increased above the baseline rate in the 3 months after delivery, eventually returning to baseline level. These and many additional studies confirm that the state of pregnancy is temporarily protective for MS and for RA. One possible explanation for these results is the high level of estriol, especially in the third trimester, which would level off after delivery, explaining the rebound effect. Progesterone is another candidate protective factor in autoimmune diseases during pregnancy. It is especially high during pregnancy via its production by the placenta. The high production in pregnancy and the alleviation of clinical signs of autoimmune diseases during that condition suggest that progesterone could be a contributing ameliorating factor.

The X Chromosome

The X chromosome carries over 1000 genes, many of which are associated with the immune response; these include CD40L, FOXP3, TLR7, TLR8, IL9R, IL2RG, and BTK. Females have two X chromosomes, whereas males have one X and one Y chromosome. To prevent a double dose of gene expression from the X chromosome, a process termed X inactivation causes one X in each female cell to be inactivated. In general, this results in a 50:50 ratio of activity from maternal and paternal X chromosomes. That is, there is an equal number of cells expressing the maternal or paternal X-linked genes. However, in some situations, a skewed pattern occurs. This skewing has been associated with several autoimmune diseases including systemic sclerosis, Hashimoto's thyroiditis, Graves' disease, and RA (reviewed in [55]). In some situations, only partial inactivation of an individual X chromosome occurs resulting in a double dose of some X-linked genes. Abnormalities in the number of sex chromosomes occur that are often not immediately apparent. These include individuals who are phenotypically male with an extra X chromosome (Klinefelter syndrome 47, XXY), women with an extra X chromosome, or women who lack a part or all of an X chromosome. Individuals with an abnormal number of X chromosomes have a high prevalence of autoimmune diseases, particularly SLE, MS, and RA. These data suggest that an imbalance in encoding of the immune system-associated genes on the X chromosome contributes to an increased risk of autoimmune diseases.

Social and Cultural Factors

In addition to biological explanations, such as hormonal differences between males and females, we also need to consider the social and cultural differences between males and females that could impact autoimmunity. Multiple large studies have investigated the role of smoking in MS and found it to be a major risk factor in disease development and progression. A recent meta-analysis of 56 case control studies found a statistically significant association with MS risk [56]. Other studies had suggested an association between smoking and MS progression or disability, but this was not borne out in this study. Interestingly, there is an increase in the incidence of MS in women and its gender disparity—from 1:1 in the 1950s to 3:1 at the present time, paralleling the increase in smoking in women. Other factors that could influence the gender skewing in autoimmunity include occupation, longevity, exposure to infection, and exposure to sunlight. Many of these will be considered in greater detail in the section below on geography.

8.4.4   Geography

With the realization that neither genes nor gender alone can explain autoimmunity, we turn to a consideration of the environment, both external and internal (microbiome). Certain countries, predominantly in the Northern latitude, have a higher prevalence of autoimmune diseases. For example, the rate of MS in Sweden is greater than 100/100,000, and in Brazil and Mexico, it is 0–5/100,000 (Fig. 8.3). Similar trends are seen for T1D. The differences in the prevalence of autoimmunity in different regions are not simply due to differences in the genetic makeup of the individuals in those countries. Studies of immigration have revealed that the rate of MS correlates with the country that one immigrates to, if the move occurs before the individual reaches the age of 15. Similarly, numerous studies have evaluated the rate of T1D in migratory populations. A study was carried out on children who migrated to the United Kingdom from India and Pakistan where the incidence was 3.1/100,000 per year. Over the 10 years of the study, the incidence of T1D in the migrated children increased to 11.7/100,000, approximately the level of the UK population [57].

   Many explanations have been put forward for the differences in autoimmune disease prevalence in different environments. A frequently suggested explanation is the difference in sunlight. Vitamin D has been shown in several studies to be protective, but at least two separate studies have indicated that sun exposure (and UV light) is more important than Vitamin D [33]. By this logic, the high prevalence in Northern latitudes could be due to less sun. However, the incidence of T1D and prevalence of MS in Australia and New Zealand are high, suggesting that a direct causal interpretation of the latitude and sunlight is simplistic. Another hypothesis is dietary practice. This has come under renewed interest as a result of recent studies that suggest that the consumption of a high salt diet could be a risk factor that predisposes to MS through the induction of Th17 cells [58] and/or suppression of Tregs [59]. However, a study that analyzed urinary sodium of 465 patients with Clinically Isolated Syndrome (an early precursor to MS) did not find an association with clinical conversion to MS [60].

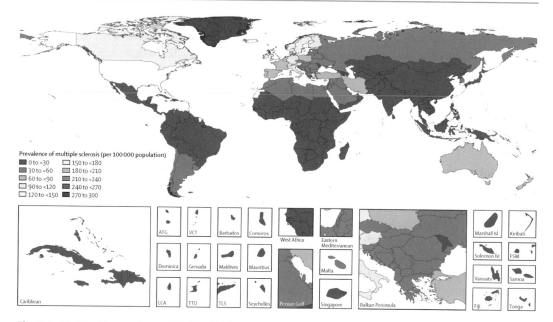

Fig. 8.3 World-wide prevalence of MS in 2016. (Global Burden of Disease 2016 Multiple Sclerosis Collaborators, Lancet Neurology 18: 269–85. Fig. 1 Creative Commons)

Another explanation for the high prevalence of autoimmunity in different geographical areas is exposure to particular microbes. One of the earliest and most thorough studies suggesting an association of a microbe with an autoimmune disease was that of Levin et al. [61], a longitudinal study of three million US military personnel. They found that the risk of MS correlated with the changes in antibody titers to Epstein–Barr virus, but not cytomegalovirus. Infection with several different viruses, including mumps, rotavirus, rubella, cytomegalovirus, and human enterovirus, have all been associated with T1D (summarized in [62]). A meta-analysis of 33 studies of human enterovirus and T1D showed an odds ratio of 9.8 between that virus and the clinical disease [63]. Another intriguing study suggests that a leveling off of an increase in T1D has occurred concomitant with the introduction of rotavirus vaccination [64]. So, what could be the mechanism of a relationship of a particular virus and an autoimmune disease? The two most likely nonexclusive explanations are (1) a cross-reactive epitope between the virus and a self-antigen and (2) the ability of viruses to induce inflammatory cytokines. In fact, an "interferon signature," that is, a heightened expression of genes induced by interferon, is characteristic of many autoimmune diseases [65].

Paradoxically, exposure to microbes could protect against autoimmunity, in addition to contributing to disease. The protective effect of a "dirty" environment has been evoked by the hygiene hypothesis to explain protection against allergic diseases through early exposure to microbes [66]. This has recently been suggested as an explanation for protection against autoimmunity [67]. A positive correlation of autoimmunity occurs in countries with a low incidence of hepatitis virus and tuberculosis and rare traveler's diarrhea [67] and high domestic product. Multiple mechanisms can be suggested, such as competition for immune products (cytokines, antibodies, MHC) and immune regulation by pathogens.

Understanding the role of the microbiome and commensal environment in autoimmunity may provide a more nuanced understanding of the role of microorganisms and predisposition or protection against autoimmunity. Several studies have demonstrated an aberrant microbiota at the onset of T1D [68]. The gut microbiota were analyzed by microarray in children aged 1–5 with new-onset T1D and compared with that of age-matched healthy controls. The predominant species varied by age group and was clearly different between diabetic children and controls. The Environmental Determinants of Diabetes in the Young (TEDDY) study, which prospectively aims to identify environmental causes of T1D, has evaluated the gut microbiomes by metagenomics in 10,913 stool samples of 783 children from 3 months of age to the development of anti-islet antibodies or T1D as compared to case controls [69] in six clinical centers in the USA and Europe. The 267 seroconverters and 101 children diagnosed with T1D were compared to the 415 controls. The most striking findings involved the dramatic changes in microbiome composition associated with breast feeding and its cessation, although these did not differ significantly between the groups. Several pathways that contribute to the synthesis of short-chain fatty acids were increased in healthy controls, although the authors indicate that "most of the taxonomic and functional signals … were modest in effect size and statistical significance." A companion study utilizing 16 s rRNA sequencing on 903 children from the same centers again revealed "subtle associations between microbial taxonomy and the development of islet autoimmunity or T1D" [70].

A recent study evaluated not only the composition of the microbiome but also the immune response to it by studying antibodies to commensal bacteria in two cohorts of individuals with autoimmune disease [71]. In the first cohort, sera were collected within 6 months of diagnosis of T1D and compared with healthy controls and individuals with Crohn's disease. The three groups could be distinguished based on their antibody responses to commensal bacteria. Another cohort was analyzed for anticommensal bacterial response of individuals before diabetes with individuals of the same HLA haplotype who were discordant for disease diagnosis. Serum IgG2 antibodies against *Roseburia faecis* and against a bacterial consortium were associated with future T1D development in an *HLA DR3/DR4* dependent manner. These results suggest that larger studies with functional analyses may shed even further insight into environmental associations with autoimmunity and provide insights into diagnosis and risk factors.

8.4.5 Lifestyle Factors

Genes, gender, and environment interact in the development of autoimmunity. Furthermore, additional lifestyle factors can contribute to the development and progression of autoimmune diseases. Risk factors include exposure to certain chemicals [72] and obesity [73]. As noted above, smoking appears to be a risk factor for MS with a 1.6 increase in incidence in a well-established longitudinal study of nurses and smoking [74] and is associated with a hazard of secondary progressive MS [75]. As noted above, protection seems to be afforded by sunlight (which must be tempered by the risk of skin cancer). In one study, Vitamin D supplementation was protective in MS in whites only [33]. The results of other studies have been contradictory [76]. Nevertheless, a healthy diet was shown to correlate with better neurological performance in MS patients [77]. In summary, these studies appear to demonstrate that lifestyle choices can influence both susceptibility and progression in some autoimmune diseases. It is clear that there is a need for more research in this area.

References

1. Picard C, Bobby Gaspar H, Al-Herz W, Bousfiha A, Casanova JL, Chatila T, et al. International Union of Immunological Societies: 2017 Primary Immunodeficiency Diseases Committee Report on Inborn Errors of Immunity. J Clin Immunol. 2018;38(1):96–128.
2. Kuehn HS, Ouyang W, Lo B, Deenick EK, Niemela JE, Avery DT, et al. Immune dysregulation in human subjects with heterozygous germline mutations in CTLA4. Science. 2014;345(6204):1623–7.

3. Villa A, Notarangelo LD. RAG gene defects at the verge of immunodeficiency and immune dysregulation. Immunol Rev. 2019;287(1):73–90.
4. Puck JM. Newborn screening for severe combined immunodeficiency and T-cell lymphopenia. Immunol Rev. 2019;287(1):241–52.
5. Zhang SY, Casanova JL. Inborn errors underlying herpes simplex encephalitis: from TLR3 to IRF3. J Exp Med. 2015;212(9):1342–3.
6. Durandy A, Kracker S, Fischer A. Primary antibody deficiencies. Nat Rev Immunol. 2013;13(7):519–33.
7. Mathis D, Benoist C. Aire. Annu Rev Immunol. 2009;27:287–312.
8. Torgerson TR, Ochs HD. Immune dysregulation, polyendocrinopathy, enteropathy, X-linked: forkhead box protein 3 mutations and lack of regulatory T cells. J Allergy Clin Immunol. 2007;120(4):744–50; quiz 51–2.
9. Bruton OC. Agammaglobulinemia. Pediatrics. 1952;9(6):722–8.
10. Cantaert T, Schickel JN, Bannock JM, Ng YS, Massad C, Delmotte FR, et al. Decreased somatic hypermutation induces an impaired peripheral B cell tolerance checkpoint. J Clin Invest. 2016;126(11):4289–302.
11. Bonilla FA, Barlan I, Chapel H, Costa-Carvalho BT, Cunningham-Rundles C, de la Morena MT, et al. International Consensus Document (ICON): common variable immunodeficiency disorders. J Allergy Clin Immunol Pract. 2016;4(1):38–59.
12. Romberg N, Chamberlain N, Saadoun D, Gentile M, Kinnunen T, Ng YS, et al. CVID-associated TACI mutations affect autoreactive B cell selection and activation. J Clin Invest. 2013;123(10):4283–93.
13. Romberg N, Le Coz C, Glauzy S, Schickel JN, Trofa M, Nolan BE, et al. Patients with common variable immunodeficiency with autoimmune cytopenias exhibit hyperplastic yet inefficient germinal center responses. J Allergy Clin Immunol. 2019;143(1):258–65.
14. Meynier S, Rieux-Laucat F. FAS and RAS related Apoptosis defects: from autoimmunity to leukemia. Immunol Rev. 2019;287(1):50–61.
15. Sepulveda FE, de Saint Basile G. Hemophagocytic syndrome: primary forms and predisposing conditions. Curr Opin Immunol. 2017;49:20–6.
16. Cicalese MP, Aiuti A. Clinical applications of gene therapy for primary immunodeficiencies. Hum Gene Ther. 2015;26(4):210–9.
17. Roth TL, Puig-Saus C, Yu R, Shifrut E, Carnevale J, Li PJ, et al. Reprogramming human T cell function and specificity with non-viral genome targeting. Nature. 2018;559(7714):405–9.
18. Baker MG, Sampson HA. Phenotypes and endotypes of food allergy: a path to better understanding the pathogenesis and prognosis of food allergy. Ann Allergy Asthma Immunol. 2018;120(3):245–53.
19. Boyce JA, Assa'ad A, Burks AW, Jones SM, Sampson HA, Wood RA, et al. Guidelines for the Diagnosis and Management of Food Allergy in the United States: summary of the NIAID-Sponsored Expert Panel Report. J Allergy Clin Immunol. 2010;126(6):1105–18.
20. Dunlop JH, Keet CA. Epidemiology of food allergy. Immunol Allergy Clin N Am. 2018;38(1):13–25.
21. Jones SM, Burks AW. Food Allergy. N Engl J Med. 2017;377(23):2294–5.
22. Lin CH. Food allergy: what it is and what it is not? Curr Opin Gastroenterol. 2019;35(2):114–8.
23. Sicherer SH. Food allergy. Mt Sinai J Med. 2011;78(5):683–96.
24. Bock SA. Prospective appraisal of complaints of adverse reactions to foods in children during the first 3 years of life. Pediatrics. 1987;79(5):683–8.
25. Chafen JJ, Newberry SJ, Riedl MA, Bravata DM, Maglione M, Suttorp MJ, et al. Diagnosing and managing common food allergies: a systematic review. JAMA. 2010;303(18):1848–56.
26. Rona RJ, Keil T, Summers C, Gislason D, Zuidmeer L, Sodergren E, et al. The prevalence of food allergy: a meta-analysis. J Allergy Clin Immunol. 2007;120(3):638–46.
27. Young E, Stoneham MD, Petruckevitch A, Barton J, Rona R. A population study of food intolerance. Lancet. 1994;343(8906):1127–30.
28. Savage J, Johns CB. Food allergy: epidemiology and natural history. Immunol Allergy Clin North Am. 2015;35(1):45–59.
29. Gupta RS, Singh AM, Walkner M, Caruso D, Bryce PJ, Wang X, et al. Hygiene factors associated with childhood food allergy and asthma. Allergy Asthma Proc. 2016;37(6):e140–e6.
30. Berin MC. Mechanisms that define transient versus persistent food allergy. J Allergy Clin Immunol. 2019;143(2):453–7.
31. Steinke JW, Platts-Mills TA, Commins SP. The alpha-gal story: lessons learned from connecting the dots. J Allergy Clin Immunol. 2015;135(3):589–96.. quiz 97
32. MacGinnitie AJ, Rachid R, Gragg H, Little SV, Lakin P, Cianferoni A, et al. Omalizumab facilitates rapid oral desensitization for peanut allergy. J Allergy Clin Immunol. 2017;139(3):873–81 e8.
33. Langer-Gould A, Lucas R, Xiang AH, Chen LH, Wu J, Gonzalez E, et al. MS sunshine study: sun exposure but not vitamin D is associated with multiple sclerosis risk in blacks and Hispanics. Nutrients. 2018;10(3).
34. Westerlind H, Ramanujam R, Uvehag D, Kuja-Halkola R, Boman M, Bottai M, et al. Modest familial risks for multiple sclerosis: a registry-based study of the population of Sweden. Brain. 2014;137(Pt 3):770–8.

35. Gough SC, Simmonds MJ. The HLA region and autoimmune disease: associations and mechanisms of action. Curr Genomics. 2007;8(7):453–65.

36. Schlosstein L, Terasaki PI, Bluestone R, Pearson CM. High association of an HL-A antigen, W27, with ankylosing spondylitis. N Engl J Med. 1973;288(14):704–6.

37. Cortes A, Pulit SL, Leo PJ, Pointon JJ, Robinson PC, Weisman MH, et al. Major histocompatibility complex associations of ankylosing spondylitis are complex and involve further epistasis with ERAP1. Nat Commun. 2015;6:7146.

38. Matzaraki V, Kumar V, Wijmenga C, Zhernakova A. The MHC locus and genetic susceptibility to autoimmune and infectious diseases. Genome Biol. 2017;18(1):76.

39. Dendrou CA, Petersen J, Rossjohn J, Fugger L. HLA variation and disease. Nat Rev Immunol. 2018;18(5):325–39.

40. Fernandes Filho JA, Vedeler CA, Myhr KM, Nyland H, Pandey JP. TNF-alpha and -beta gene polymorphisms in multiple sclerosis: a highly significant role for determinants in the first intron of the TNF-beta gene. Autoimmunity. 2002;35(6):377–80.

41. Hajeer AH, Hutchinson IV. TNF-alpha gene polymorphism: clinical and biological implications. Microsc Res Tech. 2000;50(3):216–28.

42. Schur PH. Genetics of systemic lupus erythematosus. Lupus. 1995;4(6):425–37.

43. International Multiple Sclerosis Genetics Consortium. Electronic address ccye, international multiple sclerosis genetics C. low-frequency and rare-coding variation contributes to multiple sclerosis risk. Cell. 2018;175(6):1679–87 e7.

44. Stanford SM, Bottini N. PTPN22: the archetypal non-HLA autoimmunity gene. Nat Rev Rheumatol. 2014;10(10):602–11.

45. International Multiple Sclerosis Genetics C, Hafler DA, Compston A, Sawcer S, Lander ES, Daly MJ, et al. Risk alleles for multiple sclerosis identified by a genomewide study. N Engl J Med. 2007;357(9):851–62.

46. De Jager PL. The era of GWAS is over - No. Mult Scler. 2018;24(3):258–60.

47. Vandenbroeck K. The era of GWAS is over - Yes. Mult Scler. 2018;24(3):256–7.

48. Ngo ST, Steyn FJ, McCombe PA. Gender differences in autoimmune disease. Front Neuroendocrinol. 2014;35(3):347–69.

49. Golden LC, Voskuhl R. The importance of studying sex differences in disease: the example of multiple sclerosis. J Neurosci Res. 2017;95(1–2):633–43.

50. Hughes GC, Choubey D. Modulation of autoimmune rheumatic diseases by oestrogen and progesterone. Nat Rev Rheumatol. 2014;10(12):740–51.

51. Voskuhl RR, Wang H, Wu TC, Sicotte NL, Nakamura K, Kurth F, et al. Estriol combined with glatiramer acetate for women with relapsing-remitting multiple sclerosis: a randomised, placebo-controlled, phase 2 trial. Lancet Neurol. 2016;15(1):35–46.

52. MacKenzie-Graham A, Brook J, Kurth F, Itoh Y, Meyer C, Montag MJ, et al. Estriol-mediated neuroprotection in multiple sclerosis localized by voxel-based morphometry. Brain Behav. 2018;8(9):e01086.

53. Wilhelmson AS, Lantero Rodriguez M, Stubelius A, Fogelstrand P, Johansson I, Buechler MB, et al. Testosterone is an endogenous regulator of BAFF and splenic B cell number. Nat Commun. 2018;9(1):2067.

54. Confavreux C, Hutchinson M, Hours MM, Cortinovis-Tourniaire P, Moreau T. Rate of pregnancy-related relapse in multiple sclerosis. Pregnancy in Multiple Sclerosis Group. N Engl J Med. 1998;339(5):285–91.

55. Orstavik KH. Why are autoimmune diseases more prevalent in women? Tidsskr Nor Laegeforen. 2017;137(12–13):866–8.

56. Degelman ML, Herman KM. Smoking and multiple sclerosis: a systematic review and meta-analysis using the Bradford Hill criteria for causation. Mult Scler Relat Disord. 2017;17:207–16.

57. Bodansky HJ, Staines A, Stephenson C, Haigh D, Cartwright R. Evidence for an environmental effect in the aetiology of insulin dependent diabetes in a transmigratory population. BMJ. 1992;304(6833):1020–2.

58. Kleinewietfeld M, Manzel A, Titze J, Kvakan H, Yosef N, Linker RA, et al. Sodium chloride drives autoimmune disease by the induction of pathogenic TH17 cells. Nature. 2013;496(7446):518–22.

59. Sumida T, Lincoln MR, Ukeje CM, Rodriguez DM, Akazawa H, Noda T, et al. Activated beta-catenin in Foxp3(+) regulatory T cells links inflammatory environments to autoimmunity. Nat Immunol. 2018;19(12):1391–402.

60. Fitzgerald KC, Munger KL, Hartung HP, Freedman MS, Montalban X, Edan G, et al. Sodium intake and multiple sclerosis activity and progression in BENEFIT. Ann Neurol. 2017;82(1):20–9.

61. Levin LI, Munger KL, Rubertone MV, Peck CA, Lennette ET, Spiegelman D, et al. Temporal relationship between elevation of epstein-barr virus antibody titers and initial onset of neurological symptoms in multiple sclerosis. JAMA. 2005;293(20):2496–500.

62. Christen U, Bender C, von Herrath MG. Infection as a cause of type 1 diabetes? Curr Opin Rheumatol. 2012;24(4):417–23.

63. Yeung WC, Rawlinson WD, Craig ME. Enterovirus infection and type 1 diabetes mellitus: systematic review and meta-analysis of observational molecular studies. BMJ. 2011;342:d35.

64. Perrett KP, Jachno K, Nolan TM, Harrison LC. Association of rotavirus vaccination with the incidence of type 1 diabetes in children. JAMA Pediatr. 2019;173:280.

65. Baechler EC, Batliwalla FM, Karypis G, Gaffney PM, Ortmann WA, Espe KJ, et al. Interferon-inducible gene expression signature in peripheral blood cells of patients with severe lupus. Proc Natl Acad Sci U S A. 2003; 100(5):2610–5.

66. Strachan DP. Hay fever, hygiene, and household size. BMJ. 1989;299(6710):1259–60.

67. Bach J-F. The hygiene hypothesis in autoimmunity:the role of pathogens and commensals. Nat Rev Immunol. 2018;18:105–20.

68. de Goffau MC, Fuentes S, van den Bogert B, Honkanen H, de Vos WM, Welling GW, et al. Aberrant gut microbiota composition at the onset of type 1 diabetes in young children. Diabetologia. 2014;57(8):1569–77.

69. Vatanen T, Franzosa EA, Schwager R, Tripathi S, Arthur TD, Vehik K, et al. The human gut microbiome in early-onset type 1 diabetes from the TEDDY study. Nature. 2018;562(7728):589–94.

70. Stewart CJ, Ajami NJ, O'Brien JL, Hutchinson DS, Smith DP, Wong MC, et al. Temporal development of the gut microbiome in early childhood from the TEDDY study. Nature. 2018;562(7728):583–8.

71. Paun A, Yau C, Meshkibaf S, Daigneault MC, Marandi L, Mortin-Toth S, et al. Association of HLA-dependent islet autoimmunity with systemic antibody responses to intestinal commensal bacteria in children. Sci Immunol. 2019;4(32).

72. Olsson T, Barcellos LF, Alfredsson L. Interactions between genetic, lifestyle and environmental risk factors for multiple sclerosis. Nat Rev Neurol. 2017;13(1):25–36.

73. Langer-Gould A, Brara SM, Beaber BE, Koebnick C. Childhood obesity and risk of pediatric multiple sclerosis and clinically isolated syndrome. Neurology. 2013;80(6):548–52.

74. Hernan MA, Olek MJ, Ascherio A. Cigarette smoking and incidence of multiple sclerosis. Am J Epidemiol. 2001;154(1):69–74.

75. Hernan MA, Jick SS, Logroscino G, Olek MJ, Ascherio A, Jick H. Cigarette smoking and the progression of multiple sclerosis. Brain. 2005;128(Pt 6):1461–5.

76. Shoemaker TJ, Mowry EM. A review of vitamin D supplementation as disease-modifying therapy. Mult Scler. 2018;24(1):6–11.

77. Fitzgerald KC, Tyry T, Salter A, Cofield SS, Cutter G, Fox R, et al. Diet quality is associated with disability and symptom severity in multiple sclerosis. Neurology. 2018;90(1):e1–e11.

IMMUNOEPIDEMIOLOGY OF INFECTIOUS DISEASES AND CANCER

Immunoepidemiology of *Mycobacterium tuberculosis*

9

Camila D. Odio and Richard J. Bucala

9.1 *Mycobacterium tuberculosis* (MTB): Disease Burden and Presentation

9.1.1 MTB Epidemiology

Mycobacterium tuberculosis (MTB) is the ninth leading cause of death globally and the leading cause of death from an infectious agent. In 2016, there were 6.3 million new cases of TB worldwide with 1.3 million deaths among HIV-negative and 374,000 deaths among HIV-positive subjects, respectively. The highest incident cases were reported in Southeast Asia (45%), Africa (25%), and the Western Pacific (17%) regions. Overall, the MTB incidence rate is decreasing by about 2% per year, and mortality rate is falling by about 3% per year [1]. However, 23% of the world's population (1.7 billion people) carry latent MTB [2], and poverty, crowding, undernutrition, HIV infection, and smoking have limited full eradication efforts.

9.1.2 MTB and the Human Immune System

Genetic analysis of MTB strains revealed that the pathogen emerged around 70,000 years ago and migrated with humans out of Africa. Thus, MTB and humans have been coevolving for tens of thousands of years. MTB is an obligate human pathogen that is primarily transmitted in aerosolized particles, allowing it to spread rapidly in areas of dense human habitation [3]. After pathogen inhalation, alveolar macrophages utilize numerous receptors to recognize and phagocytize the bacteria. MTB prevents its own destruction inside the macrophage by blocking fusion with toxin-containing lysosomes. The pathogen then disturbs the phagosomal membrane, allowing bacterial products and DNA to move into the

C. D. Odio
Department of Internal Medicine, Yale School of Medicine,
New Haven, CT, USA
e-mail: camila.odio@yale.edu

R. J. Bucala (✉)
Departments of Medicine (Rheumatology), Pathology, and Epidemiology, Yale School of Medicine,
New Haven, CT, USA
e-mail: richard.bucala@yale.edu

© Springer Nature Switzerland AG 2019
P. J. Krause et al. (eds.), *Immunoepidemiology*, https://doi.org/10.1007/978-3-030-25553-4_9

cytosol for growth and reproduction. As the bacteria spread to alveolar epithelium and lung parenchyma, dendritic cells and inflammatory monocytes transport MTB antigens to lymph nodes for antigen presentation and T-cell priming. Primed T cells recruit immune cells to the site of infection for the generation of granulomas that serve to contain and limit the spread of the pathogen. Immune signaling molecules maintain the integrity of these granulomas, and MTB sequestered inside granulomas is known as latent MTB. If the granulomas fail, MTB activates and can disseminate to virtually any host organ, causing the deadly, contagious form of the disease. MTB phagocytosis, T-cell priming, granuloma formation, and maintenance depend on a large network of immune cascades [4].

Once infected, individuals can eliminate the pathogen, develop latent TB, or progress to active TB [4]. Latency allows the pathogen to coexist within the host for decades. Reactivation can lead to pathogen transmission to others, with infection of an entirely new population; for instance, children, who were not born at the time of initial infection [5]. Only 5–15% of individuals progress to active TB over a lifetime, but once active, untreated TB can kill up to half of those afflicted [4]. The determinants of host response are numerous and not entirely understood; however, a number of environmental, inherited, and innate factors have been identified. This chapter explores the immunoepidemiology of MTB through the discussion of representative molecules and pathways.

9.2 Impact of Other Pathogens on the Host Response to MTB

9.2.1 Malaria, MTB, and Human Immunology

Over thousands of years of evolution, infectious diseases have shaped the human genome by selective pressure. Genetic variants that confer protection against one pathogen may influence susceptibility to another. Alleles associated with the variable expression of the innate cytokine macrophage migration inhibitory factor (MIF) illustrate this phenomenon. MIF is an upstream regulator of macrophage activation, and allelic variations in its promoter, the -794 base pair CATT microsatellite, determine *MIF* expression. The microsatellite has five to eight CATT repeats. Longer length ($CATT_6$, $CATT_7$, or $CATT_8$) results in increased gene expression compared with shorter length ($CATT_5$). Although early in vitro experiments indicated that MIF inhibited the migration of inflammatory cells, such as neutrophils, we now know that MIF actually enhances the movement and activity of inflammatory cells such that higher *MIF* expression results in increased inflammatory responses. Thus, -794 $CATT_{6-8}$ alleles are associated with high *MIF* expression and stronger inflammatory responses [6]. Geographic region is significantly correlated with variant *MIF* alleles, as sub-Saharan Africa has the highest global prevalence of the low-expression -794 $CATT_5$, *MIF* allele. Specifically, -794 $CATT_5$ *MIF* alleles were reported in 78% of a Zambian population compared to only 46% of North American Caucasians [7]. These differences in allelic frequency may be due to selective pressure against lethal malaria in sub-Saharan populations, where death ensues from complications, such as cerebral disease or severe anemia, which arise as a consequence of an excessive inflammatory response. In one study of Kenyan children, those with high expression alleles were 70% more likely to develop severe malarial anemia [8]. As may occur with other pathogens, a stronger MIF-dependent inflammatory response may cause more severe disease and lethal end-organ damage in high genotypic *MIF* expressors.

While the -794 $CATT_{6-8}$ *MIF* alleles are associated with more inflammatory, severe malaria, they may also increase susceptibility to pulmonary MTB. Studies from across the globe have observed an increased risk of pulmonary MTB in individuals with high-expression *MIF* alleles. Two meta-analyses have reviewed all the largely HIV-negative subjects in these studies, each with about 1000 cases of pulmonary MTB [9, 10]. Both analyses report that -794 $CATT_{6-8}$ alleles are associated with developing pulmonary MTB, with odds ratios (ORs) that ranged from 1.5 to 1.8. By increasing local tissue

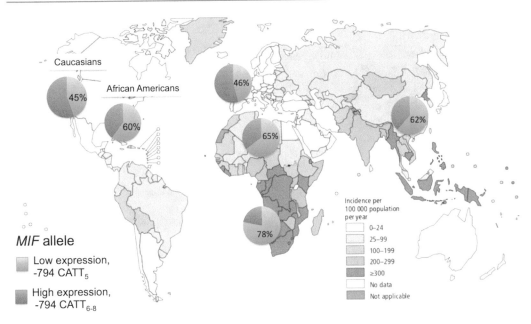

Fig. 9.1 MTB incidence rates and *MIF* allele frequencies. Superimposed MTB incidence rates, and *MIF* allele frequencies illustrate that areas with the highest MTB incidence rates (dark green) coincide with increased prevalence of low-expression *MIF* alleles

inflammation, high-expression *MIF* alleles promote alveolar lung damage, mycobacterial dissemination, and progression to active pulmonary MTB.

Notably, geographic areas with the highest incidence of MTB have the highest global prevalence of low-expression *MIF* alleles (Fig. 9.1), as has been observed with malaria. Thus, selective pressure on the immune system by regional infectious diseases likely contributes to the variability of the host response to other infections, including MTB. Although the studies discussed above suggest that the high prevalence of CATT₅ *MIF* alleles should protect against MTB, the opposite trend is depicted in Fig. 9.1. This is likely related to high HIV prevalence in the MTB endemic areas. Specifically, while high MIF levels worsen MTB infection in otherwise healthy individuals, those immunosuppressed by HIV may benefit from MIF's inflammatory effects for protection against MTB.

9.2.2 HIV May Alter the Role of MIF in MTB

Studies of MIF expression in HIV-infected patients suggest a distinct interaction between *MIF* alleles and MTB severity. In a South African cohort of HIV+ patients, there was a greater frequency of the low expression *MIF* allele (-794 CATT5) among MTB patients compared to HIV+ patients without MTB (OR 2.03), suggesting that the low expression allele increases the risk for MTB in HIV positive patients [11]. In a Ugandan cohort with HIV/MTB coinfection, a third of subjects with the −794 CATT₅ allele had MTB bacteremia, a severe form of infection, compared to only 18% of subjects with the −794 CATT₆₋₈ alleles. This represented an odds ratio of 2.4 even after controlling for age, sex, and severity of human immunodeficiency virus (HIV) infection [12]. Thus, high-expression *MIF* alleles may confer a survival advantage in patients with immune compromise due to HIV. While MIF's inflammatory effects may contribute to MTB progression in patients with intact immune systems, those with HIV-associated immune suppression may benefit from MIF's augmentation of host defenses to MTB.

Text Box: HIV and MTB

The emergence of the human immunodeficiency virus (HIV) dramatically altered the immunoepidemiology of MTB. In the United States, the incidence of MTB infection decreased by 6% per year between 1953 and 1985 but rose by 20% between 1985 and 1992. There was significant overlap between the patients with MTB infection and HIV, including their age, gender, and geographic location. At least half of new MTB cases were attributable to HIV [14]. In developing nations prior to the emergence of HIV, almost half the adult population harbored latent MTB and had a 1–3% risk of MTB infection per year. After 1985, there was a 6% annual rate increase in the number of MTB cases, and the hardest hit nations reported 5–8% of adults had MTB/HIV coinfection. Coinfection was associated with more severe MTB with 70% developing extrapulmonary disease compared to only 20% of HIV-negative patients. MTB associated mortality was 33% despite antibiotics versus 2% in HIV-negative people [15]. This high mortality rate was linked to synergy between the two pathogens. In vitro studies demonstrate that MTB increases HIV replication by stimulating the expression of HIV cell entry receptors and cytokines that promote viral production and decreasing protective immune signals [16]. Simultaneously, by depleting CD4 T cells, HIV cripples the immune response, facilitating granuloma degradation and MTB dissemination. HIV also inhibits immune cell migration necessary for MTB containment [13].

The rising incidence of MTB infection in settings with limited treatment management options has resulted in multidrug-resistant tuberculosis (MDR-TB). This infection is defined by mycobacterial strains resistant to at least one of the first-line antibiotics and requires longer, more expensive, and more toxic treatments. HIV infection is a major risk factor for MDR-TB with one meta-analysis reporting a 24% higher odds of developing MDR-TB in HIV-positive versus HIV-negative patients [17]. Outbreaks of MDR-TB often occurred when patients with MTB and HIV were housed together, and one hospital outbreak accounted for a quarter of MDR-TB in the United States over a 4-year period. HIV/MDR-TB coinfection had a mortality rate of 72% compared to 20% for MDR-TB alone [18]. HIV infection is associated with decreased antibiotic absorption, which further complicates treatment regimens [19]. By impacting susceptibility, antibiotic absorption, and mortality, HIV has dramatically altered the immunoepidemiology of MTB and poses a significant challenge for public health systems across the globe.

Antiretroviral therapy for the treatment of HIV reversed the grim trends of coinfection. For instance, in Atlanta, Georgia, the 1-year survival rate for patients with HIV/MTB coinfection improved from 58% in 1991 to 83% in 1997 largely due to therapeutic advances [20]. The World Health Organization (WHO) reports that 6.2 million people with coinfection were saved between 2005 and 2016, but more than a third of deaths in HIV-positive people are still due to MTB. Delay in HIV/MTB treatment is a top risk factor for developing MDR tuberculosis, and 490,000 cases of resistant MTB occurred in 2016 [1]. Overall, HIV has forever changed how MTB interacts with humanity, and global collaboration is critical to eradicating both infections.

The emergence of the human immunodeficiency virus (HIV) has had an unparalleled effect on the global burden of MTB (see text box). By impairing the "helper" CD4 T-cell response, HIV disrupts granuloma integrity and the host's ability to maintain MTB latency, accelerating MTB reactivation [13]. Indeed, while the lifetime risk of MTB reactivation is ~10% in immunocompetent individuals [4], that risk increases to 10% per annum in HIV-infected individuals [13]. In sum, the interactions between the immune system and human pathogens are complex, and the selective pressures imposed by regional infectious diseases contribute to the immunoepidemiology of MTB.

9.3 Environmental Determinants of Host Response

9.3.1 Nutrition and MTB Susceptibility

Nutrient and micronutrient availability accounts for some diversity in the host immune response to MTB. One population-based study in the USA followed 14,279 patients over 20 years, and 61 subjects developed tuberculosis. Prior to MTB infection, 11% had low albumin, a marker of poor nutritional status, compared to only 0.5% with low albumin among those who did not develop MTB. Subjects with low body mass index (BMI) had 12.4-fold greater hazard for developing MTB versus those with normal BMI even after controlling for demographic, socioeconomic, and medical factors [21]. Gastric bypass surgery, which is used to treat obesity, intentionally decreases nutrient absorption. Those treated with this procedure have a tenfold greater risk than the general population of developing MTB, and the incidence of new or progressive infection in these patients is reported at 0.4–5% [22]. Despite these findings, nutrition intervention trials have had mixed results. A number of studies have examined the effects of macro- and micronutrient supplementation in subjects receiving treatment for tuberculosis, and no improvements in mortality or cure rates were identified [23]. It may be that nutritional status is more important for MTB infection prevention than eradication.

9.3.2 Vitamin D and Host Defense

The mechanisms whereby nutrients support immune function have not been fully elucidated but some supplements appear more central to host defense. For instance, in vitro, vitamin D has been shown to support macrophage-mediated killing of MTB [24]. In both European [25] and African [26] cohorts, vitamin D deficiency was associated with MTB infection. In a study of South African subjects, those with active MTB were significantly more likely to be vitamin D deficient than those with latent infection (OR 5.2). Moreover, seasonal variation in MTB incidence appeared to be causally related to varying vitamin D levels with significantly more MTB cases reported during the winter months [26]. In a study of Brazilian prisoners, those with active and latent MTB had significantly lower vitamin D levels than healthy controls even after adjusting for drug use, previous imprisonment, and black race (OR 3.71). However, vitamin D deficiency was not associated with progression from uninfected to latent MTB or from latent to active disease [27]. Thus, these authors conclude that vitamin D deficiency does not contribute to the development of MTB infection, but rather active MTB disease may disrupt vitamin D metabolism. In contrast, a Spanish study of subjects exposed to MTB reported that those who developed infection had significantly lower vitamin D levels than those who did not (20 ng/mL vs 27 ng/mL, $p = 0.028$) [28]. Similarly, a Pakistani study of patients exposed to MTB reported that those with low vitamin D levels had a fivefold greater risk for progressing to active disease as compared to those with normal levels [29]. In sum, these studies suggest that vitamin D levels play a role in the development of MTB infection and that MTB disease may disturb vitamin D metabolism. Interestingly, vitamin D supplementation as part of MTB treatment has not shown definitive improvement in mortality or cure rates [23]. The inconsistencies between observational and interventional trials may be related to varying doses and formulations of vitamin D supplementation, different baseline vitamin D levels among subjects, and variety in body composition that may impact vitamin D absorption and response [29].

Aside from vitamin D levels, genetic differences in the vitamin D receptor have been associated with the development of MTB. Immune cells express the vitamin D receptor, and infections stimulate its production. When bound by vitamin D, this receptor activates immune signaling pathways that support host defense. Genetic variations that decrease vitamin D receptor activity are linked to greater

MTB susceptibility. One meta-analysis of 65 articles reported a 70–90% increased risk of MTB in patients with vitamin D receptor polymorphisms that diminished downstream signaling, but these results varied by ethnicity [30]. In a separate meta-analysis, one variant of the vitamin D receptor increased the risk of MTB in a Chinese cohort, while a different polymorphism was protective against MTB in a European group [31]. Moreover, a double-blind randomized trial of vitamin D supplementation showed shorter time to MTB cure only in patients with specific vitamin D receptor variants [32]. Thus, inconsistencies in the efficacy of vitamin D supplementation may be partially related to the genetic variability of the receptor. Overall, differences in vitamin D availability and receptor genetics likely contribute to the diversity of immune responses to MTB, but more studies are needed to confirm these relationships.

9.4 Inherited Determinants of Host Response

9.4.1 Human Leukocyte Antigen (HLA) and MTB

Twin studies have demonstrated that the concordance of MTB disease is significantly higher for monozygotic (66%) vs. dizygotic (23%) twins, indicating that there is a strong genetic component to disease presentation, some of which is inherited [33]. Human leukocyte antigen (HLA) molecules are involved in antigen presentation for immune cell priming, and inherited variations in these proteins influence host defense. There are two classes of HLA genes that serve separate roles in stimulation of the immune system. Class I consists of six different isotypes that can be inherited (HLA-A, HLA-B, HLA-C, HLA-E, HLA-F, HLA-G), and class II has five isotypes (HLA-DM, HLA-DO, HLA-DP, HLA-DQ, HLA-DR). In each class, there is genetic diversity that influences the immune response by affecting antigen presentation and signaling functions. These changes are annotated according to a nomenclature of letters and numbers that will be used throughout this section. Numerous studies have identified associations between HLA types and MTB infection by assessing the frequency of each HLA type in subjects with and without disease [34]. The HLA antigens more highly represented in patients with MTB are considered risk factors for the development of infection, while those more frequently found in the healthy controls are protective. A few illustrative studies are shown in Table 9.1.

The immunogenic diversity provided by small genetic changes in HLA molecules is notable even within isotypes. One study of HLA-DRB1 reported that the HLA-DRB1*04:11:01 subtype was associated with increased risk of pulmonary MTB (OR 2.23, $p = 0.0019$), while the DRB1*04:07:01 subtype was highly protective against infection (OR 0.02, $p < 0.0001$) [39]. This was consistent with the low binding affinity of HLA-DRB1*04:11:01 to MTB proteins, which limits the molecule's ability to present pathogen fragments for immune cell priming. In contrast, DRB1*04:07:01 has high

Table 9.1 HLA classes described according to function and isotypes. HLA isotypes associated with MTB risk are listed along with the associated statistical significance

	HLA class I	HLA class II
Function	Displays intracellular antigens to CD8 T cells	Displays extracellular antigens to CD4 T cells
Isotypes	Six isotypes: HLA-A, HLA-B, HLA-C, HLA-E, HLA-F, HLA-G	Five isotypes: HLA-DM, HLA-DO, HLA-DP, HLA-DQ, HLA-DR
Increase risk of MTB	HLA-B51 ($p = 0.001$) [35]	HLA-DR8 ($p = 0.003$) [34] HLA-DQA1 ($p = 9.3 \times 10^{-9}$) [36]
Decrease risk of MTB	HLA-B13 ($p \leq 0.0001$) [34] HLA-B27 ($p = 0.006$) [37] HLA-B52 ($p = 0.003$) [35]	HLA-DR3 ($p = 0.002$) [34] HLA-DR7 ($p \leq 0.0001$) [34] HLA-DQB1 ($p = 0.018$) [38]

binding affinity for MTB proteins allowing it to stimulate immune cells against the pathogen, which improves eradication. Other data suggest that various HLA types may have evolved to bind to specific MTB strains. One study reported that the *HLA-B*14:01* and *HLA-B*1402* alleles were associated with both Caucasian individuals and the Euro-American strain of MTB. In contrast, the *HLA-A*23:01* and *HLA-C*16:01* alleles, also more common in Caucasians, were protective against the Euro-American MTB but increased the risk of East Asian MTB strains [38]. Thus, it appears that HLA alleles associated with various ethnicities may have evolved to protect against regional MTB strains. Simultaneously, MTB strains may have mutated to evade the predominant HLA types of the region. HLA molecules provide a window into the complicated interactions between MTB and the human immune system and add to the immunoepidemiology of MTB.

9.5 SNP Polymorphisms and the Immune Response

9.5.1 Single-Nucleotide Polymorphisms (SNPs) Overview

Single-nucleotide polymorphisms (SNPs) are changes at single nucleotides in the genome and are the biggest source of genetic sequence variations in humans. When SNPs affect coding or promoter regions, which occurs in only a small minority of instances, they can alter the structure, function, and/or efficacy of proteins, thereby impacting immune responses. For example, thousands of SNPs within the HLA coding genes create the diversity of molecules discussed in the previous section. SNPs in other key immunoregulatory molecules have been associated with more severe MTB presentations contributing to the diversity of responses to infection.

9.5.2 Toll-like Receptors (TLRs) and MTB

Toll-like receptors (TLRs) bind microbial antigens and prime T cells to produce cytokines and microbicidal molecules. These receptors stretch across cell membranes with the outer portion binding proteins from viruses, bacteria, and fungi. Once activated by pathogens, the intracellular portion of the receptor is activated and initiates the innate immune system's defense against the infections (Fig. 9.2). TLRs were the first infection response proteins discovered, and nine types have subsequently been described (numbered 1–9). Given their centrality to immune function, it is not surprising that TLR SNPs have been associated with variations in MTB susceptibility.

A 16 study meta-analysis from 2013 reported that a SNP in TLR2 increased the risk of MTB (OR 5.82, $p = 0.02$), while a SNP in TLR6 decreased it (OR 0.61, $p = 0.04$) [40]. Stratification revealed that a SNP in TLR1 was associated with MTB in Africans (OR 2.47, $p < 0.01$) and American Hispanics (OR 2.12, $p < 0.01$), but these trends were not observed in Europeans or Asians. In contrast, a SNP in TLR2 increased MTB risk in Asians (OR 2.95, $p < 0.001$) and Europeans (OR 2.73, $p = 0.002$), but was not significantly associated with disease in Hispanic or Africans. Variations in immune responses by ethnicity could reflect differences in SNP frequencies among groups. Interactions between regional MTB strains and the human immune system over time could also be contributing. One research group explored these ethnic and regional differences by stimulating cells from Chinese, Filipino, and Caucasian subjects with TLR-binding proteins from four different MTB strains [41]. They reported that cells from Filipino subjects produce less inflammatory signaling molecules regardless of MTB strain. Additionally, one MTB strain elicited fewer immune responses in all cells regardless of ethnicity. Thus, both the host and pathogen play a central role in the immunoepidemiology of MTB, and further studies are needed to confirm these relationships.

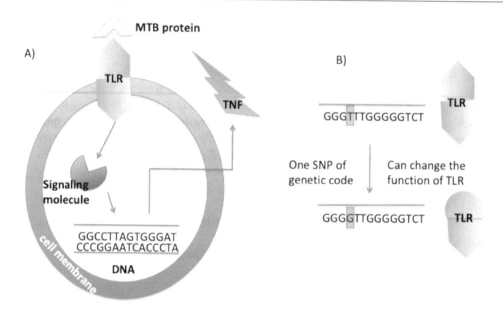

Fig. 9.2 Toll-like receptors and TB. (**a**) When TLRs bind pathogens, they change shape and stimulate signaling molecules. These activate DNA to promote the production of inflammatory cytokines like TNF for host defense. (**b**) SNPs change one nucleotide in the genetic code, and this can alter the structure and function of defense molecules

Aside from ethnicity, interesting trends in gender-related MTB susceptibility are associated with TLR SNPs. Men have a higher risk of MTB than women in large studies reporting prevalence ratios of 2.21. Reasons for this disparity likely include men having decreased access to or engagement with healthcare [42]. However, biological causes have also been discovered. In particular, because TLR8 is inherited on the sex-determining X chromosome, TLR8 SNPs are associated with gender susceptibility. One study reported that a TLR8 SNP increased with risk of MTB in women (OR = 1.41) but decreased it in men (OR = 0.72). Thus, other sex-associated signaling molecules likely interact with TLR8 variants and contribute to MTB susceptibility [43]. More gender-stratified research is needed to elucidate the biological mechanisms associated with MTB immunity.

9.5.3 Tumor Necrosis Factor (TNF) and MTB

As alluded to in the previous section, MTB binding to TLRs produces inflammatory and microbicidal pathways, which are critical for host defense. For instance, increased MTB infection rates have been documented in patients treated with blockers of the innate cytokine TNF, which is widely used for the management of autoimmune diseases. SNPs in *TNF* genes have been linked to MTB risk. A meta-analysis of 2735 cases and 3177 controls reported that two *TNF* SNPs were associated with pulmonary TB regardless of ethnicity [44]. Interestingly, separate studies linked one of these SNPs with decreased TNF expression [45] and the other with increased TNF production [46]. Thus, the associations between *TNF* genetic changes and MTB disease are likely more complicated than variations in TNF levels influencing immunity. Again, more work is needed to clarify these associations and their underlying mechanisms.

9.6   Determinants of Extrapulmonary MTB

9.6.1   IL-12-IFN-γ Pathway and Extrapulmonary MTB

Of the 10% of patients who progress to active MTB, about 20% develop extrapulmonary disease, which includes infections of the brain, bones, and liver, among other organs. The mechanisms of extrapulmonary spread are a subject of continued study. Immunosuppression, such as by HIV, cancer, and medications, is an established risk factor [47]. Extrapulmonary disease in otherwise immunocompetent hosts is still not understood, but SNPs in key genes have explained some of these cases (Tables 9.2a and 9.2b).

The most common genetic mutations associated with severe MTB occur in the IL-12Rβ1. This receptor binds the immune signaling molecule IL-12 that is produced by MTB-stimulated macrophages. When IL-12 binds to the IL-12Rβ1 receptor on T cells, IFN-γ is produced that induces free radicals to kill MTB and activates surrounding immune cells to do the same. One study of 50 children with severe MTB reported that 4% had mutations in this receptor [48]. Identifying IL-12Rβ1 mutations can have therapeutic implications since treating affected patients with IFN-γ has shown potential for curing severe MTB [49].

Given the importance of IFN-γ to host defense, a number of studies have examined IFN-γ SNPs in MTB patients. One group compared patients with extrapulmonary MTB ($n = 33$) and pulmonary MTB ($n = 129$) with healthy controls ($n = 156$) and reported that a *IFN-γ* SNP was more common in the MTB patients ($p < 0.0001$), although no difference in SNP frequency was observed between the pulmonary and extrapulmonary MTB cohorts. Notably, IFN-γ levels were significantly lower in the extrapulmonary MTB group as compared to the other two cohorts. This *IFN-γ* SNP occurs at an important binding site on the *IFN-γ* gene and limits the production of IFN-γ [50]. Low IFN-γ levels in

Table 9.2a SNPs affecting the IL-12-IFN-γ pathway. These have been significantly associated with severe, extrapulmonary MTB. Their function and notable lessons from their study are documented

Molecules	Function	Notable points
IL-12Rβ1 [48]	Stimulates T cells to produce IFN-γ, which is critical for MTB eradication	Patients with these mutations and severe MTB have been successfully treated with IFN-γ [49]
IFN-γ [50]	Stimulates the production of free radicals to kill MTB and activates other cells to do the same	IFN-γ SNPs and neutralizing autoantibodies increase the risk of extrapulmonary MTB. Autoantibodies against other key molecules may contribute to severe MTB
STAT1 [53]	Transmits the IFN-γ signal within the cell facilitating immune activation	Mutations in this protein highlight the IFN-γ pathway as central to preventing severe MTB

Table 9.2b SNPs affecting non-IL-12-IFN-γ pathways. SNPs in the listed molecules have been significantly associated with severe, extrapulmonary MTB. Their function and notable lessons from their study are documented

Molecules	Function	Notable points
MIF [54]	Released by infection stimulated cells; promotes inflammation	MIF associated inflammation may damage granulomas facilitating the progression to active and extrapulmonary MTB
TLR2 [55]	Cell surface receptor that binds MTB and initiates the immune response	Interactions between MTB strain and SNPs influence disease presentation
TGF-β1 [54]	Produced when TLRs bind pathogens and amplifies the immune response	The degree of infection associated inflammation may vary by SNP
P2X7 [47]	Purine binding receptor on macrophages that promotes mycobacterial killing when activated	Studying the cells from subjects with these SNPs can help identify the mechanisms whereby the mutations increase infection risk

patients with this SNP were observed in a study comparing stimulated cells with and without the SNP [51]. Another study reported IFN-γ neutralizing autoantibodies in one patient with disseminated MTB, further confirming the importance of IFN-γ in host defense [52]. Separately, SNPs in molecules downstream of IFN-γ have also been associated with disseminated MTB. Specifically, IFN-γ stimulates immune cells by activating the signal transduction and activator of transcription 1 (STAT1) protein. Mutations in this protein have been discovered in patients with severe MTB and other disseminated infections highlighting the importance of this pathway in infection control [53].

9.6.2 Other SNPs Associated with Severe MTB

Analyses of patients with MTB of the spine ($n = 110$) [54] and meninges ($n = 187$) [55] revealed associations with SNPs in two proteins already discussed in this chapter, MIF and TLR2. The high-expression *MIF* allele increased the odds of spinal MTB by 47% ($p < 0.01$), and a *TLR2* SNP increased the odds of MTB meningitis by 51% ($p = 0.006$). Notably, the TLR2 SNP association was only observed in patients with a particular MTB strain. Thus, the interaction between various MTB strains and immune system SNPs is an important contributor to extrapulmonary disease.

Activation of TLRs stimulates the production of the inflammatory cytokine transforming growth factor (TGF)-β1. The spinal tuberculosis study reported higher rates of two TGF-β1 SNPs in cases vs controls with odds ratios of 2.3 ($p \leq 0.04$). These alleles also were associated with higher inflammatory markers suggesting that genetic changes can worsen inflammation. Separately, a meta-analysis of 18 studies examined risk factors for extrapulmonary MTB and reported that a SNP in the macrophage purinergic receptor protein P2X7 was the most strongly associated with severe MTB (OR 2.28). This receptor is present on macrophages and promotes mycobacterial killing when activated. P2X7 SNP is a loss-of-function mutation, thereby explaining how the SNP increases risk for MTB spread [47]. Interestingly, this meta-analysis also combined the data from four studies examining the aforementioned *IFN-γ* SNP and did not find an association between the SNP and extrapulmonary disease (OR 1.03). Specifically, a Columbian study reported that the rate of extrapulmonary infection was higher without the *IFN-γ* SNP, while an Egyptian study reported the opposite [47]. Moreover, a Brazilian [50] and a Tunisian study reported no significant association between extrapulmonary disease and the *IFN-γ* SNP [47]. Of note, none of these studies controlled for race or MTB strain, although the Tunisian study did report a "predominant" MTB strain in the population. These analyses also were limited by small sample sizes (ranging from 30 to 50) with the largest cohort ($n = 84$) reporting the only positive association between the *IFN-γ* SNP and extrapulmonary disease. This group of studies demonstrates the challenges of identifying significant SNP-infection associations. Future studies should attempt to stratify data by race, gender, and MTB strain. Sample sizes may be enlarged by collaborative efforts among MTB treatment centers.

9.7 Conclusions

The clinical presentation of MTB is affected by a variety of host immune factors.

MTB has a large spectrum of presentation from subclinical microbe eradication to generalized dissemination, and phenotype is determined by host–pathogen interaction. A number of factors contribute to the diversity of presentations including selective pressure on immunity by other pathogens, environmental influences, inherited factors, pathogen strain, and inborn variations of the immune system. Given the complex, multifaceted interactions, it has been difficult to develop a complete picture of the immunoepidemiology of MTB. Until now, seminal discoveries have been piecemeal and highlight the importance of generating large, clinically well-characterized cohorts that can be stratified according to influential demographics. Armed with this knowledge, we expect more comprehensive studies will produce prognostic and therapeutic response algorithms to improve preventative and curative treatments. Lessons learned also inform the general study of host–pathogen interactions and the mechanisms underlying diverse disease presentations.

References Cited

1. WHO | Global tuberculosis report 2017. WHO. 2017 [cited 2018 Mar 23]. Available from: http://www.who.int/tb/publications/global_report/en/.
2. Houben RMGJ, Dodd PJ. The global burden of latent tuberculosis infection: a re-estimation using mathematical modelling. PLoS Med. 2016;13(10):e1002152.
3. Comas I, Coscolla M, Luo T, Borrell S, Holt KE, Kato-Maeda M, et al. Out-of-Africa migration and Neolithic coexpansion of *Mycobacterium tuberculosis* with modern humans. Nat Genet. 2013;45(10):1176–82.
4. Pai M, Behr MA, Dowdy D, Dheda K, Divangahi M, Boehme CC, et al. Tuberculosis. Nat Rev Dis Primer. 2016;2:16076.
5. Levy S. The Evolution of TuberculosisGenetic analysis offers new insight on the spread of an ancient disease. Bioscience. 2012;62(7):625–9.
6. Yao J, Leng L, Sauler M, Fu W, Zheng J, Zhang Y, et al. Transcription factor ICBP90 regulates the MIF promoter and immune susceptibility locus. J Clin Invest. 2016;126(2):732–44.
7. Zhong X, Leng L, Beitin A, Chen R, McDonald C, Hsiao B, et al. Simultaneous detection of microsatellite repeats and SNPs in the macrophage migration inhibitory factor (MIF) gene by thin-film biosensor chips and application to rural field studies. Nucleic Acids Res. 2005;33(13):e121.
8. Awandare GA, Martinson JJ, Were T, Ouma C, Davenport GC, Ong'echa JM, et al. Macrophage Migration Inhibitory Factor (MIF) promoter polymorphisms and susceptibility to severe malarial anemia. J Infect Dis. 2009;200(4):629–37.
9. Ma M, Tao L, Liu A, Liang Z, Yang J, Peng Y, et al. Macrophage migration inhibitory factor-794 CATT microsatellite polymorphism and risk of tuberculosis: a meta-analysis. Biosci Rep. 2018;38(4):BSR20171626.
10. Areeshi MY, Mandal RK, Dar SA, Jawed A, Wahid M, Lohani M, et al. MIF -173 G > C (rs755622) gene polymorphism modulates tuberculosis risk: evidence from a meta-analysis and trial sequential analysis. Sci Rep. 2017;7(1):17003.
11. Reid D, Shenoi S, Singh R, Wang M, Patel V et al. Low expression macrophage migration inhibitory factor alleles and tuberculosis in HIV infected South Africans. Cytokine: X. 2019 Feb 11; 100004.
12. Das R, Koo M-S, Kim BH, Jacob ST, Subbian S, Yao J, et al. Macrophage migration inhibitory factor (MIF) is a critical mediator of the innate immune response to *Mycobacterium tuberculosis*. Proc Natl Acad Sci U S A. 2013;110(32):E2997–3006.
13. Pawlowski A, Jansson M, Sköld M, Rottenberg ME, Källenius G. Tuberculosis and HIV co-infection. PLoS Pathog. 2012;8(2):e1002464.
14. Cantwell MF, Snider DE, Cauthen GM, Onorato IM. Epidemiology of tuberculosis in the United States, 1985 through 1992. JAMA. 1994;272(7):535–9.
15. Corbett EL, Watt CJ, Walker N, Maher D, Williams BG, Raviglione MC, et al. The growing burden of tuberculosis: global trends and interactions with the HIV epidemic. Arch Intern Med. 2003;163(9):1009–21.
16. Rosas-Taraco AG, Arce-Mendoza AY, Caballero-Olín G, Salinas-Carmona MC. *Mycobacterium tuberculosis* upregulates coreceptors CCR5 and CXCR4 while HIV modulates CD14 favoring concurrent infection. AIDS Res Hum Retrovir. 2006;22(1):45–51.
17. Mesfin YM, Hailemariam D, Biadglign S, Kibret KT. Association between HIV/AIDS and multi-drug resistance tuberculosis: a systematic review and meta-analysis. PLoS One. 2014;9(1):e82235.
18. Frieden TR, Sherman LF, Maw KL, Fujiwara PI, Crawford JT, Nivin B, et al. A multi-institutional outbreak of highly drug-resistant tuberculosis: epidemiology and clinical outcomes. JAMA. 1996;276(15):1229–35.
19. Gurumurthy P, Ramachandran G, Hemanth Kumar AK, Rajasekaran S, Padmapriyadarsini C, Swaminathan S, et al. Malabsorption of rifampin and isoniazid in HIV-infected patients with and without tuberculosis. Clin Infect Dis. 2004;38(2):280–3.

20. Leonard MK, Larsen N, Drechsler H, Blumberg H, Lennox JL, Arrellano M, et al. Increased survival of persons with tuberculosis and human immunodeficiency virus infection, 1991--2000. Clin Infect Dis. 2002;34(7):1002–7.
21. Cegielski JP, Arab L, Cornoni-Huntley J. Nutritional risk factors for tuberculosis among adults in the United States, 1971–1992. Am J Epidemiol. 2012;176(5):409–22.
22. Khiria LS, Narwaria M. Tuberculosis after laparoscopic Roux-en-Y gastric bypass for morbid obesity. Surg Obes Relat Dis. 2011;7(3):323–5.
23. Grobler L, Nagpal S, Sudarsanam TD, Sinclair D. Nutritional supplements for people being treated for active tuberculosis. Cochrane Database Syst Rev. 2016;6:1–195.
24. Martineau AR, Wilkinson KA, Newton SM, Floto RA, Norman AW, Skolimowska K, et al. IFN-gamma- and TNF-independent vitamin D-inducible human suppression of mycobacteria: the role of cathelicidin LL-37. J Immunol. 2007;178(11):7190–8.
25. Ustianowski A, Shaffer R, Collin S, Wilkinson RJ, Davidson RN. Prevalence and associations of vitamin D deficiency in foreign-born persons with tuberculosis in London. J Infect. 2005;50(5):432–7.
26. Martineau AR, Nhamoyebonde S, Oni T, Rangaka MX, Marais S, Bangani N, et al. Reciprocal seasonal variation in vitamin D status and tuberculosis notifications in Cape Town, South Africa. Proc Natl Acad Sci U S A. 2011;108(47):19013–7.
27. Maceda EB, Gonçalves CCM, Andrews JR, Ko AI, Yeckel CW, Croda J. Serum vitamin D levels and risk of prevalent tuberculosis, incident tuberculosis and tuberculin skin test conversion among prisoners. Sci Rep. 2018;8(1):997.
28. Arnedo-Pena A, Juan-Cerdán JV, Romeu-García MA, García-Ferrer D, Holguín-Gómez R, Iborra-Millet J, et al. Vitamin D status and incidence of tuberculosis infection conversion in contacts of pulmonary tuberculosis patients: a prospective cohort study. Epidemiol Infect. 2015;143(8):1731–41.
29. Talat N, Perry S, Parsonnet J, Dawood G, Hussain R. Vitamin D deficiency and tuberculosis progression. Emerg Infect Dis. 2010;16(5):853–5.
30. Sutaria N, Liu C-T, Chen TC. Vitamin D status, receptor gene polymorphisms, and supplementation on tuberculosis: a systematic review of case-control studies and randomized controlled trials. J Clin Transl Endocrinol. 2014;1(4):151–60.
31. Chen C, Liu Q, Zhu L, Yang H, Lu W. Vitamin D receptor gene polymorphisms on the risk of tuberculosis, a meta-analysis of 29 case-control studies. PLoS One. 2013;8(12):e83843.
32. Martineau AR, Timms PM, Bothamley GH, Hanifa Y, Islam K, Claxton AP, et al. High-dose vitamin D3 during intensive-phase antimicrobial treatment of pulmonary tuberculosis: a double-blind randomised controlled trial. Lancet. 2011;377(9761):242–50.
33. Meyer CG, Thye T. Host genetic studies in adult pulmonary tuberculosis. Semin Immunol. 2014;26(6):445–53.
34. Kettaneh A, Seng L, Tiev KP, Tolédano C, Fabre B, Cabane J. Human leukocyte antigens and susceptibility to tuberculosis: a meta-analysis of case-control studies. Int J Tuberc Lung Dis. 2006;10(7):717–25.
35. Vijaya Lakshmi V, Rakh SS, Anu Radha B, Hari Sai Priya V, Pantula V, Jasti S, et al. Role of HLA-B51 and HLA-B52 in susceptibility to pulmonary tuberculosis. Infect Genet Evol. 2006;6(6):436–9.
36. Sveinbjornsson G, Gudbjartsson DF, Halldorsson BV, Kristinsson KG, Gottfredsson M, Barrett JC, et al. HLA class II sequence variants influence tuberculosis risk in populations of European ancestry. Nat Genet. 2016;48(3):318–22.
37. Salie M, van der Merwe L, Möller M, Daya M, Spuy VD, D G, et al. Associations between human leukocyte antigen class I variants and the *Mycobacterium tuberculosis* subtypes causing disease. J Infect Dis. 2014;209(2):216–23.
38. Wamala D, Buteme HK, Kirimunda S, Kallenius G, Joloba M. Association between human leukocyte antigen class II and pulmonary tuberculosis due to *Mycobacterium tuberculosis* in Uganda. BMC Infect Dis. 2016;16:23.
39. de LDS, Ogusku MM, dos SMP, Silva CM de M, de AVA, Antunes IA, et al. Alleles of HLA-DRB1*04 associated with pulmonary tuberculosis in Amazon Brazilian population. PLoS One. 2016;11(2):e0147543.
40. Zhang Y, Jiang T, Yang X, Xue Y, Wang C, Liu J, et al. Toll-like receptor −1, −2, and −6 polymorphisms and pulmonary tuberculosis susceptibility: a systematic review and meta-analysis. PLoS One. 2013;8(5):e63357.
41. Nahid P, Jarlsberg LG, Kato-Maeda M, Segal MR, Osmond DH, Gagneux S, et al. Interplay of strain and race/ethnicity in the innate immune response to M. tuberculosis. PLoS One. 2018;13(5):e0195392.
42. Horton KC, MacPherson P, Houben RMGJ, White RG, Corbett EL. Sex differences in tuberculosis burden and notifications in low- and middle-income countries: a systematic review and meta-analysis. PLoS Med. 2016;13(9):e1002119.
43. Salie M, Daya M, Lucas LA, Warren RM, van der Spuy GD, van Helden PD, et al. Association of toll-like receptors with susceptibility to tuberculosis suggests sex-specific effects of TLR8 polymorphisms. Infect Genet Evol. 2015;34:221–9.
44. Yi Y-X, Han J-B, Zhao L, Fang Y, Zhang Y-F, Zhou G-Y. Tumor necrosis factor alpha gene polymorphism contributes to pulmonary tuberculosis susceptibility: evidence from a meta-analysis. Int J Clin Exp Med. 2015;8(11):20690–700.

45. Kaluza W, Reuss E, Grossmann S, Hug R, Schopf RE, Galle PR, et al. Different transcriptional activity and in vitro TNF-alpha production in psoriasis patients carrying the TNF-alpha 238A promoter polymorphism. J Invest Dermatol. 2000;114(6):1180–3.
46. Louis E, Franchimont D, Piron A, Gevaert Y, Schaaf-Lafontaine N, Roland S, et al. Tumour necrosis factor (TNF) gene polymorphism influences TNF-alpha production in lipopolysaccharide (LPS)-stimulated whole blood cell culture in healthy humans. Clin Exp Immunol. 1998;113(3):401–6.
47. Webster AS, Shandera WX. The extrapulmonary dissemination of tuberculosis: a meta-analysis. Int J Mycobacteriol. 2014;3(1):9–16.
48. Boisson-Dupuis S, Baghdadi JE, Parvaneh N, Bousfiha A, Bustamante J, Feinberg J, et al. IL-12Rβ1 deficiency in two of fifty children with severe tuberculosis from Iran, Morocco, and Turkey. PLoS One. 2011;6(4):e18524.
49. Alangari AA, Al-Zamil F, Al-Mazrou A, Al-Muhsen S, Boisson-Dupuis S, Awadallah S, et al. Treatment of disseminated mycobacterial infection with high-dose IFN-γ in a patient with IL-12Rβ1 deficiency. Clin Dev Immunol. 2011;2011:1.
50. Vallinoto ACR, Graça ES, Araújo MS, Azevedo VN, Cayres-Vallinoto I, Machado LFA, et al. IFNG +874T/A polymorphism and cytokine plasma levels are associated with susceptibility to *Mycobacterium tuberculosis* infection and clinical manifestation of tuberculosis. Hum Immunol. 2010;71(7):692–6.
51. López-Maderuelo D, Arnalich F, Serantes R, González A, Codoceo R, Madero R, et al. Interferon-gamma and interleukin-10 gene polymorphisms in pulmonary tuberculosis. Am J Respir Crit Care Med. 2003;167(7):970–5.
52. Browne SK, Burbelo PD, Chetchotisakd P, Suputtamongkol Y, Kiertiburanakul S, Shaw PA, et al. Adult-onset immunodeficiency in Thailand and Taiwan. NEJM. 2012;367:725–34.
53. Pedraza-Sánchez S, Lezana-Fernández JL, Gonzalez Y, Martínez-Robles L, Ventura-Ayala ML, Sadowinski-Pine S, et al. Disseminated tuberculosis and chronic mucocutaneous candidiasis in a patient with a gain-of-function mutation in signal transduction and activator of transcription 1. Front Immunol. 2017;8:1651.
54. Wang J, Zhan X-L, Liu C, Zhang D, Meng L, Deng LMIF. TGF-β1, IFN-γ and NRAMP1 gene polymorphisms in relation to the clinicopathological profile of spinal tuberculosis in Chinese Han population. Int J Clin Exp Path. 2016;9(4):4438–47.
55. Caws M, Thwaites G, Dunstan S, Hawn TR, Thi Ngoc Lan N, Thuong NTT, et al. The influence of host and bacterial genotype on the development of disseminated disease with *Mycobacterium tuberculosis*. PLoS Pathog. 2008;4(3):e1000034.

Reference Reviews

Dorman SE, Holland SM. Interferon-gamma and interleukin-12 pathway defects and human disease. Cytokine Growth Factor Rev. 2000;11(4):321–33.
Meyer CG, Thye T. Host genetic studies in adult pulmonary tuberculosis. Semin Immunol. 2014;26(6):445–53.
Pai M, Behr MA, Dowdy D, Dheda K, Divangahi M, Boehme CC, et al. Tuberculosis. Nat Rev Dis Primer. 2016;2:16076.
Pawlowski A, Jansson M, Sköld M, Rottenberg ME, Källenius G. Tuberculosis and HIV co-infection. PLoS Pathog. 2012;8(2)
Webster AS, Shandera WX. The extrapulmonary dissemination of tuberculosis: a meta-analysis. Int J Mycobacteriol. 2014;3(1):9–16.

Immunoepidemiology of Human Immunodeficiency

10

Elijah Paintsil

10.1 The Origin of the Acquired Immunodeficiency Syndrome Pandemic

10.1.1 Introduction to HIV/AIDS

Acquired immunodeficiency syndrome (AIDS) was officially acknowledged as a new disease in 1981 by the US Center for Disease Control and Prevention (CDC) based on a constellation of symptoms observed in previously healthy men who had sex with men (MSM) [1]. Shortly thereafter, investigators in France and the USA discovered the etiologic agent of AIDS as a retrovirus – human immunodeficiency virus (HIV) [2, 3]. The advent of highly active antiretroviral therapy (HAART) in 1995 changed the trajectory of HIV-1 infection from a death sentence to a chronic and treatable disease. With the current armamentarium of antiretroviral therapy (ART), it is estimated that complete eradication of HIV-1 virus in an infected individual will take over 70 years. A curative ART and a preventative vaccine continue to elude the scientific community. HIV persists as a major global public health issue, having claimed more than 35 million lives since the beginning of the epidemic. According to UNAIDS 2018 data (Fig. 10.1), there were approximately 36.9 million people throughout the world living with HIV at the end of 2017, with 1.8 million of them being new infections or about 5000 new cases a day. Nearly 1.0 million people died from HIV-related causes globally in 2017. As illustrated in Fig. 10.2, the epidemic has disproportionately affected Africa; 70% of the global burden of HIV is in Africa, with 66% in sub-Saharan Africa.

10.1.2 The Origin of AIDS: Cross-Species Transmission of Simian Immunodeficiency Virus

HIV-1 infection is a prototypical example of how the host immune system can modulate cross-species transmission and spread of an infectious disease agent. The first lead to the origin of HIV came in 1986 from the isolation of another retrovirus, HIV-2, in AIDS patients in West Africa. HIV2 is mor-

E. Paintsil (✉)
Departments of Pediatrics, Pharmacology, and Epidemiology of Microbial Diseases, Yale School of Medicine and Yale School of Public Health, New Haven, CT, USA
e-mail: elijah.paintsil@yale.edu

© Springer Nature Switzerland AG 2019
P. J. Krause et al. (eds.), *Immunoepidemiology*, https://doi.org/10.1007/978-3-030-25553-4_10

Fig. 10.1 People living with HIV (PLWH) of all ages from 1990 to 2017. Black dots represent average estimate, and bars represent lower and upper estimates. (Adapted and modified from UNAIDS 2018 estimates (http://aidsinfo.unaids.org/))

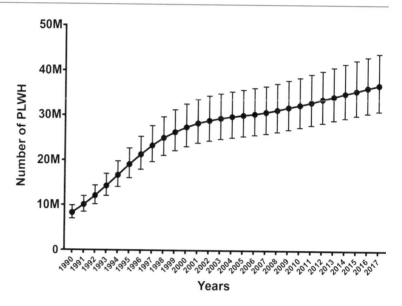

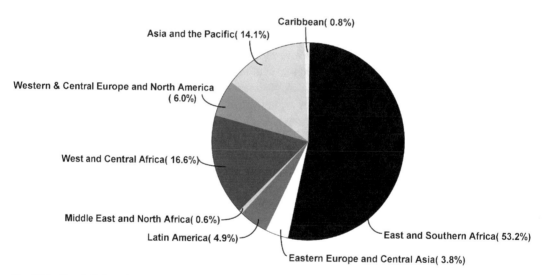

Fig. 10.2 People living with HIV by region. Pie chart depicts proportion of people living with HIV in WHO regions at the end of 2017. (Adapted and modified from UNAIDS 2018 estimates (http://aidsinfo.unaids.org/)

phologically similar to, but genetically distinct from HIV-1, the causative agent of AIDS [4]. These two isolates became known as HIV-1 and HIV-2 based on chronological time of isolation. HIV-2 was found to be genetically closer to a simian virus that caused immunodeficiency in captive macaques [5]. Subsequently, several strains of simian immunodeficiency viruses (SIVs) were isolated from different primates in sub-Saharan Africa, including African green monkeys, sooty mangabeys, mandrills, chimpanzees, and others. Old World monkeys were found to be the natural host for different strains of SIV. Subspecies of nonhuman primates from different geographic regions have been infected with the same type of SIV for at least 30,000 years [6]. The name of an SIV strain is derived from the primate species that it infects and a suffix that is added to SIV to denote their primate species of origin (e.g., SIV_{sm} from sooty mangabeys [SM]) [7]. These SIVs are generally nonpathogenic in their natural hosts but can become pathogenic when they cross species. Cross-species transmission of SIV_{sm} from sooty mangabeys (their natural host) to different species of macaques resulted in the emergence of the SIV$_{mac}$ strain and its related SIVs [8]. SIV$_{mac}$ is the only SIV that is pathogenic in rhesus macaques; it causes symptoms akin to AIDS disease in humans [8].

HIV-1 and HIV-2 in humans resulted from zoonotic transfers of SIVs infecting chimpanzees (SIVcpz) and sooty mangabeys (SIVsmm), respectively [9]. HIV-1, HIV-2, and SIV are lentiviruses. Lentiviruses cause persistent and chronic infections in susceptible hosts. Lentiviruses are transmitted vertically within species and horizontally between species. Vertical transmission of lentiviruses results in invasion of the germ-line of their hosts, meaning that some viral DNA is incorporated into host DNA and is transmitted from generation to generation of hosts [10]. Although most primate species are infected with a specific strain of SIV, several SIV mosaic lineages have emerged through cross-species transmissions, superinfections, and recombinations of different virus strains [11]. Not all cross-species transmissions result in successful infections in the receiving host; some transmissions lead to dead-end infections [12]. Cross-species transmission of chimpanzee virus, SIVcpz, from chimpanzees to humans resulted in the HIV-1 virus [13]. This accession is supported by the close genetic relationship between SIVcpz and HIV-1 (Fig. 10.3) [14] and the similar clinical manifestations of SIVcpz infection and disease progression in chimpanzees to those of HIV-1 infection in humans [15]. HIV-1 is comprised of four distinct lineages known as groups M, N, O, and P, each of which is believed to have resulted from an independent cross-species transmission event from the common chimpanzee. There are two main species of chimpanzees: common, *Pan troglodytes*, and bonobo, *Pan paniscus*, species. *Pan troglodytes* species is further grouped into four subspecies – western (*P. t. verus*), Nigeria-Cameroonian (*P. t. ellioti*), central (*P. t. troglodytes*), and eastern (*P. t. schweinfurthii*) chimpanzees. SIVcpz infects only central and eastern chimpanzees [16] found in central and eastern Africa, the epicenter of the HIV epidemic. Transmission of SIVcpz to humans might have occurred through cutaneous or mucosal membrane exposure to the blood and/or other

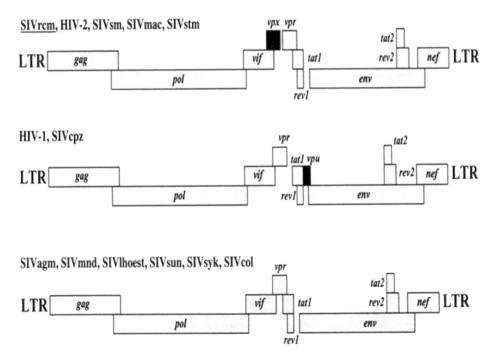

Fig. 10.3 Genomic maps of HIV and SIV. (Adapted and modified from Hirsch et al. 14])

body fluids of chimpanzees infected with SIVcpz during hunting activities [17]. Researchers found SIVcpz-specific antibodies and nucleic acids in fecal and urine samples of wild-living central and eastern chimpanzees but not in western and Nigeria-Cameroonian chimpanzees [16].

10.1.3 Molecular Adaptations for Successful Cross-Species Transmission of SIV

Primates have evolved an innate immune response to protect against infection with viral pathogens [18, 19]. However, viruses have evolved strategies to counteract host immune responses to produce successful infections. SIV and HIV interact with several host proteins for a successful infection. For SIVcpz to adapt to its new human host, the viral matrix protein came under intense host-specific selection pressure that resulted in an amino acid substitution (Met to Arg or Lys) in the viral matrix protein (Gag-30) [20]. Interestingly, the adaptive SIVcpz virus with a basic residue at Gag-30 can no longer establish an infection in its original chimpanzee host unless the basic residue is changed back to Met [21]. Lentiviruses had to overcome several adaptive bottlenecks posed by restriction factors in the new primate host to establish infection. Three classes of restriction factors serve as barriers to SIV cross-species transmission: (1) apolipoprotein B mRNA editing enzyme catalytic polypeptide-like 3G (APO BEC3G), which interferes with reverse transcription [22]; (2) tripartite motif 5α protein (TRIM5α), which interferes with viral uncoating [23]; and (3) tetherin, which inhibits the budding and release of virions from infected cells [24]. Among these three restriction factors, tetherin has had the greatest impact on SIV precursors of HIV-1 and HIV-2. Most SIVs use their viral Nef protein to remove tetherin from the host cell surface [25] or use viral Vpu protein to degrade tetherin (Fig. 10.4a) [26]. Other SIVs use their envelope glycoprotein to interfere with tetherin [27, 28]. These SIV proteins have less effect on human tetherin. Human tetherin, unlike that of primates, has a five-codon deletion in the region encoding the cytoplasmic domain (Fig. 10.4b) [29]. SIV Nef and envelope

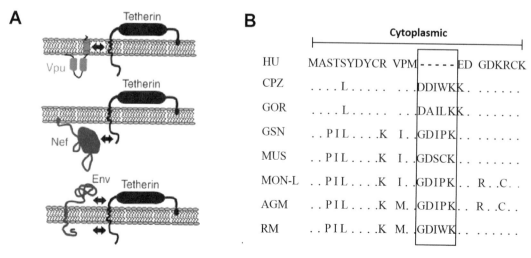

Fig. 10.4 Tetherin function and interactions with HIV and SIV proteins. (**a**) Viral antagonists of tetherin and their sites of interaction (indicated by arrows). Vpu associates with the transmembrane domain of tetherin, Nef targets the cytoplasmic domain, and Env interacts with the extracellular or cytoplasmic domain. (**b**) Amino acid sequence of the cytoplasmic domain of tetherin of various primates. HU human, with 5-codon deletion, CPZ chimpanzee, GOR gorilla, GSN greater pot-nosed monkey, MUS mustached monkey, MON-L mona monkey, AGM African green monkey, and RM rhesus macaque. (Adapted and modified from Paul Sharp et al. [7])

glycoprotein interact with the cytoplasmic domain of tetherin. SIV Nef and envelope glycoprotein cannot interact properly with the human tetherin cytoplasmic domain because of the deletion of five codons in the cytoplasmic domain of human tetherin. Therefore, SIVs are rendered inactive on transmission to humans resulting in no sustained infection. In sum, the deletion of the cytoplasmic domain of human tetherin has successfully averted transmission of most SIV strains to humans. However, SIVcpz established a successful infection in humans using its Vpu protein. SIVcpz Vpu binds to human tetherin membrane-spanning domain and degrades tetherin to allow budding and release of new virions leading to sustained infections in humans.

10.2   Host Immune Restriction of HIV-1 Acquisition and Transmission

10.2.1 Variable Host Susceptibility

A successful HIV-1 infection is dependent on interactions among HIV-1, immune factors of the human host, and the mode of transmission of the virus. This section focuses on how host immune factors modify susceptibility to HIV-1 infection and the likelihood of transmission of HIV-1 to another person. Even though all human beings are theoretically susceptible to infection with HIV-1, a minority of people are resistant to HIV-1 infection even when exposed multiple times to the virus [30, 31]. Genes encoding a chemokine receptor (the C-C motif receptor 5 gene [CCR5]) and the human major histocompatibility complex (MHC) class I human leukocyte antigens (HLA) were identified early in the HIV pandemic as genetic variants that impact susceptibility to HIV-1 infection. HIV-1 requires co-receptors, in addition to the CD4+ receptor, to enter target cells. CCR5 binds to the HIV-1 gp120 envelope glycoprotein to allow HIV entry into a host cell. A 32-base-pair deletion within the coding region of CCR5 (CCR5Δ32) results in a frame shift and generates a nonfunctional receptor that does not support membrane fusion or infection by HIV-1 strains that use CCR5 as a co-receptor. CCR5Δ32 and a much rarer m303 T > A point mutation in CCR5 when present in either homozygous or combined heterozygous form confer complete resistance to infection by HIV-1 viruses that use CCR5 as a co-receptor for entry into host cells. The allele frequency for CCR5Δ32 ranges from 5% to 15% in individuals of European decent. The CCR5Δ32 homozygous genotype is found in about 1% of individuals of European descent but is rare in non-European populations. Genome-wide association studies (GWAS) have failed to detect this allele in individuals of African descent. Persons homozygous for CCR5Δ32 mutation are highly protected from HIV-1 infection, while relative protection is conferred by the heterozygous state (Fig. 10.5) [32].

  The discovery of the protective effect of CCR5Δ32 to acquisition of HIV-1 was made possible by an experiment of nature. During the early days of the HIV-1 epidemic, hemophiliacs were disproportionally affected. These individuals received pooled concentrates of plasma-derived clotting factor VIII and clotting factor IX, which were not screened for HIV-1 at the time. A single exposure to blood or blood products contaminated with HIV-1 carries a 90% risk of infection. In the National Cancer Institute-sponsored multicenter hemophilia cohort, almost all individuals with severe disease (95% risk) who received several infusions of pooled plasma concentrates before 1985 acquired HIV-1. The risk of HIV-1 infection in this cohort correlated with severity of disease and frequency and quantity of concentrates given. A study of the 5% ($n = 43$) who received several pooled concentrate infusions but did not acquire HIV-1 found that seven were homozygous for CCR5Δ32 and another seven were heterozygous for CCR5Δ32 [33]. This observation suggested that CCR5Δ32 might confer protection from HIV-1 infection. The CCR5Δ32 mutant encodes a receptor with only four transmembrane segments. This truncated protein loses its function as a co-receptor because it is not expressed on the host cell surface. The CCR5 expression level at the cell surface in heterozygote CCR5Δ32 is about 50% of

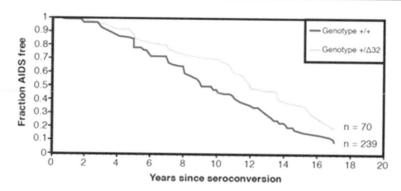

Fig. 10.5 Kaplan-Meier survival distribution curves demonstrating the dependence of disease progression on CKR5 (CCR5) genotype in seroconverters among hemophiliacs and homosexual men. A total of 309 patients with known seroconversion dates and for which long-term data were available were followed for development of AIDS. The curves were significantly different ($x2 = 8.1$, 1 degree of freedom (df), $P = 0.005$). Relative hazard equals 0.61 in a Cox proportional hazards model. (Reprinted with permission from AAAS, [32])

the expression level in homozygote wild type allele. Other mutations affecting the coding sequence of CCR5 have been described. However, these are rare and are heterozygous with no identified effect on susceptibility to HIV-1 infection. Some of these variants were found in Asian populations (e.g., G106R, C178R, R223Q, K26R, FS299) and others in African populations (e.g., Y339F, R60S). CCR2 is a mutant allele of another CC-chemokine receptor (CCR2-64I) in which a valine within the first transmembrane segment of the receptor is replaced by an isoleucine. CCR2 is used as a co-receptor by only a few strains of HIV-1. The allele frequency is about 10–20%, and it does not vary much among different populations. This allele does not confer protection against HIV-1 infection.

Co-receptor ligands can also resist HIV-1 infection. Besides acting as a co-receptor for HIV-1 gp120 envelope glycoprotein, CCR5 is also a receptor for other related CC-chemokines. These CCR5 chemokine agonists can bind to CCR5 leading to steric hindrance and rapid internalization of the co-receptor resulting in reduced numbers of co-receptors available on the cell surface to support HIV-1 entry. Examples of CCR5 ligands are macrophage inflammatory proteins (MIP-1α, MIP-1β) and "regulated upon activation normal T-cell-expressed and T-cell-secreted" (RANTES) proteins. These have been found to be major HIV-1 suppressive factors. Monoclonal antibodies that block various regions of CCR5 and compete with these endogenous ligands block infection with HIV-1 R5 strains [34]. The efficiency with which these ligands block HIV-1 entry does not correlate directly with their affinity for CCR5 but rather with their capacity to down-regulate CCR5 expression on the cell surface [35]. Also, CXCR4 ligand, SDF-1, can bind to CXCR4 thereby preventing entry of HIV-1 X4 strains. Analogs of CCR5 and CXCR4 ligands can remove CCR5 and CXCR4 co-receptors from the cell surface.

Other host factors have varied roles in susceptibility or resistance to HIV-1 infection. One of these is HLA protein (MHC protein in vertebrates). HLA proteins on the surface of host cells present antigen to immune cells. The specificity and diversity of HLA reflect the interplay between infection and immunity throughout human evolution. Because antigen presentation is a very basic immune function, HLA genes affect regulation of immunity, production of cytokines, and other immune responses. HLA proteins are highly polymorphic and can present various types of viral antigens/epitopes. The ability to present foreign antigens is limited to the genetic composition of an individual. No two persons (except identical twins) have the same HLA proteins, but individuals with similar HLA genotypes will recognize and display similar foreign antigens/epitopes with similar effectiveness. Certain HLA alleles have been associated with resistance to HIV-1 infection. There are exposed uninfected individuals who are resistant to HIV-1 infection even after multiple, high-risk, and continued exposures to HIV-1, i.e., repeatedly exposed seronegative (ESN) individuals. They make up about 10–15% of exposed individuals. Some of these individuals produce HIV-1-specific HLA-restricted cytotoxic CD8 T-lymphocyte (CTL) responses even in the absence of HIV-1 specific antibodies. HLA-A and HLA-B are involved in CD8 T-lymphocyte recognition, whereas HLA-C and HLA-E are involved in natural killer (NK) cell recognition. HIV-1 amino acids are displayed on HLA-A and HLA-B molecules, which can then be recognized and destroyed by cytotoxic CD8 T-lymphocytes. HIV-1 Nef protein can selectively downregulate HLA-A and HLA-B so that HIV-infected cells are not recognized by CD8 T-lymphocytes and hence escape destruction. Certain HLA alleles, including *HLA-B*57*, *HLA-B*58*, *HLA-B*27*, *HLA-B*4*, and *HLA-A*11*, have been associated with resistance to HIV-1 infection in Southeast Asians, whereas *HLA-B*07* increases susceptibility to HIV-1 infection. In a cohort of sex workers in Kenya, MHC class I A2/6802 supertype was associated with HIV-1 resistance, whereas MHC class I A∗2301 allele was associated with HIV-1 susceptibility. The MHC class II allele HLA-DRB∗01 is also associated with resistance to HIV-1 infection. These associations are consistent with HLA restriction of cytotoxic CD8 T-lymphocyte responses to HIV-1, HLA restriction of helper CD8 T-cell responses to HIV-1, or an interaction of these alleles with other genetic factors. In the Kenyan cohort, it was observed that HIV-1-resistant sex workers produced significantly higher levels of IL-2 in response to HIV Env peptides and gp120 compared to unexposed controls or HIV-1 infected women. Interestingly, when ESN sex workers interrupted their sexual practices, they became susceptible to HIV-1 [36]. Thus, repeated exposure to HIV-1 may be required to maintain the ESN phenotype. In some ESN individuals, potential immune protection against HIV-1 infection is provided by HIV-1-specific mucosal immunoglobulin and NK cells [37, 38]. There is compelling epidemiologic evidence to suggest that a number of additional host factors may protect individuals from acquisition of HIV-1 infection (see Table 10.1).

10.2.2 Mother-to-Child Transmission of HIV

Transmission of HIV-1 from an infected mother to her child can occur in utero, peripartum, and postpartum. Two significant milestones in the pediatric HIV epidemic are (1) the landmark Pediatric AIDS Clinical Trials group study (PACTG 076) in 1994 that demonstrated a 67% reduction in perinatal HIV transmission with the administration of a combination of prenatal, intrapartum, and neonatal zidovudine and (2) the introduction of highly active antiretroviral therapy (HAART) in the 1990s. Without the use of antiretroviral therapy (ART) during pregnancy for prevention of transmission, the rate of mother-to-child transmission (MTCT) of HIV-1 ranges from 12% to 40% [39]. MTCT rates as low as <1% have been achieved with the use of combination ART and appropriate management of labor and delivery. The birth of a child infected with HIV-1 in a high-income country is a sentinel event representing system failures and missed opportunities during pregnancy, labor, and delivery. However, MTCT of HIV-1 continues to fuel the HIV epidemic in low- and middle-income countries, particularly in sub-Saharan African countries [40]. Despite the promotion of prevention of MTCT (PMTCT) programs, several countries in sub-Saharan Africa have not achieved the World Health Organization (WHO) target of virtual elimination, i.e., less than 5% MTCT of HIV-1.

Several mechanisms and risk factors have been associated with MTCT of HIV-1, including host genetics and immunity. MHC is an important determinant of resistance and/or susceptibility of a fetus to transmission of HIV-1 from the mother. In a study of MTCT of HIV-1 in Nairobi, it was found that class I HLA concordance in mother-child pair was independently associated with increased risk of

Table 10.1 Host factors associated with susceptibility to HIV-1 infection

Gene	SNP reference number and name	Effect
HIV entry		
CCR5	Δ32, rs3333	Prevent HIV acquisition
CCL5	rs2280789 rs2107538 3′222C	Increase risk of HIV acquisition
CCL2-CCL17-CCL11	Hap 7 (31 kb) at 17q11.2-q12	Prevent HIV acquisition
DC-SIGN	rs4804803, −336G	Increase risk of HIV acquisition
Cellular viral cofactor		
PPIA/CypA	rs6850, 1650G	Increases risk of HIV acquisition
APOBEC3G	C40693T	Increases risk of HIV acquisition
APOBEC3B	Δ3B/ Δ3B	Increases risk of HIV acquisition
TRIM5	rs16934386, promoter SNP2, rs7127617 Promoter SNP 3	Increase risk of HIV acquisition
	rs10838525, R136Q rs3740996, H43Y	Prevent HIV acquisition
Cytokines		
IRF-1	rs17848395, 619A	Prevents HIV acquisition
HLA system		
HLA	*HLA* class I concordance	Increases risk of HIV acquisition
Others		
Chr.22q13	Microsatellite D22S423 at 22q13	Prevents HIV acquisition

Adopted and modified from An and Winkler [53]

HLA human leukocyte antigen, *SNP* single-nucleotide polymorphism

MTCT (Table 10.1) [41]. Thus, discordant HLA may protect the infant from infection because of allogeneic infant anti-maternal MHC immune responses. Maternal HLA-A∗2301 has been associated with MTCT of HIV, independent of maternal HIV viral load [42]. HLA-A2 in the infant has been associated with a ninefold reduction in risk of MTCT [41]. Moreover, there are reports of an association between β-defensins and MTCT [43–45]. Human β-defensins are expressed on epithelial cells and defend the host against microbes at host-environmental interfaces [46]. Two single-nucleotide polymorphisms (SNPs) in β-defensin-1 (-44C/G and -52G/A) in infants exposed to HIV-1 are protective against transmission of HIV-1 from the mother [45]. Maternal neutralizing antibodies (NAbs) cross the placenta beginning at 18 weeks of gestation, peak at delivery, and persist in the infant for as long as 18 months. Therefore, NAbs to maternal HIV-1 variants could potentially limit the transmission of neutralization-sensitive maternal HIV-1 variants [47]. However, there have been inconsistent reports on the role of maternal Nabs in reducing MTCT [48]. There are reports that maternal Nabs may act to prevent exposure of the infant to sensitive variants in utero and that NAb escape viral variants maybe responsible for MTCT [47, 49].

10.3   Immunoepidemiology of HIV-1 Disease Progression

There are three main phenotypes of HIV-1 disease progression: (1) long-term nonprogressors (LTNP) are individuals infected with HIV-1 but who maintain stable CD4+ T-cell levels and low viremia for 10 or more years; (2) fast progressors are individuals infected with HIV-1 who cannot control viremia and develop AIDS within 3 years; and (3) elite controllers (EC) are individuals infected with HIV-1 but are

Table 10.2 Host factors associated with HIV-1 disease progression

Gene	SNP reference number and name	Effect
HIV entry		
CCR5	Δ32/+	Delays AIDS
	rs1799987	Accelerates AIDS
CCR2	rs1799864, V64I	Delays AIDS
CXCR6	rs2234355, E3K	Increases survival after PCP
SDF1	rs1801157, 3′A (3′UTR)	Delays AIDS
CCL5	rs2280789	Accelerates AIDS
	rs1800825, −28	Delays progression
CCL18-CCL3-CCL4	rs1719153, rs1719134, 47 kb haplotype at 17q12	Accelerate AIDS
Cellular viral cofactor		
CUL5	rs7117111, SNP5	Accelerates AIDS
	rs11212495, SNP6	Accelerates AIDS
	rs7103534, SNP4	Delays AIDS
PPIA/CypA	rs817826, 1604G	Accelerates AIDS
Tsg101	Haplotype C	Delays progression
APOBEC3G	rs8477832, H186R	Accelerates AIDS
	rs3736685, 197193C	Accelerates AIDS
Cytokines		
IL10 (Th2 cytokine)		Accelerates AIDS
IFNG (TH1 cytokine)	rs2069709, −179 T	Accelerates AIDS
CXCR1 (IL8 receptor)	Haplotype Ha	Delayed progression
HLA system		
HLA	Class I A, B, C homozygotes	Accelerate AIDS
	B*35-Px	Accelerates AIDS
	B*27	Delays AIDS
	B*57	Delays AIDS
KIR	*KIR*3DS1 + *HLA* Bw4−801	Delays AIDS
	*KIR*3DS1 in absence of ligand	Accelerates AIDS
Others		
ZNRD1	rs9261174	Delays AIDS
Prox1	rs17762192-C	Delays progression

Adopted and modified from An and Winkler [53]
HLA human leukocyte antigen, *SNP* single-nucleotide polymorphism, *PCP Pneumocystis jirovecii* pneumonia, *UTR* untranslated region

able to control HIV-1 replication to <50 copies/ml without ART and consist of about 1% of all HIV-1 infected individuals. The heterogeneity in disease phenotypes has been attributed to host genetics and immune surveillance. Several genetic variants that contribute to HIV-1 disease phenotype have been discovered through candidate gene analysis (CGA) and unbiased genome-wide association studies (GWAS) (Table 10.2). *HLA* class I genes encode cell surface molecules that present antigenic epitopes of the virus to CD8+ T cytotoxic lymphocytes. The presentation of HIV-1 peptides by HLA class I is the main determinant of HIV-1 disease progression because different HLA proteins present antigen with varying degrees of success. *HLA* gene homozygosity for 1, 2, or 3 class I loci has a positive correlation with HIV-1 disease progression, and individuals homozygous at *HLA-A*, *HLA-B*, and *HLA-C* genes have the shortest AIDS-free survival time. Diversity at the HLA-B gene has been identified as the primary host genetic influence on HIV-1 disease progression, and key amino acid positions in the peptide binding groove of HLA-B are strongly associated with HIV-1 control. *HLA-B*57* and *HLA-B*27* gene alleles have been consistently associated with delayed disease progression. *HLA-B*57* is associated with low HIV-1 viral load and slow decline of CD4+ T cells. However, some individuals with *HLA-B*57* may progress to disease at a similar rate as HIV-1-infected individuals without *HLA-B*57*. Thus, no single genetic variant confers elite control of HIV-1. Additive or synergistic effects of multiple genetic variants are required for HIV-1 control. *HLA-B*35* Px allele is associated with a more rapid HIV-1 disease progression because of a limited repertoire of HIV-1 epitope recognition. In addition to HLA-B, a variant located 35 kb upstream of *HLA-C* gene (rs9264942) contributes independently to set point of viral load and to HIV-1 control. This SNP results in increased expression levels of *HLA-C* mRNA and HLA-C on the cell surface.

The chemokine receptor CCR5Δ32 on CD4 helper T cells is associated with delayed progression of HIV-1 disease in both HIV-1 treatment-naïve and treatment-experienced individuals. Genetic variation in the promoter region and infrequent nonsynonymous mutations in *CCR5* modify the rate of HIV-1 disease progression. The *CCR5* gene (rs1799987) upregulates CCR5 expression and accelerates HIV-1 disease progression. Other SNPs and mutations in other chemokine receptors on CD4 helper T cells (*CCR2*[rs1799864, V64I] and *CXCR6*[rs2234355, E3K]) have been associated with delayed HIV-1 disease progression. Chemokines that bind to HIV-1 coreceptors have been associated with HIV-1 disease modification. SNPs that downregulate CCL5 levels are associated with higher viral load and rapid HIV-1 disease progression (Table 10.2).

APOBEC3 family members are cytidine deaminases that are produced by host cells and mutate pathogen DNA. As such, they play an important role in host innate immune system responses to infection by retroviruses, including HIV-1. APOBEC3 family genes (A, B, C, D, E, F, G, and H) are located in a tandem array on chromosome 22q12-q13. APOBEC3 enzymes edit newly synthesized viral DNA by deaminating dC to dU, resulting in lethal G-to-A hypermutations. The hypermutations have been associated with decreased fitness of HIV-1 virions. HIV-1 has evolved to encode a protein called viral infectivity factor (Vif) that targets APOBEC3 for proteasomal degradation through a ubiquitination pathway that involves the host proteins Cullin5, elongins B and C, and Rbx1. Thus, Vif protein negates the effect of APOBEC3G and APOBEC3F on HIV-1 replication. Several APOBEC3G haplotypes comprised of promoter and intronic SNPs influence HIV-1 disease progression (Table 10.2). Variants of APOBEC3G that influence HIV-1 disease progression are associated with increased *APOBEC3 G*expression levels that overcome HIV-1 Vif-mediated degradation. *APOBEC3G* mRNA expression levels have positive correlation with disease progression; nonprogressors have high expression, while rapid progressors have low expression. APOBEC3B is resistant to Vif-mediated degradation and shows moderate to strong anti-HIV activity. Complete deletion of the *APOBEC3B* gene is associated with greater risk of acquisition of HIV-1, higher viral load, and faster disease progression. Heterozygous null *APOBEC3B* has no effect on HIV-1. The homozygous *APOBEC3B* gene is common, with allele frequencies ranging from greater than 27% in Asians to 4% or less in Africans.

10.4 Lessons from HIV-1 Immunoepidemiology Leading to Therapeutic Cure and Preventative HIV-1 Vaccines

Despite important scientific advancements in the field of HIV-1 research in the last three decades, the search for cure and preventative vaccines for HIV-1 continues to elude the scientific community. These breakthroughs may not come serendipitously, and the time to the attainment of these breakthroughs has been shortened by developing a better understanding of the interactions between HIV-1 and human immunity in different populations. Important lessons have been learned from observations and natural experiments of immunity to HIV-1 that have resulted in several near eradications of HIV-1 virus (functional cure) and one instance of complete HIV-1 eradication (cure). Functional cure is the state when there is persistentlow-level HIV-1 viremia in the absence of antiretroviral therapy (ART). Thus, functional cure results in long-term, drug-free HIV-1 remission.

There are reports of cohorts of HIV-infected patients who initiated ART during the acute phase of infection and controlled viral replication for several years following discontinuation of ART. A good example is the case of "the Mississippi baby" [50]. A woman who had received no prenatal care presented in labor to a hospital in Mississippi. She was diagnosed with HIV-1 at the time of delivery and therefore did not receive antiretroviral prophylaxis to prevent maternal-child transmission of HIV-1. ART was initiated in the infant at 30 hours of age. A three-drug regimen of zidovudine, lamivudine, and nevirapine in therapeutic doses was administered to provide prophylaxis for high-risk HIV-1 exposure. At day 7 of life, HIV-1 infection was confirmed in the baby, and she was continued on the therapeutic regimen. She was lost to follow-up between 15 months and 18 months of age. During this period, the caregiver stopped giving ART to the baby. When the child returned to care, blood samples obtained at 23 and 24 months of age were undetectable for HIV-1 RNA. A repeat HIV-1 DNA test at 24 months of age was negative, as well as an HIV-1 antibody test. She had no virus replicating in her bloodstream or detectable replication-competent viral reservoirs. It was concluded that she was probably functionally cured. Unfortunately, at about 46 months of age, HIV-1 RNA was detected in her plasma.

Of the nearly 70 million persons who have acquired HIV-1 infection since the beginning of the epidemic, there has been documented "cure" in only one person – "the Berlin patient" [51]. This patient was a 40-year-old white man diagnosed with HIV infection in 1995 and subsequently initiated on ART. In 2007, he was diagnosed with acute myelogenous leukemia (AML) and underwent treatment with total ablative chemotherapy, radiation therapy, and stem cell transplantation with donor cells homozygous for CCR5Δ32. His CCR5 receptor status was tested because of previous work that had shown that human subpopulations with CCR5 receptor malfunction had an improved outcome after HIV infection. At the time he was diagnosed with AML, his CD4 T-cell count was 415 per cubic millimeter, and HIV-1 RNA was not detectable. His AML relapsed 332 days after transplantation. He underwent reinduction therapy with cytarabine and gemtuzumab and received a second transplant from the same donor, after treatment with a single dose of whole-body irradiation (200 cGy). The second procedure led to a complete remission of the AML and coincidentally remission of his HIV-1 infection. Twenty months after discontinuation of ART, HIV-1 virus could not be detected in his peripheral blood, bone marrow, or rectal mucosa, as assessed with RNA and proviral DNA PCR assays. These observations underscore the central role of the CCR5 receptor during HIV-1 infection and disease progression. Although allogeneic stem cell transplantation from an HLA-matched donor is a feasible option for patients with hematologic neoplasms, it has not been established as a therapeutic option for HIV-1 infected individuals without malignancies. The approach presents several significant hurdles: (i) the cost is prohibitive, and most PLWH will not be able to afford this treatment, (ii) the toxicity from pretransplant conditioning results in high rates of morbidity and mortality, (iii) the ethical dilemma of subjecting an otherwise healthy HIV-1 infected individual to allogeneic hematopoietic cell transplantation (HCT) with high risk of serious side effects when HIV infection is most often controlled effectively with contemporary ART, and (iv) a limited donor pool of HLA-matched donors who are also homozygous for CCR5Δ32. However, lessons learned from the Berlin patient have led to further investigations into the development of cost-effective CCR5-targeted treatment options. Since the successful outcome of the Berlin patient, several attempts of allogeneic HCT in HIV-1-infected individuals with malignancies have resulted in mixed outcomes. The most recent success story (March 2019) from London, UK, is HIV-1 remission in an HIV-infected individual with Hodgkin's lymphoma who underwent allogeneic HCT with homozygous CCR5Δ32 donor cells [52]. Instead of allogeneic transplantation, recent advances in the field of gene therapy have evolved methods to generate a functional knockout of CCR5 expression from an HIV-1-infected individual's own cells, known as autologous transplantation. These methods include designer nuclease platforms, such as zinc finger nucleases (ZFNs) and clustered regularly interspaced short palindromic repeat 9

(CRISPR/Cas9). There are several ongoing clinical trials using the concept of engineered viral resistance in a patient's own cells, although early outcomes have been mixed. A better understanding of the roles genetics and host immunity play in HIV-1 infection and disease progression could help in the development of vaccines that will elicit robust and effective immune responses in certain populations.

10.5 Conclusions

Immunoepidemiologic findings of genetic polymorphisms in HIV-infected populations have been linked to improved or worsening outcome from HIV infection. These observations have provided important insights into variations in HIV acquisition, control of virus set point, and HIV-1 disease progression. To date, genetic association studies using candidate-gene approaches and more recently GWAS have attributed only about 20% of HIV acquisition, control, and disease progression to genetic variants. The most important predictors have been common gene variants affecting the chemokine system involved in HIV-1 cell entry and HLA class I alleles involved in host defenses. Further studies are needed to clarify the association between other genetic variants and HIV-1 acquisition, disease progression, and transmission. The case of the Berlin patient demonstrates that long-lived, replication-competent HIV-1 reservoirs can be reduced or cleared sufficiently to permit the discontinuation of ART without subsequent viral rebound. Further research and clinical trials are ongoing to replicate the success story of the Berlin patient. Of note, the longer it takes to find a cure for HIV-1, the more likely that the HIV-1-host interaction will result in the selection of other genetic variants and novel innate immune responses to protect against HIV-1 infection in humans. Following the successful establishment of HIV-1 infection in humans, we should be cognizant of the fact that other nonhuman primate viruses may with time overcome human host genetics and immune resistance and establish new zoonotic infections in humans.

References

1. Centers for Disease C. Kaposi's sarcoma and Pneumocystis pneumonia among homosexual men–New York City and California. MMWR Morb Mortal Wkly Rep. 1981;30(25):305–8.
2. Barre-Sinoussi F, Chermann JC, Rey F, Nugeyre MT, Chamaret S, Gruest J, et al. Isolation of a T-lymphotropic retrovirus from a patient at risk for acquired immune deficiency syndrome (AIDS). Science. 1983;220(4599):868–71.
3. Popovic M, Sarngadharan MG, Read E, Gallo RC. Detection, isolation, and continuous production of cytopathic retroviruses (HTLV-III) from patients with AIDS and pre-AIDS. Science. 1984;224(4648):497–500.
4. Clavel F, Guetard D, Brun-Vezinet F, Chamaret S, Rey MA, Santos-Ferreira MO, et al. Isolation of a new human retrovirus from West African patients with AIDS. Science. 1986;233(4761):343–6.
5. Chakrabarti L, Guyader M, Alizon M, Daniel MD, Desrosiers RC, Tiollais P, et al. Sequence of simian immunodeficiency virus from macaque and its relationship to other human and simian retroviruses. Nature. 1987;328(6130):543–7.
6. Sharp PM, Bailes E, Gao F, Beer BE, Hirsch VM, Hahn BH. Origins and evolution of AIDS viruses: estimating the time-scale. Biochem Soc Trans. 2000;28(2):275–82.
7. Sharp PM, Hahn BH. Origins of HIV and the AIDS pandemic. Cold Spring Harb Perspect Med. 2011;1(1):a006841.
8. Daniel MD, Letvin NL, King NW, Kannagi M, Sehgal PK, Hunt RD, et al. Isolation of T-cell tropic HTLV-III-like retrovirus from macaques. Science. 1985;228(4704):1201–4.
9. Hahn BH, Shaw GM, De Cock KM, Sharp PM. AIDS as a zoonosis: scientific and public health implications. Science. 2000;287(5453):607–14.
10. Katzourakis A, Tristem M, Pybus OG, Gifford RJ. Discovery and analysis of the first endogenous lentivirus. Proc Natl Acad Sci U S A. 2007;104(15):6261–5.
11. Aghokeng AF, Bailes E, Loul S, Courgnaud V, Mpoudi-Ngolle E, Sharp PM, et al. Full-length sequence analysis of SIVmus in wild populations of mustached monkeys (Cercopithecus cephus) from Cameroon provides evidence for two co-circulating SIVmus lineages. Virology. 2007;360(2):407–18.

12. van Rensburg EJ, Engelbrecht S, Mwenda J, Laten JD, Robson BA, Stander T, et al. Simian immunodeficiency viruses (SIVs) from eastern and southern Africa: detection of a SIVagm variant from a chacma baboon. J Gen Virol. 1998;79(Pt 7):1809–14.
13. Gao F, Bailes E, Robertson DL, Chen Y, Rodenburg CM, Michael SF, et al. Origin of HIV-1 in the chimpanzee Pan troglodytes troglodytes. Nature. 1999;397(6718):436–41.
14. Hirsch VM, Dapolito G, Goeken R, Campbell BJ. Phylogeny and natural history of the primate lentiviruses, SIV and HIV. Curr Opin Genet Dev. 1995;5(6):798–806.
15. Keele BF, Jones JH, Terio KA, Estes JD, Rudicell RS, Wilson ML, et al. Increased mortality and AIDS-like immunopathology in wild chimpanzees infected with SIVcpz. Nature. 2009;460(7254):515–9.
16. Keele BF, Van Heuverswyn F, Li Y, Bailes E, Takehisa J, Santiago ML, et al. Chimpanzee reservoirs of pandemic and nonpandemic HIV-1. Science. 2006;313(5786):523–6.
17. Peeters M, Courgnaud V, Abela B, Auzel P, Pourrut X, Bibollet-Ruche F, et al. Risk to human health from a plethora of simian immunodeficiency viruses in primate bushmeat. Emerg Infect Dis. 2002;8(5):451–7.
18. Malim MH, Emerman M. HIV-1 accessory proteins--ensuring viral survival in a hostile environment. Cell Host Microbe. 2008;3(6):388–98.
19. Kajaste-Rudnitski A, Pultrone C, Marzetta F, Ghezzi S, Coradin T, Vicenzi E. Restriction factors of retroviral replication: the example of Tripartite Motif (TRIM) protein 5 alpha and 22. Amino Acids. 2010;39(1):1–9.
20. Wain LV, Bailes E, Bibollet-Ruche F, Decker JM, Keele BF, Van Heuverswyn F, et al. Adaptation of HIV-1 to its human host. Mol Biol Evol. 2007;24(8):1853–60.
21. Mwaengo DM, Novembre FJ. Molecular cloning and characterization of viruses isolated from chimpanzees with pathogenic human immunodeficiency virus type 1 infections. J Virol. 1998;72(11):8976–87.
22. Sheehy AM, Gaddis NC, Choi JD, Malim MH. Isolation of a human gene that inhibits HIV-1 infection and is suppressed by the viral Vif protein. Nature. 2002;418(6898):646–50.
23. Stremlau M, Owens CM, Perron MJ, Kiessling M, Autissier P, Sodroski J. The cytoplasmic body component TRIM5alpha restricts HIV-1 infection in Old World monkeys. Nature. 2004;427(6977):848–53.
24. Neil SJ, Zang T, Bieniasz PD. Tetherin inhibits retrovirus release and is antagonized by HIV-1 Vpu. Nature. 2008;451(7177):425–30.
25. Jia B, Serra-Moreno R, Neidermyer W, Rahmberg A, Mackey J, Fofana IB, et al. Species-specific activity of SIV Nef and HIV-1 Vpu in overcoming restriction by tetherin/BST2. PLoS Pathog. 2009;5(5):e1000429.
26. Iwabu Y, Fujita H, Kinomoto M, Kaneko K, Ishizaka Y, Tanaka Y, et al. HIV-1 accessory protein Vpu internalizes cell-surface BST-2/tetherin through transmembrane interactions leading to lysosomes. J Biol Chem. 2009;284(50):35060–72.
27. Bour S, Schubert U, Peden K, Strebel K. The envelope glycoprotein of human immunodeficiency virus type 2 enhances viral particle release: a Vpu-like factor? J Virol. 1996;70(2):820–9.
28. Gupta RK, Mlcochova P, Pelchen-Matthews A, Petit SJ, Mattiuzzo G, Pillay D, et al. Simian immunodeficiency virus envelope glycoprotein counteracts tetherin/BST-2/CD317 by intracellular sequestration. Proc Natl Acad Sci U S A. 2009;106(49):20889–94.
29. Sauter C. Adjuvant therapy for breast cancer. N Engl J Med. 1994;331(11):742; author reply 4–5.
30. Horton RE, McLaren PJ, Fowke K, Kimani J, Ball TB. Cohorts for the study of HIV-1-exposed but uninfected individuals: benefits and limitations. J Infect Dis. 2010;202(Suppl 3):S377–81.
31. Detels R, Liu Z, Hennessey K, Kan J, Visscher BR, Taylor JM, et al. Resistance to HIV-1 infection. Multicenter AIDS Cohort Study. J Acquir Immune Defic Syndr. 1994;7(12):1263–9.
32. Dean M, Carrington M, Winkler C, Huttley GA, Smith MW, Allikmets R, et al. Genetic restriction of HIV-1 infection and progression to AIDS by a deletion allele of the CKR5 structural gene. Hemophilia Growth and Development Study, Multicenter AIDS Cohort Study, Multicenter Hemophilia Cohort Study, San Francisco City Cohort, ALIVE Study. Science. 1996;273(5283):1856–62.
33. Kroner BL, Rosenberg PS, Aledort LM, Alvord WG, Goedert JJ. HIV-1 infection incidence among persons with hemophilia in the United States and western Europe, 1978–1990. Multicenter Hemophilia Cohort Study. J Acquir Immune Defic Syndr. 1994;7(3):279–86.
34. Osbourn JK, Earnshaw JC, Johnson KS, Parmentier M, Timmermans V, McCafferty J. Directed selection of MIP-1 alpha neutralizing CCR5 antibodies from a phage display human antibody library. Nat Biotechnol. 1998;16(8):778–81.
35. Signoret N, Pelchen-Matthews A, Mack M, Proudfoot AE, Marsh M. Endocytosis and recycling of the HIV coreceptor CCR5. J Cell Biol. 2000;151(6):1281–94.
36. Kaul R, Rowland-Jones SL, Kimani J, Dong T, Yang HB, Kiama P, et al. Late seroconversion in HIV-resistant Nairobi prostitutes despite pre-existing HIV-specific CD8+ responses. J Clin Invest. 2001;107(3):341–9.
37. Mazzoli S, Trabattoni D, Lo Caputo S, Piconi S, Ble C, Meacci F, et al. HIV-specific mucosal and cellular immunity in HIV-seronegative partners of HIV-seropositive individuals. Nat Med. 1997;3(11):1250–7.
38. Devito C, Hinkula J, Kaul R, Lopalco L, Bwayo JJ, Plummer F, et al. Mucosal and plasma IgA from HIV-exposed seronegative individuals neutralize a primary HIV-1 isolate. AIDS. 2000;14(13):1917–20.

39. Bryson YJ, Luzuriaga K, Sullivan JL, Wara DW. Proposed definitions for in utero versus intrapartum transmission of HIV-1. N Engl J Med. 1992;327(17):1246–7.

40. Paintsil E, Andiman WA. Update on successes and challenges regarding mother-to-child transmission of HIV. Curr Opin Pediatr. 2009;21(1):94–101.

41. MacDonald KS, Embree J, Njenga S, Nagelkerke NJ, Ngatia I, Mohammed Z, et al. Mother-child class I HLA concordance increases perinatal human immunodeficiency virus type 1 transmission. J Infect Dis. 1998;177(3):551–6.

42. Mackelprang RD, Carrington M, John-Stewart G, Lohman-Payne B, Richardson BA, Wamalwa D, et al. Maternal human leukocyte antigen A*2301 is associated with increased mother-to-child HIV-1 transmission. J Infect Dis. 2010;202(8):1273–7.

43. Braida L, Boniotto M, Pontillo A, Tovo PA, Amoroso A, Crovella S. A single-nucleotide polymorphism in the human beta-defensin 1 gene is associated with HIV-1 infection in Italian children. AIDS. 2004;18(11):1598–600.

44. Milanese M, Segat L, Pontillo A, Arraes LC, de Lima Filho JL, Crovella S. DEFB1 gene polymorphisms and increased risk of HIV-1 infection in Brazilian children. AIDS. 2006;20(12):1673–5.

45. Ricci E, Malacrida S, Zanchetta M, Montagna M, Giaquinto C, De Rossi A. Role of beta-defensin-1 polymorphisms in mother-to-child transmission of HIV-1. J Acquir Immune Defic Syndr. 2009;51(1):13–9.

46. Pazgier M, Hoover DM, Yang D, Lu W, Lubkowski J. Human beta-defensins. Cell Mol Life Sci. 2006;63(11):1294–313.

47. Samleerat T, Thenin S, Jourdain G, Ngo-Giang-Huong N, Moreau A, Leechanachai P, et al. Maternal neutralizing antibodies against a CRF01_AE primary isolate are associated with a low rate of intrapartum HIV-1 transmission. Virology. 2009;387(2):388–94.

48. Barin F, Jourdain G, Brunet S, Ngo-Giang-Huong N, Weerawatgoompa S, Karnchanamayul W, et al. Revisiting the role of neutralizing antibodies in mother-to-child transmission of HIV-1. J Infect Dis. 2006;193(11):1504–11.

49. Wu X, Parast AB, Richardson BA, Nduati R, John-Stewart G, Mbori-Ngacha D, et al. Neutralization escape variants of human immunodeficiency virus type 1 are transmitted from mother to infant. J Virol. 2006;80(2):835–44.

50. Persaud D, Gay H, Ziemniak C, Chen YH, Piatak M Jr, Chun TW, et al. Absence of detectable HIV-1 viremia after treatment cessation in an infant. N Engl J Med. 2013;369(19):1828–35.

51. Hutter G, Nowak D, Mossner M, Ganepola S, Mussig A, Allers K, et al. Long-term control of HIV by CCR5 Delta32/Delta32 stem-cell transplantation. N Engl J Med. 2009;360(7):692–8.

52. Gupta RK, Abdul-Jawad S, McCoy LE, Mok HP, Peppa D, Salgado M, et al. HIV-1 remission following CCR5Delta32/Delta32 haematopoietic stem-cell transplantation. Nature. 2019;568:244.

53. An P, Winkler CA. Host genes associated with HIV/AIDS: advances in gene discovery. Trends Genet. 2010;26(3):119–31.

Fungal Immunoepidemiology

11

Marwan M. Azar

11.1 Introduction

The kingdom Fungi is comprised of biologically distinct, single or multicellular eukaryotic organisms and stands alongside the kingdoms Animalia and Plantae in complexity. Fungi serve as major decomposers of organic material, digesting large polysaccharide, protein, or lipid molecules via efficient exoenzymatic activity. As a result of fungal metabolism, large quantities of nitrogen, phosphorus, and carbon are released into the surrounding environment, enabling plants and animals to utilize previously inaccessible nutrients. As such, fungi play a vital role in supporting a sustainable ecosystem [1].

There are an estimated 2.2 to 5.1 million species of fungi in total, but only approximately 300 species are known to be pathogenic in humans [2]. Although fungi have often been regarded as mainly causing nuisance diseases, including unpleasant but harmless ailments such as athlete's foot, ringworm, or mucosal candidiasis, the true pathogenic potential of fungi is much more serious and far-reaching. The Global Action Fund for Fungal Infections (GAFFI) has estimated that over 300 million people are affected by serious fungal infections annually and 1.6 million people succumb to fungal disease every year, a staggering death toll that is on par with that of tuberculosis and surpasses that of malaria [3].The rise in the global burden of serious fungal disease has been closely associated with an increasingly large at-risk population of hosts that is particularly susceptible to invasive fungal infection. The advent of the HIV/AIDS pandemic in the 1980s and more recently the widespread use of life-saving solid-organ and hematopoietic stem cell transplantation, cytotoxic chemotherapy for malignancies, and immunomodulating medications for various autoimmune disorders have culminated in an at-risk population of many millions worldwide, including over ten million patients who are at risk of invasive aspergillosis in Europe, the USA, and Japan alone [3]. Although many pathogenic fungi cause deep-seated disease only in highly immunocompromised individuals, some can infect fully immunocompetent hosts or those with chronic disease or with specific risk factors such as intravascular devices or other foreign body implants. Infection with *Candida* species, a pathogenic yeast, is the fourth most common cause of bloodstream infection in hospitalized patients and the fifth most common nosocomial pathogen overall [4]. In areas endemic for *Histoplasma capsulatum*, such as the Ohio and Mississippi River valleys, up to 90% of the population has been exposed to this fun-

M. M. Azar (✉)
Department of Medicine (Infectious Diseases), Yale University School of Medicine,
New Haven, CT, USA
e-mail: Marwan.azar@yale.edu

© Springer Nature Switzerland AG 2019
P. J. Krause et al. (eds.), *Immunoepidemiology*, https://doi.org/10.1007/978-3-030-25553-4_11

gus during their lifetime. In the year 2012, there were more than 5000 histoplasmosis-related hospital admissions [5].

The magnitude of the public health impact of fungal infections has prompted a surge in mycology research aiming to better understand fungal pathogenesis and immunology, spanning from molecular and genetic to translational and clinical investigation. The study of fungal immunoepidemiology aims to characterize the range of host immune responses in populations to various fungal infections, to understand how genetic and environment factors affect these responses, and to examine how specific innate and acquired immune dysfunction predisposes to particular types of fungal infections. Insights gained from immunoepidemiology are key to defining the geographic distribution of fungi and serve as the building blocks for targeted therapeutic and preventative modalities that may one day revolutionize the treatment of fungal infections.

11.2 Fungal Classification and Morphology

As with other life forms, fungi are grouped using a phylogenetic classification scheme. Seven phyla currently exist, although the current classification is in flux. Medical mycology has adopted a more pragmatic approach to classification, dividing medically important fungi into yeasts, dimorphic fungi, and molds [6]. Yeasts are unicellular organisms that most commonly divide by budding, while molds are multicellular and produce elongated structures called hyphae that are either septated (contain cross-walls) or aseptated. Septated molds include the nonpigmented hyaline molds (such as *Aspergillus*) and the dematiaceous molds, whose hyphae are melanized. Aseptate molds, also known as coenocytic molds (such as *Rhizopus*), contain few or no septae. Molds exist predominantly in asexual form but produce sexual structures including conidia in order to reproduce. Dimorphic fungi can exist in both yeast and mold forms depending on the ambient temperature. These fungi are often endemic to the terrain of certain parts of the USA and the world.

Fungi possess a thick cell wall composed of glycoproteins and polysaccharides located outside the plasma cell membrane (Fig. 11.1) [7]. The inner cell wall typically consists of a chitin layer, with a thick middle layer of glucan components and an outer layer of extensively mannosylated proteins. In some fungi such as *Cryptococcus*, an additional thick outer polysaccharide layer, mainly composed of glucuronoxylomannan, is present. The biologic makeup of the cell wall has important implications for fungal immunology and virulence as well as the development of diagnostic [8], therapeutic [9], and preventative [10] modalities for fungal infections. The cryptococcal capsule, for example, has been shown to act as a potent anti-phagocytic barrier. By virtue of its thickness, the fungal cell wall is resistant to damage by antibody-mediated complement activation. Assays that detect circulating cell wall components (such as 1,3 β-D glucan and galactomannan) are now widely used in the diagnosis of invasive fungal infections. The three main classes of antifungal medications inhibit fungal growth by interfering with specific components of the fungal cell wall (ergosterol: azoles and polyenes; glucan: echinocandins).

11.3 The Innate Immune Response to Fungi

11.3.1 Fungal Recognition by Antigen-Presenting Cells

In immunocompetent hosts, the innate immune system responds to, and effectively eliminates, the vast majority of fungal pathogens. If fungi succeed in breaching primary protective skin and mucosal barriers, they are met and recognized by cells of the innate immune system, including dendritic cells, macrophages, and monocytes. Innate immune cells carry mammalian signaling receptors, also known

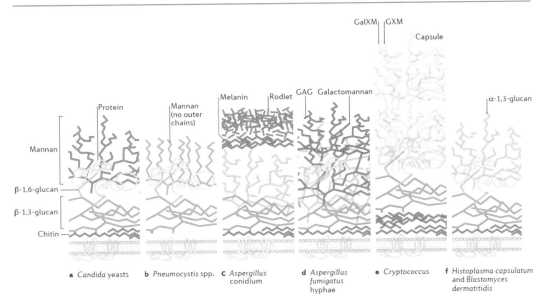

Fig. 11.1 Components of the fungal cell wall. (Adapted from Ewing and Gow [7])

as fungal pattern recognition receptors (PRRs) that bind fungal ligands, also known as fungal pathogen-associated molecular patterns (PAMPs) [11]. Fungal PAMPs are often fungal cell wall components, including glucans, α-mannans, and O-linked and N-linked mannans. Nucleic acid ligands (fungal DNA and RNA) have also been described (Table 11.1). The process of fungal recognition is mediated by binding of PAMPs to PRRs on innate immune cells. Once this interaction occurs, downstream intracellular-signaling pathways are activated within the immune cell. Multiple PRRs that mediate fungal recognition have been described, including C-lectin-type receptors (CLR), toll-like receptors (TLRs), NOD-like receptors, and others. Different families or types of PRRs can recognize the same fungal ligand. For example, both TLR-2 and CD14 can recognize α-(1,4)-Glucans. Alternatively, a PRR can recognize several different fungal ligands. For example, Dectin-2 is cognate with both α-Mannans and O-linked mannoproteins. There are fungal strain-specific PAMPs that are differentially recognized by PRRs, and absence of those PRRs has been shown to lead to strain-specific susceptibility. Sensing by multiple PRRs at once can lead to synergistic downstream signaling. The CLR are the most important PRR family for the detection of fungi. Inherited disorders in CLR lead to particular vulnerability to fungal infections. The CLR family is comprised of two groups based on intracellular-signaling motifs: (i) CLRs with immunoreceptor tyrosine-based activation motifs (ITAMs) or ITAM-like domains such as Dectin-1 and (ii) CLRs containing non-immunoreceptor tyrosine-based motifs including DC-SIGN and MR. Among the CLRs, Dectin-1 mediates recognition of multiple clinically important fungi including *Candida*, *Aspergillus*, and *Histoplasma* by binding to B-glucan on the fungal cell wall [12]. An example of CLR-mediated signal transduction via Dectin-1 is shown in Fig. 11.2.

11.3.2 Fungal Killing by Innate Immune Cells

After recruitment to inflammatory sites, effector innate immune cells including monocytes, neutrophils, and natural killer (NK) cells engage fungal pathogens and kill them [13]. Monocytes and macrophages produce cytokines and chemokines that are directly fungicidal but also enhance neutrophil

Table 11.1 Pathogen-associated molecular patterns (PAMPs), pattern recognition receptors (PRRs), and immune deficiencies associated with medically important fungi

Fungal pathogen	Fungal PAMP	Fungi-specific PRR	Selected associated immunodeficiencies [immunologic defect]
Candida	*Glucans*: β-glucan, α-glucans *Mannans*: Mannans, α-mannans, O-linked mannans, N-linked mannans, β-mannosides, α-mannose, galactomannan, phospholipomannan, Glucuronoxylomannan *Other*: N-acetyl-D glucosamine, glyceroglycolipids, Glycoprotein A, chitin, HSP60, BAD-1, DNA, RNA	*CLR*: Dectin-1, Dectin-2, Dectin-3, Mincle, DC-SIGN, mannose receptor *TLR*: TLR-2, TLR-4, TLR-6, TLR-7, TLR-9 *NOD*-like receptors: NOD2, NLRC4, NLRP3, NLRP10 *Integrins*: CR3 *Other*: CD23, CD36, surfactant proteins A and D, galectin-3, FcγR	*CMC* [IL17F, IL17RA, IL17RC, ACT1, STK4, IRF8, CARD9, STAT1, STAT3, RORC, AIRE, anti–IL-17 auto-antibodies] *Invasive candidiasis/CMC* [CARD9, MPO] *Chronic granulomatous disease* [NADPH oxidase] *Severe congenital neutropenia* [ELA2, HAX1]
Cryptococcus	*Glucans*: β-glucan, α-glucans *Mannans*: Mannans, glucuronoxylomannan, phospholipomannan, O-linked mannans, rhmanomannans *Other*: Glycoprotein A	*CLR*: Dectin-1, mincle, mannose receptor *TLR*: TLR-1 TLR-2, TLR-4, TLR-6, TLR-9 *Other*: CD14, CD36, surfactant proteins A and D, FcγR	*IL-12 receptor deficiency* [IL-12R] *Autoantibodies* [to GM-CSF or IFN-γ] *Job's syndrome/CMC* [STAT3] *MonoMAC syndrome* [GATA2] *Humoral deficiencies* [Fcγ receptor polymorphisms]
Pneumocystis	*Glucans*: β-glucan *Mannans*: Mannans, α-mannose, N-linked mannans *Other*: Glyceroglycolipids, N-acetyl-D glucosamine, Glycoprotein A, chitin	*CLR*: Dectin-1, mincle, mannose receptor *Other*: Lactosylceramine	*Severe lymphopenia* [IL2RG, IL7RA, ADA, RAG1, RAG2, JAK3, ZAP70, ARTEMIS, NEMO/IKBKG, IKBA] *T-cell dysfunction* [CD40L, IL21R] *Job's syndrome/CMC* [STAT3] *Wiskott-Aldrich syndrome* [WAS] *B-cell dysfunction* [BTK]
Aspergillus	*Glucans*: β-glucan *Mannans*: Mannans, α-mannans, O-linked mannans, galactomannan, glucuronoxylomannan *Other*: Glycoprotein A, HSP60, BAD-1, DNA	*CLR*: Dectin-1, Dectin-2, DC-SIGN, MBL *TLR*: TLR-2, TLR-4, TLR-9 *NOD*-like receptors: NOD1, NLRP3 *Integrins*: CR3 *Other*: Pentraxin-3, surfactant proteins A and D	*Chronic granulomatous disease* [NADPH oxidase] *Job's syndrome/CMC* [STAT3] *Extrapulmonary aspergillosis/ CMC* [CARD9] *MonoMAC syndrome* [GATA2] *Leukocyte adhesion deficiency* [CD18] *Severe congenital neutropenia* [ELA2, HAX1]
Histoplasma	*Glucans*: β-glucan *Mannans*: Mannans, glucuronoxylomannan *Other*: HSP60, BAD-1	*CLR*: Dectin-1 *Integrins*: CR3	*IFN-γ deficiency* [IFNGR1] *IL-12 receptor deficiency* [IL-12R] *Job's syndrome/CMC* [STAT3, DOCK8] *CMC* [STAT1] *MonoMAC syndrome* [GATA2] *T-cell dysfunction* [CD40L]

Abbreviations: *CLR* C-type lectin receptors, *CMC* Chronic mucocutaneous candidiasis, *TLR* Toll-like receptors, *PAMP* pathogen associated molecular patterns, *PRR* pattern recognition receptors

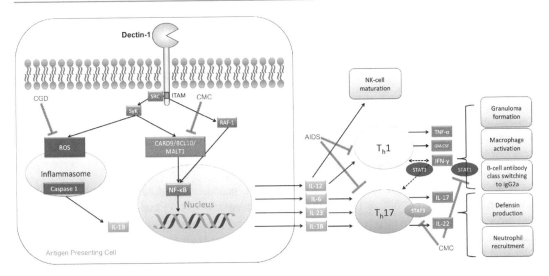

Fig. 11.2 Dectin-1 signaling pathway and associated immunodeficiencies. β-glucan binding to Dectin-1 receptor induces displacement of CD45 and CD148 phosphatases promoting SRC-dependent phosphorylation of the intracellular ITAM-like motif, which leads to Syk kinase recruitment then PKCδ phosphorylation of CARD9. CARD9 then complexes with BCL10 and MALT1 producing a CARD9/BCL1−/MALT1 complex that activates NF-κB (subunits p65 and c-REL), a protein, and possibly complex that controls DNA transcription and cytokine production. Syk-dependent signaling also leads to production of reactive oxygen species (ROS) that induce caspase-1 activation then assembly of the NLRP3 inflammasome. The inflammasome, a multiprotein intracellular complex, promotes maturation and secretion of the pro-inflammatory cytokine Interleukin 1β (IL-1β). Dectin-1 binding also activates NF-κB through a Syk-independent pathway, mediated by RAF-1 kinase phosphorylation and deacetylation. Activation of NF-κB via both pathways ultimately leads to the production of inflammatory cytokines such as IL-1β, IL-6, IL-12, and IL-23. IL-1β and IL-23 promote T-helper 17 cell differentiation. T_h17 cells then secrete IL-17A that along with chemokines such as CXCL1 and CXCL2 stimulates neutrophil recruitment to sites of inflammation and activates T and B cells against the fungal insult. IL-12 induces T_h1 cell differentiation then IFN-γ release, which activates macrophages, promoting fungal eradication

fungal killing. Activated monocytes can differentiate into macrophages capable of phagocytosing yeasts and also into dendritic cells that transport fungal antigens to regional lymph nodes where they stimulate adaptive immune cell responses to fungal invasion. Dendritic cells secrete IFN-α and IL-23 that activate NK cells to produce GM-CSF, prompting the production of neutrophils in the bone marrow. Various chemokine receptor/ligand combinations regulate monocyte recruitment during different fungal infections. For example, CCL20-CCR6 activation leads to recruitment of monocytes in the setting of invasive pulmonary aspergillosis, while CX3CL1-CX3CR1 signaling mediates kidney macrophages killing of *Candida* yeasts in a mouse model [14]. Monocytes play an important role in mucosal immunity. After fungal recognition, monocytes secrete inflammatory cytokines (IL-1β, IL-6, IL-23, and TNF-α) that promote T-cell differentiation to Th17 lymphocytes. Th17 cells secrete IL-17 and IL-22 that direct production of antifungal molecules such as defensins. Monocytes and macrophages can build lymphocyte-independent immunologic memory (or trained immunity) against fungi and other pathogens via epigenetic reprogramming that involve histone modifications, DNA methylation, and other mechanisms. For example, trained immunity ensues from β-glucan-Dectin-1 interaction and is associated with a shift of cellular metabolism from oxidative phosphorylation to aerobic glycolysis, which is thought to enhance the capacity of monocytes to respond to fungal rechallenge [15].

Neutrophils clear fungal cells differentially according to pathogen size. Neutrophils are able to ingest yeast cells and other small fungal structures such as conidia and then exert fungicidal activity via NADPH oxidase-mediated intracellular ROS production within phagolysosomes. ROS production also downregulates IL-1β production to limit disproportionate neutrophil recruitment and reduces detrimental effects of an excessive inflammatory response. In response to larger microbes such as mold hyphae that are too big for phagocytosis, neutrophils release neutrophil extracellular traps (NET) and produce ROS extracellularly to induce killing. NET are extracellular filaments composed of neutrophil nucleic acids and antimicrobial granule proteins (including neutrophil elastase, cathepsin G, myeloperoxidase, and calprotectin) that trap and kill fungal elements and may also act as physical barriers that impede pathogen movement. NET may reduce collateral tissue damage by diffusing cytotoxic granules proteins away from host cells. In a mouse model of *A. fumigatus* infection, neutrophil calprotectin was crucial in effective killing of hyphae but nonessential for control of smaller *A. fumigatus* conidia [16].

In addition to activating neutrophils through GM-CSF production, NK cells exhibit direct antifungal activity. Activation of NK cell natural cytotoxicity receptors (NCR) such as NKp30 (by an as of yet unidentified fungal PAMP) triggers release of perforin, a cytotoxic molecule that leads to fungal death by forming pores in the fungal plasma cell membrane [17]. Downregulation of NKp30 via blocking antibodies or siRNA results in decreased release of perforin and impaired fungal killing. In addition, NK cells directly damage fungal cells by inducing apoptosis via the Fas-FasL or the TNF pathway. NK cells recruited via the CCL2-CCR2 chemokine axis produce IFN-γ, which is protective in some fungal infections such as aspergillosis but has been shown to be detrimental during infection with *Candida* and *Cryptococcus* [18].

Other innate immune cells have important roles in antifungal immunity. Gamma-delta (γδ)T cells play an important role in mucocutaneous immunity by producing IL-17 and inducing defensin production by epithelial cells. Epithelial and endothelial cells often serve as the first line of antifungal defense. After fungal recognition, epithelial cells produce inflammatory cytokines such as IL-1 that promote neutrophil activation and influx. Eosinophils kill fungi by releasing cytotoxic granule proteins, such as eosinophil-derived neurotoxin and major basic protein, but are also implicated in maladaptive allergic responses to environmental fungi as in allergic bronchopulmonary aspergillosis (ABPA) [19].

11.4   The Adaptive Immune Response to Fungi

11.4.1 T-Cell Response: Proinflammatory Responses

Adaptive immune responses to fungi come into play when initial defenses of the innate immune system have been overcome or dampened by immunosuppression [20]. The T-cell-mediated response is essential for adequate control of invasive fungal infections. After recognizing fungal ligands via PRRs, dendritic cells migrate to local lymph nodes where they orchestrate a subsequent phase of immunity, governed by pathogen-specific effector B and T cells. Dendritic cells prime naïve T cells through presentation of pathogen-associated antigens on MHC class I or class II molecules combined with co-stimulatory molecule expression. Several subsets of specialized dendritic cells that differ based on anatomical location and surface marker expression cooperate to stimulate T-cell responses. Dendritic cells stimulate naïve CD8+ T cells via MHC class I and CD4+ T cells via MHC class II. CD8+ T cells, especially the Th1 and Th17 subsets, contribute to fungal eradication, but it is not yet clear if they are indispensable to antifungal immunity. Dendritic cell and macrophage-secreted IL-12 promote development into Th1 cells, a T-cell subset that is highly effective in antifungal defense. Th1 cells produce TNF-α, GM-CSF, and especially the critical IFN-γ. IFN-γ binds to the IFN-γ receptor on macrophages and leads to JAK1-/JAK2-mediated activation of STAT1, a signal transducer and transcription protein that recruits NRAMP1 to the phagolysosome. This allows for more effective killing of fungi within the phagolysosome so that macrophages are turned into voracious phagocytes capable of abrogating fungal invasion. IFN-γ also prompts B-cell antibody class switching to IgG2a, which is more effective at neutralizing fungi, and augments antigen presentation in antigen-presenting cells. A dominant Th1 adaptive response is associated with protective immunity against fungi. Th17 cells are generated after TGF-β and IL-6 priming of naïve CD4+ T cells. IL-6 activates STAT3, which is important for RORγt-dependent Th17 cell development, whereas IL-23 is critical for adequate expansion and functioning. Th17 cells operate in concert with Th1 cells, secreting IL-17 and IL-22 that promote defensing production and are especially important in antifungal mucosal immunity. They also upregulate Th1 response and dampen Th2 suppressive responses.

11.4.2 T-Cell Response: Regulatory Responses

Secretion of IL-4 and IL-13 induces differentiation of naïve CD4 T cells into Th2 cells. Th2-based immunity serves to dampen Th1 response and counteract excessive inflammation that is associated with tissue damage. Th2 cells play a critical role in response to extracellular parasitic infections such as helminths by regulating B-cell class switching to IgE and recruiting antiparasitic eosinophils and mast cells by secretion of IL-4, IL-5, and IL-13. However, a Th2-dominant response is detrimental in the setting of fungal infection, favoring progression of fungal infection and decreased pathogen clearance. Th2 cells are also involved in development of non-protective inflammatory allergic responses. As with Th2 cells, regulatory T cells (Treg) suppress the pro-inflammatory cascade through multiple pathways in order to control collateral tissue damage, but Th1 suppression can lead to loss of fungal control. Conversely, Treg may be involved in pro-inflammatory responses. Promotion of Th17 cell differentiation via IL-2 sequestration enhances mucosal immunity against oral candidiasis. Although these regulatory responses may be detrimental in some cases of fungal infection, they serve a useful purpose during the late phase of fungal infections by allowing the immune response to return to baseline after fungi have been cleared.

11.4.3 B-Cell Response

Humoral immunity is less central to control of fungal infections. In fact, most patients with inherited and acquired hypogammaglobulinemia are not at significantly increased risk for fungal infections. However, B-cell-depleting therapies such as rituximab (monoclonal antibody to CD20) have been associated with increased risk for invasive fungal disease, indicating some protective role for B cells that is not necessarily antibody-mediated. Moreover, studies in mouse models have demonstrated that monoclonal antibodies are protective against otherwise devastating *Cryptococcus* and *Pneumocystis* infections [21]. Additional investigation has shown that antibodies can be protective, non-protective, or even disease-enhancing, perhaps explaining the conflicting findings on the role of antibodies in antifungal immunity [22]. Antibodies clearly exhibit several antifungal properties. Antibodies enhance phagocytosis via opsonization. However, the fungal cell wall is resistant to complement so antibody-mediated complement activation does not result in cell wall damage. Antibody-mediated opsonization can enhance phagosome activation in macrophages and result in more efficient antigen presentation to T cells. Some antibodies mediate direct antifungal activity, including antibody-mediated iron starvation and aspartyl proteinase inhibition in *Candida* infections. Similarly anti-β-glucan antibodies interfere with cell wall remodeling and adherence in *Candida* and *Cryptococcus* infections leading to fungal death, while yeast killer toxin-like antibodies can bind killer toxin receptors on the fungal cell wall and result in damage [23]. Antibodies, particularly of the IgE class, have been implicated in allergic responses to fungi, including allergic bronchopulmonary aspergilliosis (ABPA).

11.5 Immunoepidemiology of Fungal Infections

11.5.1 Introduction

The immune response to fungal infection described above occurs in the great majority of people even though every person has a unique immune response. The study of immunoepidemiology examines subpopulations that have distinctly different responses to fungal infection from the general population and from each other. These consist of people with well-recognized immune deficiencies. Immunoepidemiology also includes the analysis of people who are relatively immunocompetent but have greater susceptibility to fungal infection based upon race, ethnicity, age, or geographical location. The remainder of the chapter will review these subpopulations.

11.5.2 Susceptibility to Fungal Infections in the Context of Immunodeficiencies

Our understanding of fungal immunology has been greatly enhanced by the study of individuals and populations at increased risk for fungal infections due to inborn or acquired immunodeficiencies. A thorough assessment of the genotypic and phenotypic profile of these populations has led to the discovery of molecular pathways critical to antifungal immunity as well as inheritable mutations and acquired susceptibilities to fungal infections. Furthermore, patients with these disorders are at risk for particular types of mycoses and exhibit certain predicable clinical manifestations, reflective of the specific underlying immune deficiency. In the section below, we examine pathways involved in immune defense against certain clinically important fungal infections by reviewing classic immunodeficiencies linked to increased disease susceptibility.

11.5.3 Chronic Mucocutaneous Candidiasis

Chronic mucocutaneous candidiasis (CMC) consists of a heterogeneous group of syndromes that usually manifest at a young age, with the common feature of chronic, protracted, noninvasive *Candida* infections of the mucous membranes, skin, nails, and hair refractory to normally effective treatments. Syndromes of CMC are caused by inherited mutations in genes involved in antifungal immunity, particularly those associated with IL-17. A subset of individuals with CMC has been found to carry autosomal dominant mutations in STAT1 [24]. As noted above, STAT1 is an important transcription factor downstream of IFN-γ signaling that primes macrophages for phagocytosis of *Candida* and that primes naïve T cells for maturation into Th17 cells. Gain-of-function STAT1 mutations lead to impaired nuclear dephosphorylation of STAT-1 resulting in decreased Th17 activation and decreased production of IL-17 and IL-22. Impaired Th17 function is thought to be the basis of increased susceptibility to mucocutaneous *Candida* infections. In Job's syndrome (also known as hyperimmunoglobulin E syndrome), a loss-of-function mutation in STAT3 impairs RORγt-dependent Th17 cell development, leading to CMC among other clinical manifestations. The syndrome of autoimmune polyendocrinopathy-candidiasis-ectodermal dystrophy (APECED), also referred to as autoimmune polyendocrine syndrome type I (APS-1), accounts for the majority of CMC cases in some populations. These include cases in Finland and Sardinia, Italy, because of the high prevalence of mutations in the *AIRE* gene, present on chromosome 21q 22.3, in those populations [25]. In the context of APECED, CMC is caused by production of autoantibodies against IL-17 and IL-22. Autoantibodies to IL-17 may also present in patients with thymoma, leading to CMC. Mutations in genes for IL-17 cytokines (IL-17F) and IL-17 receptors (IL-17 RA and RC) are associated with CMC. Many other inborn errors of IL-17 immunity have been linked to development of CMC.

In contradistinction to other forms of CMC, CARD9 deficiency is caused by loss-of-function mutations and predisposes to both mucocutaneous and invasive candidiasis, particularly CNS tropism, but not bacterial or viral infections [26]. As noted above, CARD9 activation leads to activation of NF-κB, a canonical protein complex that controls DNA transcription and cytokine production. The precise immunologic impairment associated with CARD9 deficiency is yet to be defined but are thought to affect separate pathways that lead to susceptibility to mucocutaneous disease (likely via IL-17 or IL-22 impairment) or to invasive disease (via impaired neutrophil function and chemotaxis).

11.5.4 Chronic Granulomatous Disease

Chronic granulomatous disease (CGD) consists of a heterogeneous group of disorders characterized by recurrent, invasive bacterial and fungal infections with formation of tissue granulomas [27]. Aspergillosis is the most common infection in patients with CGD, with an incidence of 2.6 cases per 100 patient-years and a prevalence of 40%. *Aspergillus nidulans*, an otherwise low-virulence species, almost exclusively affects patients with this syndrome. CGD is caused by inherited mutations in NAPDH oxidase. The NADPH oxidase complex consists of five proteins (gp91phox, p22pho, p47phox, p67phox, and p40phox), all of which are necessary for adequate generation of superoxide. Conversion of NADPH to NADP+ produces superoxide that is catalyzed into hydrogen peroxide via the action of superoxide dismutase then into hypochlorite and hydroxyl radicals.These reactive oxygen species activate granule proteases, including elastase and cathepsin G that are directly toxic to *Aspergillus*. Mutations in genes for all five components lead to impaired superoxide production and to CGD, with the most common form being X-linked (mutation in gp91phox), while other forms are later in onset and autosomal recessive. The absence of an NADPH-based respiratory burst is associated with decreased killing of catalase positive organisms including fungi, setting the stage for invasive and recurrent forms of aspergillosis.

11.5.5 Acquired Immunodeficiency Syndrome with HIV Infection

If left untreated, infection with HIV leads to gradual depletion of CD4+ T cells and the development of an acquired cellular immune deficiency syndrome. AIDS is defined as peripheral CD4+ T cell count <200 cells/μL or the presence of AIDS-defining conditions, one of which is extrapulmonary cryptococcosis (especially CNS involvement). People living with HIV/AIDS are at significant risk for cryptococcal infection. During the height of the AIDS epidemic in the early 1990s, the incidence of cryptococcosis was approximately 5 cases per 100,000 persons per year in some large urban centers [28]. The risk of infection strongly correlates with the absolute number of circulating CD4+ T cells and a dramatic increase in susceptibility at levels below 100 cells/μL. The absence of sufficient circulating CD4+ T cells leads to decreased secretion of TNF-α, GM-CSF, and IFN-γ, decreased recruitment of phagocytes and lymphocytes, and decreased granuloma formation. This allows the fungus to disseminate most commonly from alveoli where it is first inhaled into the blood then the CNS. *C. neoformans* is thought to escape phagolysosomal killing within macrophages via phagosomal extrusion, after which it is transported across the blood-brain-barrier as a "Trojan horse" where it causes meningoencephalitis [29]. The cryptococcal capsule has been shown to enhance HIV-1 replication and infectivity by promoting increased cellular NF- κB activation, a key step in the antifungal response that also results in stimulation of the latent HIV-infected pro-virus. If immune function recovers rapidly, as with the initiation of effective antiretroviral therapy, a reinvigorated CD4+ T-cell population can orchestrate an influx of inflammatory cells into sites of infection. This leads to the immune reconstitution inflammatory syndrome (IRIS), a paradoxical clinical worsening that can sometimes be life-threatening.

11.6 Susceptibility to Fungal Infections in the Context of Immunocompetent Populations

Increased susceptibility to fungal infections has clearly been documented in certain immunocompetent populations, most often based on ethnicity. A racial predisposition toward severe infection is most evident with *Coccidioides immitis/Coccidioides posadasii*, a dimorphic fungus endemic to the arid landscapes of the Southwestern USA and the agent of coccidioidomycosis [30]. Based on cases occurring in Kern County, California, between 1901 and 1936, researchers noted that persons of Filipino, African American, and Mexican American descent were significantly more likely (176, 14, and 3 times, respectively) than Caucasians to develop disseminated coccidioidomycosis [30]. More recent studies have replicated these findings, described increased predilections in other populations including Asians, and excluded occupational exposure as the sole underlying driver of risk. The genetic basis of increased susceptibility is unknown but may be associated with ABO blood group B and HLA class II antigens (HLA-A9 and HLA-B9 antigens) that are more common in Filipinos and African Americans, although this association may be not be causal. Some markers, such as the HLA class II-DRB1∗1301 allele, have been associated with severe coccidioidomycosis regardless of ethnicity [31]. An immunologic basis for increased susceptibility has been entertained, possibly due to an intrinsic inability to produce an effective cellular immune response to *Coccidioides*. Indeed, mutations in IFN-γ and IL-12 receptor β1 deficiency have been reported in some patients with disseminated coccidioidomycosis. However, in a study of patients with active coccidioidomycosis, skin reactivity after inoculation with *Coccidioides* antigen was similar in Caucasians and African Americans. Likewise, Filipinos and African Americans developed comparable T-cell reactivity to Caucasians after immunization with a formalin-killed spherule (FKS) *Coccidioides* vaccine [32]. Studies have also indicated that males exhibit increased risk for infection, but the effect is much less pronounced than that of race. Asian ethnicity may also be associated with increased risk for blastomycosis, an endemic fungal infection caused by *Blastomyces dermatitidis* and endemic to the Midwestern USA. In a 2009 outbreak of blastomycosis in Wisconsin, Asian residents, most of whom were of Hmong ethnicity, developed symptomatic infection at a rate 12 times higher than non-Asians [33]. Though the underlying mechanisms remain a mystery at present, it is likely that future immunoepidemiologic studies will unravel the genetic basis of these predilections.

11.7 Immunoepidemiologic Tools for Characterization of Fungal Geographic Distribution

Immunoepidemiologic tools have strongly informed our knowledge of the global distribution of medically important fungi. These include measures of cellular immunity via testing for skin reactivity, lymphocyte stimulation assays, and measures of humoral immunity via detection of specific antibodies. Skin-testing studies for *H.capsulatum* performed in the 1950s–1970s were key in defining the geographic distribution of this fungus [34]. They documented a high prevalence of histoplasmin skin sensitivity of more than 20% in the Midwestern USA, Central America, and parts of South America, some positivity in northern India (10–20%), and very low prevalence in Africa and Europe (<2%), except for Italy. In the USA, subsequent skin test surveys of newly recruited individuals to the US Navy mapped the endemic area with added precision. More recent studies have described areas of high endemicity in Asia; a study from China reported a prevalence of positive histoplasmin skin test of up to 50%. In highly endemic areas, skin and serologic reactivity testing has demonstrated that around 90% of the population acquire for *H. capsulatum* by age 18, though the vast majority of these infections are subclinical. Conversely, a seroprevalence study of Burmese, Hmong, and Somali refugee immigrants to the USA found an anti-*H. capsulatum* IgG positivity rate of ≤1%, suggesting that histoplasmosis is rare in these populations [35]. Skin-reactivity surveys for *C. neoformans* have indicated that it is widely present in nature and global in distribution. *C.neoformans* is also frequently isolated from habitats replete with bird excreta, suggesting an avian environmental reservoir and a possible risk factor for exposure. These findings were substantiated by serological surveys that found a significantly higher prevalence of *C. neoformans* antibodies in pigeon fanciers as compared to control groups [36]. Immunologic surveys have also contributed to defining areas of endemicity for *B. dermatitidis* [37]. In a study of forestry workers in the USA, a *B. dermatitidis* antigen-specific lymphocyte stimulation assay was positive in 30% of workers in endemic areas of Northern Wisconsin and Northern Minnesota, as compared to 0% in Washington State. None of the individuals in the study reported symptomatic disease, indicating that the majority of cases of blastomycosis are subclinical. Seroepidemiologic studies of animal populations have shed light on the geographic distribution and life cycles of fungi, including avian *Aspergillus* exposure and canine paracoccidioidomycosis and blastomycosis. As the effects of global warming begin to take effect, fungal immunoepidemiology will be instrumental in defining evolving geographic ranges of known pathogenic fungi and those of emerging pathogenic species [38].

11.8 Vaccines Against Fungi

The advent of immunization in the late eighteenth century led to a marked decline of several devastating infectious diseases, revolutionized the practice of medicine, and made great contributions to global health. Despite their widespread geographic distribution and the significant morbidity and mortality associated with mycoses, there are no currently available commercial vaccines against fungi [10]. An important barrier to the development of such vaccines is related to the population at risk. Whereas some invasive mycoses can affect fully immunocompetent persons such as those caused by endemic fungi and some dematiaceous molds, the majority infections occur in highly immunocompromised individuals. Because intact immunity is required for an appropriate response to vaccination and building of immunological memory, vaccination is often ineffective in this population [39]. Additionally, although live attenuated vaccines often elicit the strongest and longest lasting immune responses, they are with few exceptions contraindicated in immunocompromised persons because of the risk of disease reactivation. If immunosuppression is planned as part of solid-organ and hematopoietic stem cell transplantation, vaccination can be administered beforehand in order to circumvent this problem. Another strategy is to employ vaccines that act on components of the immune system that are intact. A requirement for most effective antifungal vaccines is the ability to trigger Th1 and/or Th17 immune responses that are needed for phagocyte activation and granuloma formation, critical steps in abrogating fungal infections. Most currently available vaccines for non-fungal pathogens elicit antibody responses, important in neutralizing viruses and bacteria but less effective in controlling fungi. Despite the lack of commercially available vaccines for humans, proof of concept has been successfully demonstrated in animal models. Immunization with 1,3 β-D glucan conjugated to diphtheria toxoid stimulated robust antibody responses and protected mice against inoculations of *Candida*, *Cryptococcus*, and *Aspergillus*. 1,3 β-D glucan is highly immunogenic and can serve as an effective adjuvant in triggering protective Th1 and/or Th17 immune responses [40]. In a newer vaccine model, antigens have been embedded within β-glucan particles, eliciting strong T_h1 and Th17 responses. Targeting pan-fungal structures like 1,3 β-D glucan also carries the potential of protection against a wide range of fungal infections. Live-attenuated vaccination of CD4+ T-cell-deficient mice against *B. dermatitidis* was effective in preventing blastomycosis and was associated with development of IL-17 secreting CD8+ T cells [41, 42]. These and other similar data are highly encouraging for vaccine development in immunocompromised persons. Some candidate vaccines have already been shown to be successful in Phase I clinical trials in humans and are on a likely path toward development for commercial use. An adjuvant vaccine against *Candida* targeting the N-terminal portion of the agglutinin like sequence 3 protein (Als3p) was tested in 73 patients [43]. All subjects developed T-cell-dependent and T-cell-independent responses, including generation of anti-Als3p antibodies, and vaccination was associated with protection against candidiasis. Extensive N-linked and/or O-linked mannosylation of antigens naturally occurs on fungal cell walls and is associated with more efficient processing by dendritic cells. Vaccines that incorporate antigen mannosylation have been shown to augment fungal vaccine immunogenicity.

11.9 Conclusion

Invasive mycoses are responsible for staggering levels of morbidity and mortality worldwide. The public health impact of fungal infections is on track to expand as the population at risk for pathogenic fungi continues to grow. A warming world is likely to result in evolving geographic ranges of known medically important fungi and in the emergence of newly pathogenic species. By characterizing antifungal host immune responses in ethnically, geographically, and immunologically diverse populations, fungal immunoepidemiology provides critical insights that can be utilized for global mapping of existing and emerging fungal pathogens and for the development of effective diagnostic, therapeutic, and preventative modalities. These will include development of new diagnostic fungal markers, new classes of antifungal agents, and first-generation antifungal vaccines.

References

1. Frac M, Hannula SE, Belka M, Jedryczka M. Fungal biodiversity and their role in soil health. Front Microbiol. 2018;9:707.
2. Blackwell M. The fungi: 1, 2, 3 ... 5.1 million species? Am J Bot. 2011;98(3):426–38.
3. Bongomin F, Gago S, Oladele RO, Denning DW. Global and multi-national prevalence of fungal diseases-estimate precision. J Fungi (Basel). 2017;3(4)
4. Hajjeh RA, Sofair AN, Harrison LH, Lyon GM, Arthington-Skaggs BA, Mirza SA, et al. Incidence of bloodstream infections due to Candida species and in vitro susceptibilities of isolates collected from 1998 to 2000 in a population-based active surveillance program. J Clin Microbiol. 2004;42(4):1519–27.
5. Armstrong PA, Jackson BR, Haselow D, Fields V, Ireland M, Austin C, et al. Multistate epidemiology of histoplasmosis, United States, 2011–2014. Emerg Infect Dis. 2018;24(3):425–31.
6. McGinnis MR, Tyring SK. Introduction to mycology. In: Baron S, editor. Medical Microbiology. Amsterdam, Netherlands: Elsevier; 1996.
7. Erwig LP, Gow NA. Interactions of fungal pathogens with phagocytes. Nat Rev Microbiol. 2016;14(3):163–76.
8. Ambasta A, Carson J, Church DL. The use of biomarkers and molecular methods for the earlier diagnosis of invasive aspergillosis in immunocompromised patients. Med Mycol. 2015;53(6):531–57.
9. Lewis RE. Current concepts in antifungal pharmacology. Mayo Clin Proc. 2011;86(8):805–17.
10. Spellberg B. Vaccines for invasive fungal infections. F1000 Med Rep. 2011;3:13.
11. Lionakis MS, Iliev ID, Hohl TM. Immunity against fungi. JCI Insight. 2017;2(11):e93156.
12. Lionakis MS, Levitz SM. Host control of fungal infections: lessons from basic studies and human cohorts. Annu Rev Immunol. 2018;36:157–91.
13. Drummond RA, Gaffen SL, Hise AG, Brown GD. Innate defense against fungal pathogens. Cold Spring HarbPerspect Med. 2014;5(6)
14. Lionakis MS, Swamydas M, Fischer BG, Plantinga TS, Johnson MD, Jaeger M, et al. CX3CR1-dependent renal macrophage survival promotes Candida control and host survival. J Clin Invest. 2013;123(12):5035–51.
15. Cheng SC, Quintin J, Cramer RA, Shepardson KM, Saeed S, Kumar V, et al. mTOR- and HIF-1alpha-mediated aerobic glycolysis as metabolic basis for trained immunity. Science. 2014;345(6204):1250684.

16. Branzk N, Lubojemska A, Hardison SE, Wang Q, Gutierrez MG, Brown GD, et al. Neutrophils sense microbe size and selectively release neutrophil extracellular traps in response to large pathogens. Nat Immunol. 2014;15(11):1017–25.

17. Schmidt S, Tramsen L, Lehrnbecher T. Natural killer cells in antifungal immunity. Front Immunol. 2017;8:1623.

18. Szymczak WA, Deepe GS Jr. The CCL7-CCL2-CCR2 axis regulates IL-4 production in lungs and fungal immunity. J Immunol. 2009;183(3):1964–74.

19. Ghosh S, Hoselton SA, Dorsam GP, Schuh JM. Eosinophils in fungus-associated allergic pulmonary disease. Front Pharmacol. 2013;4:8.

20. Romani L. Immunity to fungal infections. Nat Rev Immunol. 2011;11(4):275–88.

21. Nabavi N, Murphy JW. Antibody-dependent natural killer cell-mediated growth inhibition of Cryptococcus neoformans. Infect Immun. 1986;51(2):556–62.

22. Li R, Rezk A, Li H, Gommerman JL, Prat A, Bar-Or A, et al. Antibody-independent function of human B cells contributes to antifungal T cell responses. J Immunol. 2017;198(8):3245–54.

23. Torosantucci A, Chiani P, Bromuro C, De Bernardis F, Palma AS, Liu Y, et al. Protection by anti-beta-glucan antibodies is associated with restricted beta-1,3 glucan binding specificity and inhibition of fungal growth and adherence. PLoS One. 2009;4(4):e5392.

24. van de Veerdonk FL, Plantinga TS, Hoischen A, Smeekens SP, Joosten LA, Gilissen C, et al. STAT1 mutations in autosomal dominant chronic mucocutaneous candidiasis. N Engl J Med. 2011;365(1):54–61.

25. De Martino L, Capalbo D, Improda N, D'Elia F, Di Mase R, D'Assante R, et al. APECED: a paradigm of complex interactions between genetic background and susceptibility factors. Front Immunol. 2013;4:331.

26. Glocker EO, Hennigs A, Nabavi M, Schaffer AA, Woellner C, Salzer U, et al. A homozygous CARD9 mutation in a family with susceptibility to fungal infections. N Engl J Med. 2009;361(18):1727–35.

27. Dunogue B, Pilmis B, Mahlaoui N, Elie C, Coignard-Biehler H, Amazzough K, et al. Chronic granulomatous disease in patients reaching adulthood: a Nationwide study in France. Clin Infect Dis. 2017;64(6):767–75.

28. Mirza SA, Phelan M, Rimland D, Graviss E, Hamill R, Brandt ME, et al. The changing epidemiology of cryptococcosis: an update from population-based active surveillance in 2 large metropolitan areas, 1992–2000. Clin Infect Dis. 2003;36(6):789–94.

29. Charlier C, Nielsen K, Daou S, Brigitte M, Chretien F, Dromer F. Evidence of a role for monocytes in dissemination and brain invasion by Cryptococcus neoformans. Infect Immun. 2009;77(1):120–7.

30. Cox RA, Magee DM. Coccidioidomycosis: host response and vaccine development. Clin Microbiol Rev. 2004;17(4):804–39, table of contents.

31. Louie L, Ng S, Hajjeh R, Johnson R, Vugia D, Werner SB, et al. Influence of host genetics on the severity of coccidioidomycosis. Emerg Infect Dis. 1999;5(5):672–80.

32. Williams PL, Sable DL, Sorgen SP, Pappagianis D, Levine HB, Brodine SK, et al. Immunologic responsiveness and safety associated with the Coccidioides immitis spherule vaccine in volunteers of white, black, and Filipino ancestry. Am J Epidemiol. 1984;119(4):591–602.

33. Roy M, Benedict K, Deak E, Kirby MA, McNiel JT, Sickler CJ, et al. A large community outbreak of blastomycosis in Wisconsin with geographic and ethnic clustering. Clin Infect Dis. 2013;57(5):655–62.

34. Mochi A, Edwards PQ. Geographical distribution of histoplasmosis and histoplasmin sensitivity. Bull World Health Organ. 1952;5(3):259–91.

35. Bahr NC, Lee D, Stauffer WM, Durkin M, Cetron MS, Wheat LJ, et al. Seroprevalence of histoplasmosis in Somali, Burmese, and Hmong refugees residing in Thailand and Kenya. J Immigr Minor Health. 2018;20(2):334–8.

36. Walter JE, Atchison RW. Epidemiological and immunological studies of Cryptococcus neoformans. J Bacteriol. 1966;92(1):82–7.

37. Vaaler AK, Bradsher RW, Davies SF. Evidence of subclinical blastomycosis in forestry workers in northern Minnesota and northern Wisconsin. Am J Med. 1990;89(4):470–6.

38. Benedict K, Richardson M, Vallabhaneni S, Jackson BR, Chiller T. Emerging issues, challenges, and changing epidemiology of fungal disease outbreaks. Lancet Infect Dis. 2017;17(12):e403–e11.

39. Levitz SM, Golenbock DT. Beyond empiricism: informing vaccine development through innate immunity research. Cell. 2012;148(6):1284–92.

40. Levitz SM, Huang H, Ostroff GR, Specht CA. Exploiting fungal cell wall components in vaccines. SeminImmunopathol. 2015;37(2):199–207.

41. Wuthrich M, LeBert V, Galles K, Hu-Li J, Ben-Sasson SZ, Paul WE, et al. Interleukin 1 enhances vaccine-induced antifungal T-helper 17 cells and resistance against Blastomyces dermatitidis infection. J Infect Dis. 2013;208(7):1175–82.

42. Nanjappa SG, Heninger E, Wuthrich M, Gasper DJ, Klein BS. Tc17 cells mediate vaccine immunity against lethal fungal pneumonia in immune deficient hosts lacking CD4+ T cells. PLoSPathog. 2012;8(7):e1002771.

43. Wang XJ, Sui X, Yan L, Wang Y, Cao YB, Jiang YY. Vaccines in the treatment of invasive candidiasis. Virulence. 2015;6(4):309–15.

Immunoepidemiology of *Plasmodium falciparum* malaria

Amy K. Bei and Sunil Parikh

12.1 Malaria Introduction

12.1.1 Global Burden of Malaria Disease

Great progress has been made in the past two decades on malaria control with the call to globally eradicate malaria [1]. In recent years, modeling has enhanced the ability to estimate (with confidence intervals and uncertainty) the global burden of malaria [1, 2] (Fig. 12.1). The global distribution of malaria is dependent on mosquito vector, human, and environmental factors. Continued transmission of the disease requires a competent *Anopheles* vector, the *Plasmodium* parasite, and a susceptible human host population.

Virtually every vertebrate species can be infected by *Plasmodium*; however, *Plasmodium* parasites exhibit a largely species-specific tropism primarily due to host-specific factors such as protein receptors and sialic acid moieties on the surface of the erythrocytes. There are five *Plasmodium* species that naturally infect humans, *P. falciparum*, *P. vivax*, *P. malariae*, *P. ovale*, and *P. knowlesi*, and the distribution of these species is dependent on the susceptibility of the available vectors as well as the human populations. In this chapter, we will primarily focus on the immunoepidemiology of *P. falciparum*.

12.1.2 Pathogenesis of Malaria in Humans

Malaria infection in humans begins with the introduction of sporozoites from the saliva of female *Anopheles* mosquitoes (Fig. 12.2). Sporozoites travel from the site of dermal inoculation to the liver, where invasion of hepatocytes results in an asymptomatic replicative stage, followed by rupture of schizonts that release numerous merozoites into the circulation. Merozoites then enter erythrocytes and undergo repetitive 48–72-hour replication cycles, changing from merozoite to trophozoite to schizont and ultimately daughter merozoites. During this stage, individuals are symptomatic, and rupture is followed by reinvasion into new erythrocytes. The transmission cycle culminates with the differentiation of a subset of blood stage parasites into gametocytes, which are ultimately ingested by

A. K. Bei (✉) · S. Parikh
Department of Epidemiology of Microbial Diseases, Yale School of Public Health,
New Haven, CT, USA
e-mail: amy.bei@yale.edu; sunil.parikh@yale.edu

© Springer Nature Switzerland AG 2019
P. J. Krause et al. (eds.), *Immunoepidemiology*, https://doi.org/10.1007/978-3-030-25553-4_12

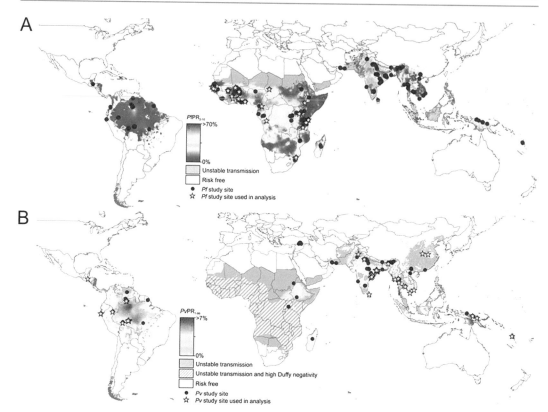

Fig. 12.1 Global malaria distribution. The geographic locations of the incidence records for *P. falciparum* (**a**) and *P. vivax* (**b**) are shown over the model-based geostatistics (MBG) point estimates of the annual mean *Pf*PR$_{2-10}$ and *Pv*PR$_{1-99}$ for 2010 within the spatial limits of stable limits of transmission (annual parasite index (API) ≥ 0.1 per 1000 per annum (p.a.)), displayed on a continuum from blue (0% PR) to red (70% PR for *P. falciparum* and >7% PR for *P. vivax*). Dark grey areas were predicted to be unstable (API ≤ 0.1 per 1000 p.a.) and light grey areas were classified as risk free. Areas in which Duffy negative allele frequency is predicted to exceed 90% are shown in hatching for additional context in the *P. vivax* map. Study sites used in the *P. falciparum* and *P. vivax* models are shown as yellow stars and other sites included in this dataset not used in the cited analyses are shown as purple points. (Reprinted from Battle et al. [3]. This work is licensed under the Creative Commons Attribution 4.0 International License. To view a copy of this license, visit http://creativecommons.org/licenses/by/4.0/ or send a letter to Creative Commons, PO Box 1866, Mountain View, CA 94042, USA)

the mosquito during a blood meal, undergoing meiotic recombination within the vector and ultimate transformation into infectious sporozoites.

The success of this cycle within the human host depends on an array of factors. Natural polymorphism in human erythrocyte receptors and intracellular proteins is one such factor that can have a profound impact on an individual's susceptibility to infection and/or the severity of disease. Red blood cell variants in both intracellular proteins and surface receptors such as glucose-6-phosphate dehydrogenase (G6PD), ABO blood group, thalassemia, sickling hemoglobin (HbS) and other hemoglobinopathies, and Duffy negativity (in the case of *P. vivax*), to name a few, all provide some degree of protection against *Plasmodium* – but may also come at a cost for the human host. There is a broad spectrum of disease pathologies including severe malaria (often including syndromes such as severe anemia, respiratory distress, and cerebral malaria), uncomplicated acute malaria, and asymptomatic malaria. In addition to human genetic polymorphisms affecting intracellular proteins and surface receptors, immunity is another key player in the pathogenesis of malaria.

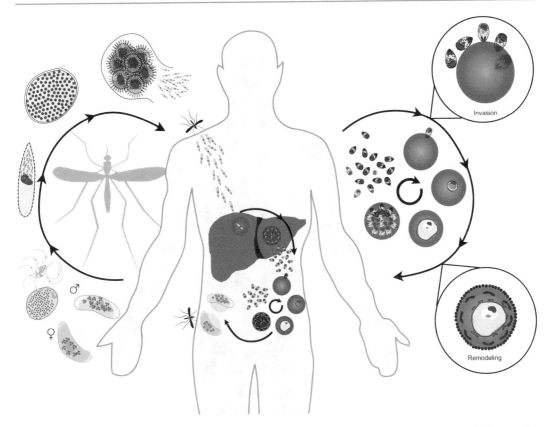

Fig. 12.2 *Plasmodium* life-cycle. The *Plasmodium* life cycle requires both a vertebrate host and an *Anopheles* mosquito vector. The life cycle consists of the asexual exoerythrocytic stage in the liver, the asexual erythrocytic stage in the blood, and sexual stage (gametocyte) conversion in the blood of the human host. The sporogonic cycle occurs in the mosquito after it ingests gametocytes during a blood meal. The two critical virulence processes of the malaria life cycle occur during the erythrocytic stage: invasion (top, right insert) and remodeling and cytoadherence (bottom, right inset). Transmission of the disease depends on the formation of gametocytes and successful infection of the mosquito vector

12.1.3 Host Immune Response to Malaria

The human immune system is able to develop functional, but non-sterilizing immunity to *Plasmodium* [4] in natural exposure settings. The immune response to malaria, as to many other pathogens, involves the innate and adaptive arms and both humoral and cellular responses. The challenge for natural immunity and vaccine design is that each stage of the life cycle is largely antigenically distinct, meaning that immune responses directed against sporozoite proteins will not cross-react with merozoite proteins or gametocyte proteins. Additionally, *Plasmodium* proteins within each stage of the life cycle are incredibly diverse. The selective pressure exerted by the human immune system has resulted in the greatest diversity within immunodominant antigens of the parasite [5]. At some stages of the parasite's life cycle, the malaria parasite is intracellular and at others, extracellular – meaning that the immune mechanisms of recognition and control will differ at each stage of the life cycle [6] (Fig. 12.3). The first stage of the parasite that enters the human host are the sporozoites, injected with the saliva by the bite of a female *Anopheles* mosquito. The immune response against these motile and extracellular parasites is largely antibody driven, although the sporozoites are transported by skin resident dendritic cells to the lymph node where they prime B- and T-cell responses. Once sporozoites travel

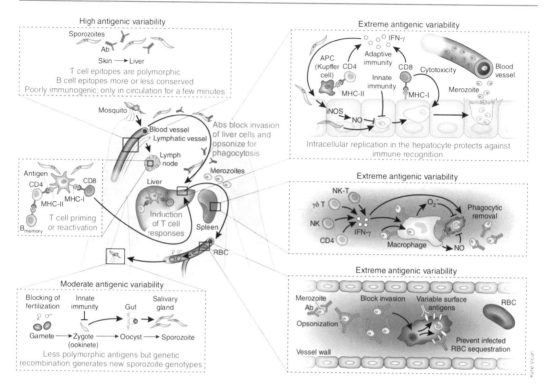

Fig. 12.3 Immune mechanisms in malaria. Life cycle of Plasmodium spp. infections, with the main immune responses that control the parasite at each stage. Sporozoites, injected into the skin by the biting mosquito, drain to the lymph nodes, where they prime T and B cells, or the liver, where they invade hepatocytes. Antibodies (Ab) trap sporozoites in the skin or prevent their invasion of liver cells. IFN-γ–producing CD4+ and CD8+ T cells inhibit parasite development into merozoites inside the hepatocyte. However, this immune response is frequently insufficient, and merozoites emerging from the liver invade red blood cells, replicate, burst out of the infected erythrocyte and invade new erythrocytes. Merozoite-specific antibodies agglutinate and opsonize the parasite and can inhibit the invasion of red blood cells through receptor blockade. Antibodies to variant surface proteins also opsonize and agglutinate infected red blood cells (RBCs) and prevent their sequestration (cytoadherence) in small blood vessels. IFN-γ–producing lymphocytes activate macrophages and enhance the phagocytosis of opsonized merozoites and iRBCs. Complement-fixing antibodies to gametocyte and gamete antigens lyse parasites inside the mosquito gut or prevent the fertilization and development of the zygote. Sporozoite, liver-stage and gametocyte and gamete antigens are somewhat polymorphic, whereas merozoite antigens and variant surface antigens are highly polymorphic. APC, antigen-presenting cell. (Reprinted by permission from Springer Nature: Springer Nature, Riley and Stewart [6], Copyright 2013)

to and take up residence in liver hepatocytes, they become intracellular and are able to trigger the cellular arm of the immune response via mechanisms such as CD4+ and CD8+ T cells, natural killer (NK) cells, NKT cells, and gamma-delta T cells. While antibodies work to block the invasion of sporozoites into the liver, cellular mediators act to target and kill the parasite in the infected hepatocyte. It is clear that vaccination with radiation-attenuated sporozoites (RAS) is able to induce sterile protection from malaria in mice [7], nonhuman primates, and humans [8] when challenged with the same strain, and this protection has been attributed to both neutralizing antibody responses and CD8+ T-cell responses, as well as CD4+ T cells, gamma-delta T cells, and natural killer (NK) cell responses [9]. Interestingly, naturally transmitted sporozoite specific memory CD8+ T cells are long-lived (6 months); however, the protection provided by RAS is much shorter [10]. As RAS are irradiated and cannot undergo DNA replication, they cease to develop beyond liver cell invasion. To strengthen the cellular immune responses at the liver stage, genetically attenuated parasite (GAP) vaccines have been developed with key liver stage developmental genes knocked out or mutated to allow for later arrest in liver stage development [11]. These vaccines induce enhanced broader antigen presentation as the parasite replicates and develops through various stages – increasing the quantity and the combined composition of parasite life-cycle stages to which the immune system is exposed.

Once the parasite matures into a liver stage schizont and releases merozoites into the blood, the parasite is again extracellular and antibody-mediated mechanisms of binding and clearance predominate, including invasion-inhibitory antibodies and antibodies that opsonize merozoites. Once inside the erythrocyte, the parasite is protected from the immune system until it exports its own proteins to the surface of the infected cell to cytoadhere to the microvasculature and prevent splenic clearance. These infected erythrocytes that expose variant surface antigens are the targets of antibodies which, in concert with cellar mediators, can lead to opsonization and killing by phagocytic cells such as macrophages and neutrophils. Interferon gamma-producing lymphocytes (such as CD4+ T cells, NK cells, NKT cells, and gamma-delta T cells) activate macrophages, which enhance the phagocytosis of opsonized extracellular merozoites and infected erythrocytes [6].

12.1.3.1 Immune Evasion: Genetic Diversity or Immune Dysfunction?

There are two prevailing hypotheses to explain the lack of sterilizing immunity to malaria infection even after a lifetime of exposure. The first hypothesis is that each parasite infection is antigenically distinct from the next and that in order to truly have sterilizing immunity, one would have to become immune to every antigenically distinct strain of *Plasmodium* that exists in the population. The second hypothesis is that while the immune system is able to respond to parasites, the *functional quality* of these responses is impaired, meaning that they are defective in some way in killing the parasite. Recent evidence suggests that a combination of these hypotheses may in fact be true and will be discussed further.

12.1.3.2 Malaria Immunoepidemiology

Immunoepidemiology combines both individual data and population level data in an effort to understand the influence of immunity on epidemiological patterns. This chapter will focus primarily on seroepidemiology, a subdiscipline of immunoepidemiology which primarily studies humoral immune markers of *exposure* and *protection*. Immune protection is necessarily linked to exposure in that protective immunity is developed over time and with multiple exposures; however, the nature, frequency, and antigenic quality of these exposure events will influence how rapidly immunity or "protection" is achieved. Seroepidemiology in the malaria field has spanned the pre-genomic and post-genomic eras, moved from low- to high-specificity assays and from low to high throughput as well. As we learn more about malaria proteins, studies have shifted from measuring immune responses to whole-parasite extract, to single proteins, to combinations of well-characterized proteins [12–14]. Recently, focused protein microarrays with over 100 well-characterized antigens "KILchip" [15] and protein microarrays which cover hundreds of malaria proteins [16, 17] have been used to study population-based immune responses. Such large-scale immune reactivity studies allow for even hypothetical proteins or proteins of unknown function to be identified as potentially important markers of exposure or protection.

12.2 Immunoepidemiology of Malaria

12.2.1 Classic Cohort Studies on Immunity and Parasite Prevalence as Transmission Intensity Changes

Before the dawn of immunoepidemiology, there was the notion that immunity to malaria could be acquired with age – an observation initially described as "premunition" [18]. This notion, even in the absence of specific immunological measurements, was based on the observations of many that the parasite positive percentage (or prevalence) fluctuated with age, with a peak in young children and a decline in older children and adults. Data from coastal Tanzania, coastal Ghana, Southern Cameroon, rural Tanzania, Madang in Papua New Guinea, rural Gambia, Kilifi in coastal Kenya (reviewed in [19]) and Dielmo and Ndiop in rural Senegal [20, 21] all showed a very similar trend – parasite prevalence was highest in young children, usually under 5 years of age, and then declined with age. These studies of parasite prevalence and age suggested the relationship between exposure and immunity even before measuring immune responses to any parasite antigen or extract was feasible.

Much of our knowledge of immunoepidemiology in malaria comes from these classic cohort studies, either cross-sectional studies in a single population as transmission changes or longitudinal cohorts following the course of exposure, infection, and immunity in the same individuals over time. The main questions addressed by these studies were: (1) Do immune responses correlate with transmission intensity? (2) Which immune responses predict protection from infection or severe disease? Early cohort studies were performed in The Gambia to determine associations between the immune response either to crude parasite extracts or to specific antigens and functional immune activity and protection from malaria infection [22, 23]. The longest standing current cohorts to date are the Dielmo [20] and Ndiop [21] longitudinal cohorts in Senegal in which patients in two villages were initially recruited in 1990 and 1993, respectively, and are still being actively followed today. Three cohorts in Kilifi were also monitored for 12 years to track febrile malaria cases, as well as asymptomatic malaria infections [24]. In this study, antibody levels to merozoite surface protein 2 (MSP2) were used to determine if seropositivity rate and seroconversion rate could predict hotspots of malaria infection. While neither seropositivity rate nor seroconversion rate predicted hotspots of malaria infection, the magnitude of the MSP2 antibody responses significantly predicted hotspots of febrile malaria and malaria infection, described by parasitemia. The magnitude of the apical membrane antigen-1 (AMA-1) antibody responses was associated with hotspots of asymptomatic infections but not febrile malaria.

12.2.2 Serological Correlates of Protection

One of the key questions surrounding the search for a serological correlate of protection is related to the *functional quality* of the immune responses we are measuring. Can we predict if levels of an antibody response will protect from malaria? When we discuss protection, are we referring to protection from infection, protection from symptomatic malaria, or protection from severe malaria? At the very outset, we need to have a clear and consistent set of definitions in order to clearly interpret data from different studies.

The notion of immunity to different disease states was first described by McGregor [25] and later expanded by Marsh and colleagues to implicate immunity to specific parasite antigens [22]. The well-accepted dogma in the field of malaria immunology is that immunity to malaria is slowly acquired and is "incomplete," meaning non-sterile. Individuals who are exposed throughout their lives are never completely protected from infection – however they will be gradually protected from the symptoms of malaria disease (Fig. 12.4a). One proposed reason for this lack of sterile, protective immunity is the diversity of strains to which an individual is exposed [28, 29]; thus, one can become completely

Fig. 12.4 (continued) at the time of sampling. In the antibody positive group, there is B – non-immune but recently treated and with high antibody titers, D1 – current acute infection in which antibody responses are actively being produced, and D2 – truly immune and asymptomatic individuals. Just as there is heterogeneity in the serological and parasitological status of an individual, at the point of analysis after follow-up, there is potential for misclassification if clinical status alone is used for interpretation of immune status. (Adapted from Kinyanjui et al. [27]. To view a copy of this license, visit https://creativecommons.org/licenses/by/2.0/).

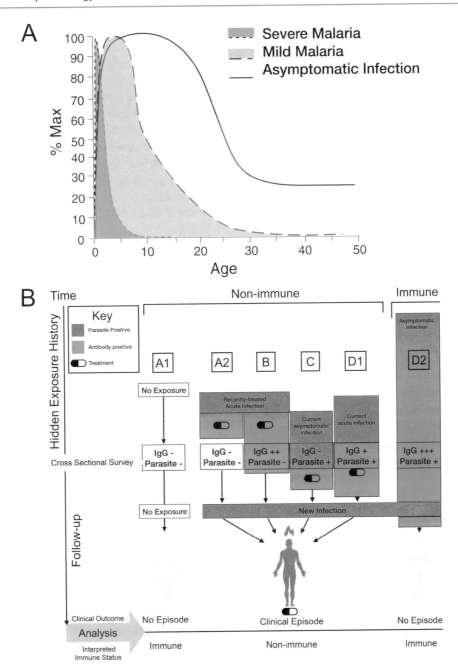

Fig. 12.4 Heterogeneity in exposure, clinical outcome, and immunity to malaria. (**a**) Classical description of population indices of immunity to malaria developed to disease states with increasing age and exposure. Immunity is first developed to severe malaria, then to mild malaria, then to asymptomatic infection, however, sterile immunity that prevents all infection is never achieved. The period prevalence of mild and severe clinical malaria as well as the age pattern of asymptomatic parasite prevalence are shown relative to maximum recorded prevalence (% Max). (Adapted from Marsh and Kinyanjui [26]). (**b**) The potential for misclassification based on "hidden exposure history." The influence of exposure history on an individual's serological and parasitological status at a cross-sectional survey and the individual's clinical history during follow-up after the cross-sectional survey. The two serological groups: antibody negative and antibody positive represent heterogenous groups. Within the antibody negative group, there is 1A – unexposed, antibody negative, 1B – exposed but antibody responses have decayed, C – exposed, but have not yet mounted antibody responses

immune to a specific strain of *Plasmodium* but not immune to others. This was described as early as 1898, when it was observed that foreign soldiers were more susceptible to malaria than members of the local police force [30]. Similarly, in India it was observed that individuals became immune to "local" strains but were susceptible when traveling to neighboring villages [30]. This was also shown experimentally in neurosyphilis patients undergoing malaria therapy, where repeated infection with the same strain (homologous infection) did not cause clinical disease upon the repeated exposure but that infection with an antigenically distinct (heterologous) strain resulted in clinical disease [30, 31]. Even with a lifetime of exposure, the extent of diversification of *Plasmodium* isolates makes it impossible to ever become truly immune to all strains as each new infection represents a new immunological challenge [5]. Gupta and Day [19] outlined a theoretical framework for different kinds of immunity, from strain-specific to strain-transcendent, in addition to the concept of "anti-infection" immunity and "anti-disease" immunity as proposed by Marsh [22]. The wealth of the evidence seems to indicate that the "anti-disease" immunity is highly strain-specific [28, 29]. There must be balance between the parasite's ability to recombine and create diverse antigenically distinct strains and the ability of the human immune response to recognize these variants [32, 33].

One of the key challenges to assessing immunological correlates of protection is that antibody classes have varying rates of decay, and individuals have a heterogeneity of malaria exposure prior to sampling, making study design a key consideration (Fig. 12.4b). Cross-sectional studies that measure antibody positive or negative responses and parasite positive and negative responses can be confounded by the "hidden exposure history" prior to the point of sampling of the individual [27] which is difficult to measure and distinguish. Antibody negativity can be due to a lack of exposure or antibody decay over time. High antibody titers can be the result of a current malaria infection boosting past exposure responses, a recently treated infection, or an immune individual. A method for adjusting for exposure differences is measurement of the antibody response to schizont extract (total parasite protein extracts from blood stage schizonts). This approach has its own caveats as well but can assist in adjusting for true and "hidden" exposure. Longitudinal studies are ideally suited to detecting exposure in that they cover a range of exposure and individuals are followed for long periods of time. Depending on when and how individuals are followed for malaria infection (clinical episode only, periodic sampling, etc.), even longitudinal studies can miss malaria exposure if it results in asymptomatic infection. Of course, these patterns will vary by age group as well as by different endemicity settings. In young children, we would expect more frequent clinical malaria episodes and fewer asymptomatic infections, while the inverse is true of adults. Likewise, in highly endemic populations, protective immunity and thus a decrease in clinical malaria and an increase in asymptomatic, antibody positive responders will be observed at younger ages than in low endemic settings, where exposure is less frequent and immunity is slower to develop. These challenges in capturing the true exposure history of individuals and their true immune status can result in misclassification for both exposure and protection and are key factors to keep in mind when designing studies aimed at identifying targets of protective immunity.

12.2.2.1 Breadth of Antibody Responses: The Whole Is Greater than the Sum of Its Parts

Recently, it was found that the intensity of antibody response to any candidate antigen was not nearly as powerful in predicting protection from malaria as the *breadth* of the immune response to many targets [14, 34]. The magnitude of immune responses to combinations of antigens was more strongly predictive of protection than responses to individual antigens alone. This finding is supported by the earlier work on strain theory and the concept that the more exposures one has (and the diversity of those exposures), the greater the protection against a broad spectrum of antigenic combinations. However, it remains difficult in epidemiological studies to disentangle exposure from protection, especially in the absence of a mechanistic measure of protection.

12.2.2.2 Mechanistic Correlates of Protection

The search for a correlate of protection from malaria is the "holy grail" in the field of malaria immunoepidemiology [35]. Having such a correlate would help stratify those that are at risk and those that are protected, even helping target interventions. However, the field is still looking for such a consistent correlate, mechanistic or otherwise. In an attempt to clarify the somewhat muddied and at times contradictory nomenclature surrounding surrogates and correlates of protection, Plotkin and Gilbert have simplified the concepts into the following terms: (1) correlate of protection (CoP), (2) mechanistic correlate of protection (mCoP), and (3) nonmechanistic correlate of protection (nCoP) [36]. A correlate of protection (CoP) is an immune marker that *statistically correlates* with vaccine efficacy and can be either mechanistic and causally responsible for protection (mCoP) or nonmechanistic and noncausal (nCoP). In past nomenclature, a nCoP was also referred to as a surrogate of protection [36]. In malaria, the ultimate goal is to identify a mCoP that can both predict and explain the cause of protection. It would be ideal if the same mCoP is equally applicable to protection from natural exposure as well as protection through vaccination; however, that might not be the case and could depend on the target antigen. A meta-analysis of correlates of protection from natural exposure demonstrates the variability and complications in trying to broadly apply such criteria to epidemiological studies [37].

In recent years, different correlates have been proposed; however, the degree of correlation with protection varies depending on the study. While immunity to the sporozoite and liver stages of malaria has been demonstrated, naturally acquired antibody to these stages have shown little correlation with protection from malaria [38], unlike what has been documented for blood stages. Moreover, the RTS,S/AS01 vaccine – which targets the circumsporozoite protein of the sporozoite – has routinely achieved ~50% protection in controlled human malaria infection (CHMI); a single mCoP has not been identified. Although antibodies are important in protection, there is a large overlap in titers between protected and unprotected individuals [6]. Mechanistic correlates of protection that can be developed into a standardized assay (in the case of neutralizing antibody) are much more challenging for the sporozoite stage, as they require both viable sporozoites and human livers – either in the context of liver culture systems or humanized mouse models. For this reason, much of this discussion will be focused on protection from *blood stage* infection, the stage of the disease which causes the clinical symptoms of malaria, and primarily mechanisms involving antibodies.

12.2.2.3 Antibody-Mediated Protection from Malaria

The main mechanisms of antibody-mediated clearance of blood stage malaria parasites include (1) direct neutralization that prevent the parasites from invading target cells, (2) antibody-dependent complement-mediated killing of parasites directly, and (3) antibody binding and opsonization and/or phagocytosis from innate immune cells (Fig. 12.5). Analysis of mechanisms of acquired immunity to malaria is a long-standing field of study. Some of the best experimental evidence for the functional importance of antibodies in protection from malaria comes from The Gambia. Nonimmune individuals were transfused with pure IgG from either Gambian "protected" adults, the IgG depleted serum from those same adults, and IgG from UK adults. The IgG from the "protected" Gambian adults reduced the risk of malaria disease and lowered parasitemia [40]. Some of the mechanisms of antibody-mediated immunity to malaria have been recapitulated by in vitro assays in the laboratory and represent candidates for mCoP. Such functional assays include invasion inhibition, the growth inhibition assay (GIA), rosette inhibition [41], inhibition of cytoadhesion from both the microvasculature and the placenta [42], and antibody-dependent cellular mechanisms such as antibody dependent cellular inhibition (ADCI), opsonophagocytosis of merozoites, and antibody-dependent respiratory burst (ADRB) [39]. While an association between GIA and vaccine-induced protection from malaria infection has been observed in non-human primate vaccination studies, the relationship between GIA and naturally acquired malaria immunity is likely more complex and dependent on the interaction of multiple immune responses, some of which are outlined in Figs. 12.3 and 12.5. Recently, Douglas

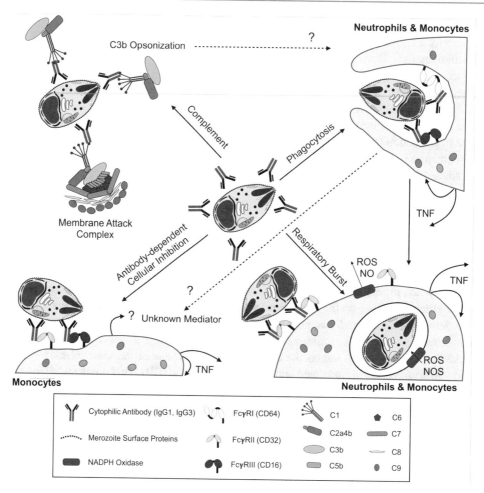

Fig. 12.5 Mechanisms of antibody mediated clearance of *Plasmodium*. Depicted here are some of the many protective immune mechanisms in response to IgG opsonized merozoites. Cytophilic antibodies (IgG1 and IgG3) bind merozoite surface proteins and trigger a number of downstream mechanisms: deposition of complement C3b, membrane attack complex formation and merozoite lysis (top left); phagocytosis of IgG-opsonized merozoites via FcγRI and FcγRIII receptors (top right); antibody-dependent "respiratory burst" via FcγRII receptors resulting in the production of reactive oxygen species or reactive nitrogen species (bottom right); and antibody-dependent cellular inhibition via FcγRII and FcγRIII receptors resulting in secretion of an unknown anti-parasitic factor. TNF is produced following FcγR-signaling and can enhance phagocyte killing functions in an autocrine, paracrine, FcγR and non-FcγR-mediated manner. Solid arrows between mechanisms indicate known relationships. Dotted lines and question marks indicate hypothesized relationships that remain to be demonstrated. It is thought that antigens localized within merozoite invasion organelles such as the rhoptries, micronemes and dense granules, are not major targets of opsonizing antibodies (Adapted from Hill et al. [39])

et al. described the mechanistic basis of GIA-mediated protection by generating chimeric human monoclonal antibodies from previously characterized anti-PfRH5 merozoite neutralizing and non-neutralizing antibodies containing IgG1 Fc regions that cannot engage complement or FcR-dependent effector mechanisms [43]. These antibodies were passively transfered into *Aotus nancymaae* monkeys and following *P. falciparum* challenge, demonstrated that complete protection could be derrived from neutralization alone for the antibodies previously associated with high GIA activity. These results offer some of the clearest mechanistic evidence published to date dissecting the quantitative relationship between *P. falciparum* vaccine candidate effector, an in vitro assay, and in vivo protection [43].

12.2.3 Immunoepidemiology to Inform Vaccine Candidates

Despite tremendous technological advances in the last few decades, 18 of the 22 current antigens under clinical development as vaccine candidates were identified before the *Plasmodium falciparum* genome was sequenced in 2002– in the "pre-genomic" era [44]. Many of these "pre-genomic" candidates were identified by classical immunoepidemiological techniques – screening unannotated genomic and cDNA libraries with serum antibodies for reactivity or functional activity and characterizing the resulting targets. The first vaccine candidates, merozoite surface protein-1 (MSP1), circumsporozoite protein (CSP), and apical membrane antigen-1 (AMA-1), were all identified in this way. Altogether, eight vaccine candidates that have been tested in clinical trials were identified in this manner [44], including a recent candidate, *Plasmodium falciparum* schizont egress antigen (PfSEA), that has not yet entered clinical testing [45]. The attractive aspect of using immunoepidemiology in vaccine discovery is that one uses the natural experiment – populations and individuals who are naturally immune and those who are not – to identify the targets.

An example of how immunological functional correlate assays inform vaccine design was the identification of MSP3 as a vaccine candidate [46]. The rationale for pursuing MSP3 came from experiments in which IgG passively transferred from immune individuals to infected individuals protected from malaria disease [40]. The mechanisms of protection provided by these passively transferred antibodies was later described as antibody-mediated cellular inhibition (ADCI) [47]. This immune correlate assay was used to screen a *P. falciparum* genomic expression library which by activity identified MSP3 as a candidate [48]. This approach is unique in that it started with a mCoP and empirically identified the target, rather than the other way around.

While nearly all current blood stage malaria vaccine candidate antigens have been identified or informed by seroepidemiology, there are challenges in using seroepidemiology to identify vaccine candidates. First, disentangling immune exposure from immune protection is a key distinction. While some vaccine candidates have been immunodominant antigens (those that generate robust immune responses with repeated exposure – such as MSP1 and AMA-1), occasionally the best candidates (or regions of candidates) are not the most naturally immunogenic; however, robust immune responses can be developed with vaccination. This phenomenon has been observed for both *Plasmodium vivax* Duffy binding protein (PvDBP) and *Plasmodium falciparum* reticulocyte binding protein homolog (PfRH5) – two candidates in early clinical development. Natural populations do not frequently make high-titer immune responses to PfRh5 [14, 49, 50]; however, IgG from endemic settings that do recognize the protein can be inhibitory [50] and predictive of protection [49] as is vaccine-induced IgG [51]. A similar observation has been observed with antibodies against PvDBP [52].

In assessing the immune response to key vaccine candidate antigens, an important consideration is the level of genetic diversity in these candidates. One of the major challenges that has limited the ability to formulate an effective vaccine is the enormous antigenic diversity of the parasite, which plays a major role in immune evasion, compromising the development of both natural and vaccine-induced protective immunity. However, these factors have not received appropriate attention in the development of malaria vaccine candidates. Failure to assess genetic diversity early in vaccine development has eliminated several malaria vaccine candidates after Phase IIb trials. It also has emerged as a potential problem for the only licensed malaria vaccine and only after a large Phase III trial involving nearly 16,000 subjects [53]. If malaria vaccine development is to be successful, new approaches need to be developed that take account the considerable natural genetic and phenotypic variation much earlier in the decision-making process before testing in costly Phase II and III trials [54]. In this post-genomic era of vaccine development, there is no longer an absence of genomic sequence data available, and consortiums such as MalariaGEN (www.malariagen.net) and initiatives such as Pf3K (www.malariagen.net/projects/pf3k) – whose goal is to make genomic sequence data from 3000 isolates around the world freely accessible to all – are making such analyses possible to perform in a robust way. In accurately measuring immune responses, it is important to consider whether measuring the response to multiple alleles of a single protein might provide different data than a single allele from a single strain, which is the standard approach. Addressing genetic diversity in vaccine candidate antigens from the perspective of accurately measuring immune responses, as well as validating vaccine candidates, remains a significant challenge for the field.

12.2.4 Serological Correlates of Exposure to Malaria

While one of the goals of immunoepidemiology studies is to define correlates and targets of protection, arguably one of the most significant advances in the field of immunoepidemiology is the definition of serological correlates of *exposure*. This is not a novel concept in the field, and the advantages of serological markers of exposure were outlined by McGregor [25]. A number of immunoepidemiological studies supported the utility of using serology as a marker of exposure. Antibody prevalence and titers were much higher in rural Gambians than in urban dwellers [55]. The use of serology delineated differences in cumulative exposure in two holoendemic Nigerian populations that appeared comparable by parasite indices [56]. Application of serology further demonstrated that after successful malaria control efforts with anti-malarial drugs in the Usambara mountains, although parasite rates had decreased, overall transmission was unaffected [57]. One of the recognized strengths of serological data to measure transmission is that serological markers are much more stable over time and are not affected by seasonality in the same way as traditional malaria indices, such as parasite prevalence or parasite rates [25]. Validation of serology as a correlate of exposure to malaria has been refined over the years, and the advantages, limitations, and areas for future development have been well-characterized [58, 59].

Using serology as a marker of transmission intensity was applied to individuals living in villages at different altitudes in the Usambara mountains of Tanzania, where transmission intensity was well-characterized and previously described with entomological metrics. Using three merozoite antigens (MSP1$_{19}$, MSP2, and AMA-1), it was observed that a single antigen (MSP1$_{19}$) could accurately predict exposure to malaria [60].

A challenge for this approach is that antibodies to each antigen have different dynamics of acquisition as well as decay [58]. Such dynamics have been described with reverse catalytic prevalence models [58], as described in detail in Boxes 12.1, 12.2, and 12.3.

Box 12.1: Why Does a mechanistic correlate of protection (mCoP) for Malaria Remain a Challenge?
The ability to culture the *Plasmodium falciparum* parasite in vitro [61] is a major advantage in the development of mCoP. However, despite the accessibility of the parasite in vitro, the published genome, and the growing field of "omics" (genomics, transcriptomics, proteomics, metabolomics, interactomics, etc.), there remain challenges in the quest for a mCoP. First, many of these correlate assays inconsistently predict protection when measured individually. Different studies present conflicting results regarding measurements of response or activity in the assay and protection from malaria. This has been observed with serological CoP [37] as well as GIA activity and protection and ADCI activity and protection [62]. There has been a growing concerted effort in the field to understand the reasons for such differences and to optimize and standardize assays as much as possible so that cross-comparable generalizable data is possible. Current efforts to standardize invasion inhibition [63], GIA [64], standard membrane feeding assays (SMFA) [65], neutrophil respiratory burst assays [66], and CSA binding inhibition

assays [42] are underway or have been successfully achieved. Another potential reason why such assays inconsistently predict protection is that it may be an oversimplification to try to distill a complex immune response to a complex parasite with a complex life cycle down to a single assay. Recently, it was shown that combining different mechanistic assays more significantly predicted protection than any assay individually [67]. In this case, GIA and respiratory burst together provided the best prediction of protection.

Box 12.2: Maximum Likelihood Fitting of Reverse Catalytic Prevalence Models [58]

$$seropositive \underset{\rho}{\overset{\lambda}{\underset{\leftarrow}{\rightarrow}}} seronegative$$

If individuals who are seronegative become seropositive at a rate of λ $year^{-1}$, and if seropositive individuals revert to seronegative at a rate of ρ $year^{-1}$, then the proportion of seropositive individuals in an initially malaria-naïve population will reach a plateau when the rate of seroconversion equals the rate or seroreversion, shown by.

$$\lambda(1 - P_\infty) = \rho(P_\infty), \text{ and } P_\infty = \frac{\lambda}{\lambda + \rho} \tag{12.1}$$

where P_t is the proportion of individuals in the cohort who are seropositive at time t. P_∞ is the final value of P achieved. If λ is small, P_∞ may never be reached. The proportion of seropositive individuals after time t is shown by

$$P_t = \frac{\lambda}{\lambda + \rho}(1 - e^{-(\lambda + \rho)t} \tag{12.2}$$

While the equation is not linear, the expected proportions can be calculated in any age group for trial values of λ and ρ and optimize the values to best fit the data. It can be assumed that errors are binomially distributed and parameters optimized by standard techniques. It is important to consider the endemicity and stability of malaria transmission when applying these models to appreciate both the power and the limitations of the estimation [68].

To address this natural variation, seroepidemiologic experiments were expanded to multiple antigens and rates of seroconversion with exposure, as well as seroreversion in the absence of re-exposure. Seroconversion was mapped and defined as rapid, moderate, and slow acquisition and reversion [69]. Having different time scales allows for a more precise mapping of exposure dynamics over time. Serological measures of transmission were used to define declining transmission in The Gambia [70].

A recent advance has been in the potential to measure exposure with fine resolution of the timing of exposure – whether an individual has been infected within the last 30 days, the last 90 days, or the last year [71]. This has been accomplished by expanding from small-scale individual protein-based approaches to protein-based microarrays covering hundreds of malaria antigens – including hypotheticals and proteins of unknown function [16]. These studies were performed using serum antibodies from two populations in Uganda, representing moderate and intense malaria transmission. Future studies in other countries and across transmission strata would be useful in further validating these markers to determine a "universal" fixed set of top antigens predictive of time-delineated exposure.

Box 12.3: Key Challenges and Future Research
Areas of future research and addressing key challenges in the field remain. These include

1. Disentangling immune markers of *exposure* from immune markers of *protection.*
2. Measuring immune responses to a pathogen with a complex life cycle and with incredibly genetically diverse antigens.
3. Identifying a true mechanistic immune correlate of protection (mCoP) – the holy grail!
4. Clearly delineating exposure and protection in different endemic populations and age groups, a continually moving target as transmission changes.
5. Identifying the diversity of immune responses in the individual over the course of infection that contribute to protection and understanding these mechanisms, as well as how they can be leveraged to improve vaccine design.
6. Integrating "omics" data (genomics, transcriptomics, proteomics, interactomics, etc.) to inform immunoepidemiology studies of exposure, protection, and to inform vaccine development.

12.2.4.1 Serologic Markers of Exposure and Implications for Public Health

Having robust serological markers of exposure would be a useful tool for evaluating the success of malaria control and elimination interventions. Being able to map hot spots of transmission would help inform where national programs could focus efforts to have the greatest impact. As multiplexed serology becomes more widely validated and adopted, it also provides opportunities to measure exposure to multiple diseases at the same time. Such multiplex seroepidemiologic approaches have been used to infer the impact of bednet use on malaria and lymphatic filariasis transmission [72]. Further, being able to assess exposure to a wide array of temporally defined markers would allow determination of whether there has been recent reintroduction of malaria into a pre-elimination zone, for example, even down to the month of exposure [71]. Further, when transmission decreases dramatically – such as in pre-elimination and elimination settings – it becomes increasingly difficult to use traditional measures of transmission intensity involving infected people and infected mosquitoes, and in this setting, serological estimates have added value [59, 73].

12.2.5 Between-Host and Within-Host Immunological Diversity: A Systems Biology Approach

In immunoepidemiology studies of malaria, the strength and functional quality of the immune response are not solely dependent on characteristics of the parasite exposure but can be affected by many host-specific factors. Some of these host factors are hardwired (or genetically determined), and others are dynamic and can change over time, such as environmental factors, nutritional status, and coinfections.

Some of these host factors may be hardwired, and others are dynamic and change over time. In a study in Kenya, host genetic factors accounted for 25% of the variation in uncomplicated malaria risk, and household factors accounted for 29% of the risk [74]. Perhaps the best known genetically determined protective factor to any infectious disease is sickle hemoglobin [75], and since this initial epidemiologic association, numerous red blood cell variants have been associated with malaria protection, including thalassemia, G6PD deficiency, hemoglobin C, and ovalocytosis. More recent work has examined the role of immunogenetic variation, the study of the genetic basis determining functional differences in how the immune system responds to the same pathogen. The earliest association in the field was that of HLA Class I (Bw53) and Class II (DRB1*1302-DQB1*0501) with malaria protection in a large study of severe malaria in The Gambia. This work was later followed by a mechanistic study suggesting that HLA-B53-restricted cytotoxic T cells recognize *P. falciparum* liver-stage Antigen-1 peptides [76, 77]. Likely due to the challenging nature of HLA studies, additional confirmatory or novel data on HLA Class I and II, malaria associations have been limited, although recent studies are exploring the role of HLA in malaria vaccine responses [78]. A larger body of literature on TNF supports a role of TNF-promoter (TNF-308A, TNF-238A, TNF-376A alleles) and inducible nitric oxide synthase (NOS2A-954C and NOS2A-1173 T alleles) polymorphisms in different manifestations of severe malaria and, less strongly, in uncomplicated malaria [79].

Immunogenetic studies that impact antibody responses have been more limited. Among the earliest studies in this area was one that demonstrated a higher concordance of levels of anti-ring-infected erythrocyte surface antigen (RESA) antibodies in monozygotic than dizygotic twins or age-/sex-matched siblings [80]. More recently, results from the Malaria GEN consortium (www.malariagen.net) have examined the genetic determinants of anti-malarial antibody responses to four well-studied antigens in a multicenter study, concluding that sickle hemoglobin was the single strongest SNP associated with merozoite antibody titers [81]. These and other studies suggest that the influence of some of the "classic" malaria resistance loci may be a result of both biochemical and immunologic impacts [82]. Beyond studies directly correlating antibody levels and SNPs, more indirect effects on antibody responses have demonstrated the impact of variants in cytokines that can influence B-cell proliferation and differentiation (such as IL-4), B-cell receptors that influence Ig class switching (such as CD40 ligand), and Ig receptors that influence the removal of Ag-Ab complexes (such as Fc gamma receptor) [79]. Among the most intriguing areas of immunoepidemiologic study relates to the differential susceptibility of the Fulani ethnic group in West Africa, as compared to other sympatric groups. Investigations into interethnic differences in cellular immune responses have been identified between these groups, and more recent studies have shown higher levels of total IgE- and *Pf*-specific IgG for several malaria antigens in the Fulani, as compared to other groups [83].

Besides genetics, additional host factors and temporal conditions can influence immune responses. The nutritional status of the human host before and after infection is a key variable in determining the immune system's capacity to mount an effective response. Further, the presence of coinfections such as viral infections (Th1) or helminth infections (Th2) can skew the immune responses in either pro-inflammatory or anti-inflammatory directions, which can alter the effector responses against the malaria parasite. These potential confounders are not always included in studies of malaria immunity and should be considered when measuring markers of immune exposure or protection from malaria.

12.2.6 Within-Host Immunological Diversity: The Next Frontier of Malaria Immunoepidemiology

The more we understand immunity to malaria, the more complex it becomes. Seroepidemiology approaches must be adapted to not just *detect* antibody to proteins but to describe *qualities* and *characteristics* of antibodies so that we may better understand their function in exposure and protection from disease [62].

With advances in both cell sorting and single-cell sequencing technologies, the ability to study B-cell affinity maturation and characterize the antibodies produced by individual B cells has revolutionized how we think about malaria immunity. B-cell cloning and sequencing, as well as phenotypic characterization with in vitro CoP, have revealed specific mutations in the antibody VDJ region that are able to produce highly strain-transcendent agglutinating antibodies [84]. Recently, studies in Mali revealed a preferential activation of inferior T follicular helper cells that are CXCR3$^+$, which provide insufficient B-cell help and result in the dysregulation of B-cell responses in malaria-exposed individuals. These atypical B cells, which express high levels of the transcription factor T-bet [85], are increasingly prevalent in high-transmission areas [86] and are elevated in individuals with more clinical episodes [85]. These cells functionally dampen productive immune responses by upregulating inhibitory Fc receptors through reduced proliferation and cytokine production and reduced antibody secretion [87]. Such results suggest that B-cell modulation could potentially improve the quality and function of immune responses, hopefully resulting in increased malaria vaccine efficiency.

Moving beyond the phenotypic varieties of B cells that secrete the antibodies to the antibodies themselves, the specific antibody isotype (IgA, IgE, IgG, IgD, and IgM) and subclass (IgG1, IgG2, IgG3, IgG4), induced by natural infection or vaccination, impact immune effector mechanisms. Within the scope of this chapter, we will focus on IgG. IgG antibodies contain two heavy chains and two light chains, which comprise two different functional domains: the Fab that binds the antigen and the constant domain (Fc). While the avidity and affinity of the Fab is often the focus of much research, the variation in the Fc region of the antibody is equally important. In the immunoepidemiology studies of malaria, the primary focus has been on IgG subclass, with opsonizing IgG1 and IgG3 often the most common isotypes for most blood-stage antigens and also associated with protection [88, 89], whereas IgG2 and IgG4 are less frequently observed, though results vary by antigen. The primary means by which diversity is generated in the Fc region is through subclass and glycosylation at the Asparagine residue 297 in the CH2 domain. Humans have 4 IgG subclasses and 36 antibody glycans, resulting in 144 possible combinations [90] (Fig. 12.6). Shifts in glycosylation during infection have been observed and imply yet another mechanism for modulation of inflammatory disease [91]. Understanding these changes in antibody composition over the course of infection and after resolution and how these dynamics influence effector function is unexplored in malaria and represents an exciting new frontier of research.

Given the degree of variation in the immune responses within an individual over the course of their infection, their nutritional status, and potentially undiagnosed coinfections, as well as genetic differences between individuals in the population, clearly delineating "protected" or "immune" is still a challenge. However, keeping these potential confounders and contributors in mind can assist in better defining the state of malaria immunity and, as such, immunoepidemiological studies of malaria.

12.3   Key Challenges and Future Directions

Immunoepidemiology studies of malaria have contributed to a better understanding of key targets and mechanisms of protective immunity and the identification of fine-resolution markers of exposure and have assisted in the identification and credentialing of vaccine candidates. This knowledge has and can be used to inform public health interventions, such as serological surveillance for reintroduction of malaria in elimination zones, mapping populations at risk for better targeting of interventions, and vaccine development.

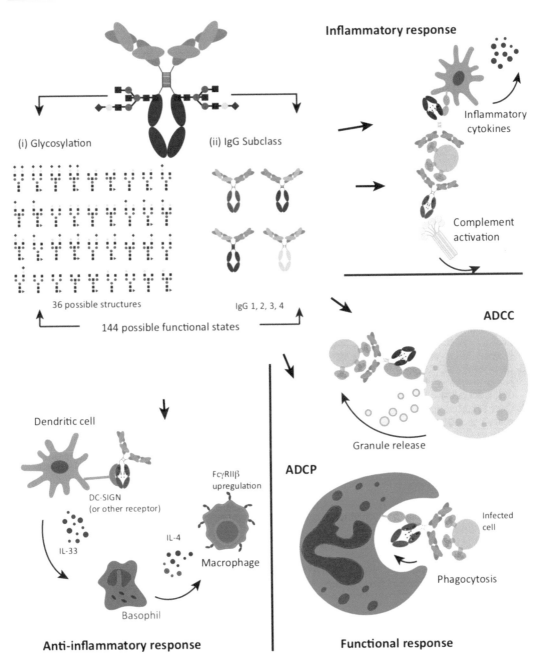

Fig. 12.6 Antibody combinatorial diversity drives antibody effector function. The IgG Fc is modified through two changes to the Fc domain of an antibody: (i) choice of glycosylation (36 options) and (ii) choice of subclass (four subclasses), creating 144 theoretical combinations and linked functional states. Depending on the antibody–glycan combination, many different functional responses may be elicited including the induction of an anti-inflammatory response; functional responses such as antibody-dependent cellular phagocytosis (ADCP), antibody-dependent cellular cytotoxicity (ADCC); or inflammatory responses including complement activation and cytokine secretion. Abbreviation: IL, interleukin. (Reprinted from Ref. [91] Copyright (2017), with permission from Elsevier)

References

1. Bhatt S, Weiss DJ, Cameron E, Bisanzio D, Mappin B, Dalrymple U, et al. The effect of malaria control on *Plasmodium falciparum* in Africa between 2000 and 2015. Nature. 2015;526(7572):207–11.
2. Gething PW, Casey DC, Weiss DJ, Bisanzio D, Bhatt S, Cameron E, et al. Mapping *Plasmodium falciparum* mortality in Africa between 1990 and 2015. N Engl J Med. 2016;375(25):2435–45.
3. Battle KE, Guerra CA, Golding N, Duda KA, Cameron E, Howes RE, Elyazar IR, Baird JK, Reiner RC Jr, Gething PW, Smith DL, Hay SI. Global database of matched *Plasmodium falciparum* and *P. vivax* incidence and prevalence records from 1985–2013. Sci Data. 2015;2:150012.
4. McGregor I. The development and maintenance of immunity to malaria in highly endemic areas. Clin Trop Med Commun Dis. 1986;1986(1):1–29.
5. Mackinnon MJ, Marsh K. The selection landscape of malaria parasites. Science. 2010;328(5980):866–71.
6. Riley EM, Stewart VA. Immune mechanisms in malaria: new insights in vaccine development. Nat Med. 2013;19(2):168–78.
7. Nussenzweig RS, Vanderberg J, Most H, Orton C. Protective immunity produced by the injection of x-irradiated sporozoites of plasmodium berghei. Nature. 1967;216(5111):160–2.
8. Seder RA, Chang LJ, Enama ME, Zephir KL, Sarwar UN, Gordon IJ, et al. Protection against malaria by intravenous immunization with a nonreplicating sporozoite vaccine. Science. 2013;341(6152):1359–65.
9. Cockburn IA, Seder RA. Malaria prevention: from immunological concepts to effective vaccines and protective antibodies. Nat Immunol. 2018;19(11):1199–211.
10. Langhorne J, Ndungu FM, Sponaas AM, Marsh K. Immunity to malaria: more questions than answers. Nat Immunol. 2008;9(7):725–32.
11. Kreutzfeld O, Muller K, Matuschewski K. Engineering of Genetically Arrested Parasites (GAPs) for a precision malaria vaccine. Front Cell Infect Microbiol. 2017;7:198.
12. Zenonos ZA, Rayner JC, Wright GJ. Towards a comprehensive *Plasmodium falciparum* merozoite cell surface and secreted recombinant protein library. Malar J. 2014;13:93.
13. Bartholdson SJ, Crosnier C, Bustamante LY, Rayner JC, Wright GJ. Identifying novel *Plasmodium falciparum* erythrocyte invasion receptors using systematic extracellular protein interaction screens. Cell Microbiol. 2013;15(8):1304–12.
14. Osier FH, Mackinnon MJ, Crosnier C, Fegan G, Kamuyu G, Wanaguru M, et al. New antigens for a multicomponent blood-stage malaria vaccine. Sci Transl Med. 2014;6(247):247ra102.
15. Kamuyu G, Tuju J, Kimathi R, Mwai K, Mburu J, Kibinge N, et al. KILchip v1.0: a novel *Plasmodium falciparum* Merozoite protein microarray to facilitate malaria vaccine candidate prioritization. Front Immunol. 2018;9:2866.
16. Crompton PD, Kayala MA, Traore B, Kayentao K, Ongoiba A, Weiss GE, et al. A prospective analysis of the Ab response to *Plasmodium falciparum* before and after a malaria season by protein microarray. Proc Natl Acad Sci U S A. 2010;107(15):6958–63.
17. Dent AE, Nakajima R, Liang L, Baum E, Moormann AM, Sumba PO, et al. *Plasmodium falciparum* protein microarray antibody profiles correlate with protection from symptomatic malaria in Kenya. J Infect Dis. 2015;212(9):1429–38.
18. Sergent E, Parrot L. L'immunité, la prémunition et la résistance innée. Archives de l'Institut Pasteur d'Algérie. 1935;13:279–319.
19. Gupta S, Day KP. A strain theory of malaria transmission. Parasitol Today. 1994;10(12):476–81.
20. Trape JF, Tall A, Sokhna C, Ly AB, Diagne N, Ndiath O, et al. The rise and fall of malaria in a West African rural community, Dielmo, Senegal, from 1990 to 2012: a 22 year longitudinal study. Lancet Infect Dis. 2014;14(6):476–88.
21. Rogier C. Natural history of *Plasmodium falciparum* malaria and determining factors of the acquisition of antimalaria immunity in two endemic areas, Dielmo and Ndiop (Senegal). Bull Mem Acad R Med Belg. 2000;155(5–6):218–26.
22. Marsh K, Otoo L, Hayes RJ, Carson DC, Greenwood BM. Antibodies to blood stage antigens of *Plasmodium falciparum* in rural Gambians and their relation to protection against infection. Trans R Soc Trop Med Hyg. 1989;83(3):293–303.
23. Marsh K, Hayes RH, Carson DC, Otoo L, Shenton F, Byass P, et al. Anti-sporozoite antibodies and immunity to malaria in a rural Gambian population. Trans R Soc Trop Med Hyg. 1988;82(4):532–7.
24. Bejon P, Williams TN, Liljander A, Noor AM, Wambua J, Ogada E, et al. Stable and unstable malaria hotspots in longitudinal cohort studies in Kenya. PLoS Med. 2010;7(7):e1000304.
25. McGregor IA. Mechanisms of acquired immunity and epidemiological patterns of antibody responses in malaria in man. Bull World Health Organ. 1974;50(3–4):259–66.
26. Marsh K, Kinyanjui S. Immune effector mechanisms in malaria. Parasite Immunol. 2006;28:51–60.
27. Kinyanjui SM, Bejon P, Osier FH, Bull PC, Marsh K. What you see is not what you get: implications of the brevity of antibody responses to malaria antigens and transmission heterogeneity in longitudinal studies of malaria immunity. Malar J. 2009;8:242.

28. Marsh K, Howard RJ. Antigens induced on erythrocytes by P. falciparum: expression of diverse and conserved determinants. Science. 1986;231(4734):150–3.
29. Newbold CI, Pinches R, Roberts DJ, Marsh K. *Plasmodium falciparum*: the human agglutinating antibody response to the infected red cell surface is predominantly variant specific. Exp Parasitol. 1992;75(3):281–92.
30. McKenzie FE, Smith DL, O'Meara WP, Riley EM. Strain theory of malaria: the first 50 years. Adv Parasitol. 2008;66:1–46.
31. Jeffery GM. Epidemiological significance of repeated infections with homologous and heterologous strains and species of Plasmodium. Bull World Health Organ. 1966;35(6):873–82.
32. Recker M, Buckee CO, Serazin A, Kyes S, Pinches R, Christodoulou Z, et al. Antigenic variation in *Plasmodium falciparum* malaria involves a highly structured switching pattern. PLoS Pathog. 2011;7(3):e1001306.
33. Buckee CO, Bull PC, Gupta S. Inferring malaria parasite population structure from serological networks. Proc Biol Sci. 2009;276(1656):477–85.
34. Osier FH, Fegan G, Polley SD, Murungi L, Verra F, Tetteh KK, et al. Breadth and magnitude of antibody responses to multiple *Plasmodium falciparum* merozoite antigens are associated with protection from clinical malaria. Infect Immun. 2008;76(5):2240–8.
35. Moormann AM, Stewart VA. The hunt for protective correlates of immunity to *Plasmodium falciparum* malaria. BMC Med. 2014;12:134.
36. Plotkin SA, Gilbert PB. Nomenclature for immune correlates of protection after vaccination. Clin Infect Dis. 2012;54(11):1615–7.
37. Fowkes FJ, Richards JS, Simpson JA, Beeson JG. The relationship between anti-merozoite antibodies and incidence of *Plasmodium falciparum* malaria: a systematic review and meta-analysis. PLoS Med. 2010;7(1):e1000218.
38. Hoffman SL, Oster CN, Plowe CV, Woollett GR, Beier JC, Chulay JD, et al. Naturally acquired antibodies to sporozoites do not prevent malaria: vaccine development implications. Science. 1987;237(4815):639–42.
39. Hill DL, Schofield L, Wilson DW. IgG opsonization of merozoites: multiple immune mechanisms for malaria vaccine development. Int J Parasitol. 2017;47(10–11):585–95.
40. Cohen S, Mc GI, Carrington S. Gamma-globulin and acquired immunity to human malaria. Nature. 1961;192:733–7.
41. Guillotte M, Juillerat A, Igonet S, Hessel A, Petres S, Crublet E, et al. Immunogenicity of the *Plasmodium falciparum* PfEMP1-VarO Adhesin: induction of surface-reactive and rosette-disrupting antibodies to VarO infected erythrocytes. PLoS One. 2015;10(7):e0134292.
42. Pehrson C, Heno KK, Adams Y, Resende M, Mathiesen L, Soegaard M, et al. Comparison of functional assays used in the clinical development of a placental malaria vaccine. Vaccine. 2017;35(4):610–8.
43. Douglas AD, Baldeviano GC, Jin J, Miura K, Diouf A, Zenonos ZA, Ventocilla JA, Silk SE, Marshall JM, Alanine DGW, Wang C, Edwards NJ, Leiva KP, Gomez-Puerta LA, Lucas CM, Wright GJ, Long CA, Royal JM, Draper SJ. A defined mechanistic correlate of protection against Plasmodium falciparum malaria in non-human primates. Nature Communications. 2019;10(1)
44. Tuju J, Kamuyu G, Murungi LM, Osier FHA. Vaccine candidate discovery for the next generation of malaria vaccines. Immunology. 2017;152(2):195–206.
45. Raj DK, Nixon CP, Nixon CE, Dvorin JD, DiPetrillo CG, Pond-Tor S, et al. Antibodies to PfSEA-1 block parasite egress from RBCs and protect against malaria infection. Science. 2014;344(6186):871–7.
46. Druilhe P, Spertini F, Soesoe D, Corradin G, Mejia P, Singh S, et al. A malaria vaccine that elicits in humans antibodies able to kill *Plasmodium falciparum*. PLoS Med. 2005;2(11):e344.
47. Bouharoun-Tayoun H, Attanath P, Sabchareon A, Chongsuphajaisiddhi T, Druilhe P. Antibodies that protect humans against *Plasmodium falciparum* blood stages do not on their own inhibit parasite growth and invasion in vitro, but act in cooperation with monocytes. J Exp Med. 1990;172(6):1633–41.
48. Oeuvray C, Bouharoun-Tayoun H, Grass-Masse H, Lepers JP, Ralamboranto L, Tartar A, et al. A novel merozoite surface antigen of *Plasmodium falciparum* (MSP-3) identified by cellular-antibody cooperative mechanism antigenicity and biological activity of antibodies. Mem Inst Oswaldo Cruz. 1994;89(Suppl 2):77–80.
49. Tran TM, Ongoiba A, Coursen J, Crosnier C, Diouf A, Huang CY, et al. Naturally acquired antibodies specific for *Plasmodium falciparum* reticulocyte-binding protein homologue 5 inhibit parasite growth and predict protection from malaria. J Infect Dis. 2014;209(5):789–98.
50. Patel SD, Ahouidi AD, Bei AK, Dieye TN, Mboup S, Harrison SC, et al. *Plasmodium falciparum* merozoite surface antigen, PfRH5, elicits detectable levels of invasion-inhibiting antibodies in humans. J Infect Dis. 2013;208(10):1679–87.
51. Payne RO, Milne KH, Elias SC, Edwards NJ, Douglas AD, Brown RE, et al. Demonstration of the blood-stage *Plasmodium falciparum* controlled human malaria infection model to assess efficacy of the P. falciparum apical membrane antigen 1 vaccine, FMP2.1/AS01. J Infect Dis. 2016;213(11):1743–51.
52. King CL, Michon P, Shakri AR, Marcotty A, Stanisic D, Zimmerman PA, et al. Naturally acquired Duffy-binding protein-specific binding inhibitory antibodies confer protection from blood-stage Plasmodium vivax infection. Proc Natl Acad Sci U S A. 2008;105(24):8363–8.

53. Neafsey DE, Juraska M, Bedford T, Benkeser D, Valim C, Griggs A, et al. Genetic diversity and protective efficacy of the RTS,S/AS01 malaria vaccine. N Engl J Med. 2015;373(21):2025–37.
54. mal ERACGoV. A research agenda for malaria eradication: vaccines. PLoS Med. 2011;8(1):e1000398.
55. Harverson G, Wilson ME. Assessment of current malarial endemicity in Bathurst, Gambia. West Afr Med J Niger Pract. 1968;17(3):63–7.
56. Voller A, Bruce-Chwatt LJ. Serological malaria surveys in Nigeria. Bull World Health Organ. 1968;39(6):883–97.
57. Draper CC, Lelijveld JL, Matola YG, White GB. Malaria in the Pare area of Tanzania. IV. Malaria in the human population 11 years after the suspension of residual insecticide spraying, with special reference to the serological findings. Trans R Soc Trop Med Hyg. 1972;66(6):905–12.
58. Corran P, Coleman P, Riley E, Drakeley C. Serology: a robust indicator of malaria transmission intensity? Trends Parasitol. 2007;23(12):575–82.
59. Tusting LS, Bousema T, Smith DL, Drakeley C. Measuring changes in *Plasmodium falciparum* transmission: precision, accuracy and costs of metrics. Adv Parasitol. 2014;84:151–208.
60. Drakeley CJ, Corran PH, Coleman PG, Tongren JE, McDonald SL, Carneiro I, et al. Estimating medium- and long-term trends in malaria transmission by using serological markers of malaria exposure. Proc Natl Acad Sci U S A. 2005;102(14):5108–13.
61. Trager W, Jensen JB. Human malaria parasites in continuous culture. Science. 1976;193(4254):673–5.
62. Teo A, Feng G, Brown GV, Beeson JG, Rogerson SJ. Functional antibodies and protection against blood-stage malaria. Trends Parasitol. 2016;32(11):887–98.
63. Authors WC, Ahouidi AD, Amambua-Ngwa A, Awandare GA, Bei AK, Conway DJ, et al. Malaria vaccine development: focusing field erythrocyte invasion studies on phenotypic diversity: the West African Merozoite Invasion Network (WAMIN). Trends Parasitol. 2016;32(4):274–83.
64. Miura K, Zhou H, Moretz SE, Diouf A, Thera MA, Dolo A, et al. Comparison of biological activity of human anti-apical membrane antigen-1 antibodies induced by natural infection and vaccination. J Immunol (Baltimore, MD: 1950). 2008;181(12):8776–83.
65. Miura K, Deng B, Tullo G, Diouf A, Moretz SE, Locke E, et al. Qualification of standard membrane-feeding assay with *Plasmodium falciparum* malaria and potential improvements for future assays. PLoS One. 2013;8(3):e57909.
66. Llewellyn D, Miura K, Fay MP, Williams AR, Murungi LM, Shi J, et al. Standardization of the antibody-dependent respiratory burst assay with human neutrophils and *Plasmodium falciparum* malaria. Sci Rep. 2015;5:14081.
67. Murungi LM, Sonden K, Llewellyn D, Rono J, Guleid F, Williams AR, et al. Targets and mechanisms associated with protection from severe *Plasmodium falciparum* malaria in Kenyan children. Infect Immun. 2016;84(4):950–63.
68. Sepulveda N, Stresman G, White MT, Drakeley CJ. Current mathematical models for analyzing anti-malarial antibody data with an eye to malaria elimination and eradication. J Immunol Res. 2015;2015:738030.
69. Ondigo BN, Hodges JS, Ireland KF, Magak NG, Lanar DE, Dutta S, et al. Estimation of recent and long-term malaria transmission in a population by antibody testing to multiple *Plasmodium falciparum* antigens. J Infect Dis. 2014;210(7):1123–32.
70. van den Hoogen LL, Griffin JT, Cook J, Sepulveda N, Corran P, Conway DJ, et al. Serology describes a profile of declining malaria transmission in Farafenni. The Gambia Malar J. 2015;14(1):416.
71. Helb DA, Tetteh KK, Felgner PL, Skinner J, Hubbard A, Arinaitwe E, et al. Novel serologic biomarkers provide accurate estimates of recent *Plasmodium falciparum* exposure for individuals and communities. Proc Natl Acad Sci U S A. 2015;112(32):E4438–47.
72. Plucinski MM, Candrinho B, Chambe G, Muchanga J, Muguande O, Matsinhe G, et al. Multiplex serology for impact evaluation of bed net distribution on burden of lymphatic filariasis and four species of human malaria in northern Mozambique. PLoS Negl Trop Dis. 2018;12(2):e0006278.
73. Alonso PL, Brown G, Arevalo-Herrera M, Binka F, Chitnis C, Collins F, et al. A research agenda to underpin malaria eradication. PLoS Med. 2011;8(1):e1000406.
74. Mackinnon MJ, Mwangi TW, Snow RW, Marsh K, Williams TN. Heritability of malaria in Africa. PLoS Med. 2005;2(12):e340.
75. Allison AC. The distribution of the sickle-cell trait in East Africa and elsewhere, and its apparent relationship to the incidence of subtertian malaria. Trans R Soc Trop Med Hyg. 1954;48(4):312–8.
76. Hill AV, Allsopp CE, Kwiatkowski D, Anstey NM, Twumasi P, Rowe PA, et al. Common west African HLA antigens are associated with protection from severe malaria. Nature. 1991;352(6336):595–600.
77. Hill AV, Elvin J, Willis AC, Aidoo M, Allsopp CE, Gotch FM, et al. Molecular analysis of the association of HLA-B53 and resistance to severe malaria. Nature. 1992;360(6403):434–9.
78. Nielsen CM, Vekemans J, Lievens M, Kester KE, Regules JA, Ockenhouse CF. RTS,S malaria vaccine efficacy and immunogenicity during *Plasmodium falciparum* challenge is associated with HLA genotype. Vaccine. 2018;36(12):1637–42.
79. Kwiatkowski DP. How malaria has affected the human genome and what human genetics can teach us about malaria. Am J Hum Genet. 2005;77(2):171–92.

80. Sjoberg K, Lepers JP, Raharimalala L, Larsson A, Olerup O, Marbiah NT, et al. Genetic regulation of human anti-malarial antibodies in twins. Proc Natl Acad Sci U S A. 1992;89(6):2101–4.

81. Shelton JM, Corran P, Risley P, Silva N, Hubbart C, Jeffreys A, et al. Genetic determinants of anti-malarial acquired immunity in a large multi-centre study. Malar J. 2015;14:333.

82. Gong L, Parikh S, Rosenthal PJ, Greenhouse B. Biochemical and immunological mechanisms by which sickle cell trait protects against malaria. Malar J. 2013;12:317.

83. Arama C, Maiga B, Dolo A, Kouriba B, Traore B, Crompton PD, et al. Ethnic differences in susceptibility to malaria: what have we learned from immuno-epidemiological studies in West Africa? Acta Trop. 2015;146:152–6.

84. Tan J, Pieper K, Piccoli L, Abdi A, Foglierini M, Geiger R, et al. A LAIR1 insertion generates broadly reactive antibodies against malaria variant antigens. Nature. 2016;529(7584):105–9.

85. Obeng-Adjei N, Portugal S, Holla P, Li S, Sohn H, Ambegaonkar A, et al. Malaria-induced interferon-gamma drives the expansion of Tbethi atypical memory B cells. PLoS Pathog. 2017;13(9):e1006576.

86. Illingworth J, Butler NS, Roetynck S, Mwacharo J, Pierce SK, Bejon P, et al. Chronic exposure to *Plasmodium falciparum* is associated with phenotypic evidence of B and T cell exhaustion. J Immunol. 2013;190(3):1038–47.

87. Portugal S, Tipton CM, Sohn H, Kone Y, Wang J, Li S, et al. Malaria-associated atypical memory B cells exhibit markedly reduced B cell receptor signaling and effector function. elife. 2015;4:e07218.

88. Bouharoun-Tayoun H, Druilhe P. *Plasmodium falciparum* malaria: evidence for an isotype imbalance which may be responsible for delayed acquisition of protective immunity. Infect Immun. 1992;60(4):1473–81.

89. Stanisic DI, Richards JS, McCallum FJ, Michon P, King CL, Schoepflin S, et al. Immunoglobulin G subclass-specific responses against *Plasmodium falciparum* merozoite antigens are associated with control of parasitemia and protection from symptomatic illness. Infect Immun. 2009;77(3):1165–74.

90. Alter G, Ottenhoff THM, Joosten SA. Antibody glycosylation in inflammation, disease and vaccination. Semin Immunol. 2018;39:102–10.

91. Jennewein MF, Alter G. The immunoregulatory roles of antibody glycosylation. Trends Immunol. 2017;38(5):358–72.

Immunoepidemiology of Cancer

13

Xiaomei Ma and Rong Wang

13.1 The Role of Immune System in Cancer Prevention and Treatment

Cancer is the second leading cause of death worldwide [1]. The human body is an exquisite system whose cells undergo constant DNA replications and cell divisions. When these processes go awry, cells may mutate and manage to achieve uncontrolled growth, leading to carcinogenesis. The hallmarks of cancer include sustaining proliferative signaling, evading growth suppressors, resisting cell death, enabling replicative immortality, inducing angiogenesis, activating invasion and metastasis, reprogramming energy metabolism, and evading immune destruction [2].

The immune system can help prevent and control cancer in multiple ways [3]. First, it can help protect against cancers that are caused or facilitated by infectious agents. Over the last few decades, it has been recognized that infections with viruses and bacteria play important roles in the etiology of various types of cancer. For example, infections with hepatitis B and hepatitis C viruses significantly increase the risk of hepatocellular carcinoma [4], and infection with certain strains of human papillomavirus (HPV) leads to almost all cervical cancers and some cancers of the vulva, vagina, penis, anus, and oropharynx [5]. As HPV infection is very common, its role in carcinogenesis was a major impetus for the development of HPV vaccines. Improving the coverage of HPV vaccination is an important preventive strategy for the many types of cancer associated with HPV infection. As for bacteria, colonization of *Helicobacter pylori* in the stomach is an established causative factor for both gastric cancer and gastric mucosa-associated lymphoid tissue lymphoma [6]. By acting as the first barrier against cancer-inducing infectious agents, the immune system serves as a gatekeeper.

Second, a functional immune system is critical for controlling an inflammatory environment that promotes carcinogenesis. As reviewed by Hanahan and colleagues, inflammation is an enabling characteristic that fosters the acquisition of core hallmark capabilities of cancer and has been demonstrated to enable the development of incipient neoplasia into full-blown cancer [2, 3]. An inflammatory environment is not necessarily caused by infection with specific pathogens; rather, it can be the result of other factors such as environmental chemical exposures and obesity. Epidemiological studies have observed a significant association between obesity and increased risks of many types of cancer, including cancer of the breast, colon, esophagus, kidney, liver, pancreas, stomach, and thyroid and multiple myeloma [7].

X. Ma (✉) · R. Wang
Department of Chronic Disease Epidemiology, Yale School of Public Health, New Haven, CT, USA
e-mail: xiaomei.ma@yale.edu; r.wang@yale.edu

© Springer Nature Switzerland AG 2019
P. J. Krause et al. (eds.), *Immunoepidemiology*, https://doi.org/10.1007/978-3-030-25553-4_13

While the underlying mechanisms are not fully understood and could be multiple, it is important to note that the chronic inflammatory state is a prominent characteristic of obesity.

Finally, a process known as cancer immunosurveillance occurs consisting of immune identification of tumor cells that express tumor-specific antigens or tumor-associated antigens and elimination of such cells, therefore stopping them from becoming overt cancer [3]. With the extremely large numbers of DNA replications and cell divisions that occur on a constant basis, it is inevitable that mistakes can appear and that mutated cells can surface. However, the mere presence of some tumor cells is far from the development of overt cancer; the real threat is the unchecked, uncontrolled overgrowth of such cells [3].

Cancer immunotherapy, i.e., the ability to harness a patient's own immune system to fight against cancer, had long been a dream of oncologists. That dream remained largely elusive until the 1990s, when the T-cell growth factor interleukin 2 (IL-2) was approved by the US Food and Drug Administration in 1991 for the treatment of metastatic kidney cancer and in 1998 for treatment of metastatic melanoma. The field of immunotherapy has witnessed substantial growth since then, especially in the last 5 years. During this time the Food and Drug Administration has approved dozens of drugs that fall into the category of cancer immunotherapy, including monoclonal antibodies, checkpoint inhibitors, immunomodulatory drugs, and viral cancer therapies.

Much of the recent development in cancer immunotherapy has been fueled by the revolutionary discovery of proteins that function as brakes on the immune system and thus stop it from doing its job of attacking cancer cells. James Allison and Tasuku Honjo were awarded the 2018 Nobel Prize in Physiology or Medicine for their work related to two brake-like proteins (CTLA-4 and PD-1), both of which are expressed on the surface of T cells. By developing antibodies or inhibitors of these proteins, scientists can release the break and unleash the immune system to fight against cancer. Clinical trials with anti-CTLA-4 antibodies and anti-PD-1 checkpoint inhibitors have generated dramatically positive results since 2010. As a group, immunotherapeutic agents have changed the paradigm for treating a variety of malignancies (e.g., melanoma, lymphoma, leukemia, and lung cancer), which tend to have many mutations that prevent them from being identified by the immune system. These agents are being actively tested for additional types of cancer (e.g., breast cancer) [8].

While different types of cancer share common characteristics, they also exhibit striking heterogeneity. In this chapter, we will cover the immunoepidemiology of two types of cancer in detail: childhood acute lymphoblastic leukemia and glioma. The former is a hematological malignancy and essentially a cancer of the immune system, while the latter is a solid tumor.

13.2 Childhood Acute Lymphoblastic Leukemia

While cancer is usually considered a disease of the elderly, children are also at risk. Despite a decrease of cancer incidence in the United States during 2001–2010, the incidence of childhood cancer (age of diagnosis, 0–14 years) increased by 0.8% per year, continuing a trend dating back to 1992 [9]. Deciphering the etiology of childhood cancer has major public health significance even as the mortality decreases with more effective treatment, because survivors face a lifelong battle with late effects of treatment such as second malignancies and many challenges while pursuing important milestones such as education attainment and employment.

In the United States, leukemia is the most common type of childhood cancer. Approximately 85% of childhood leukemia is acute lymphoblastic leukemia (ALL), which accounts for one-fourth of all cancers diagnosed in children 0 to 14 years of age, with a sharp incidence peak at age 2–5 years [10]. A similar incidence peak of childhood ALL has been observed in other industrialized nations but not in developing countries. These data, along with other findings such as some evidence of spatial and temporal clustering in ALL incidence, has prompted the delayed infection hypothesis proposed by Mel Greaves from the United Kingdom [11]. The essence of the Greaves hypothesis is that two genetic events may be responsible for the development of common ALL; the first occurs spontaneously in utero, while the second occurs in the same mutated clone following antigenic challenge after birth [11]. Children who have a delayed exposure to infectious agents and an improper developmental modulation of the immune system due to the early-life immunologic isolation may experience greater cell proliferation following their exposure to pathogens later in childhood (e.g., when they attend daycare or grade school). Aberrantly strong reactions to infections later in childhood may increase the risk of the second mutation and lead to childhood ALL [11].

Another scientist from the United Kingdom, Leo Kinlen, proposed that childhood leukemia might result from a rare response to a common but unidentified infection (or infections) and that increased risks would occur when populations were mixed so that infected and susceptible individuals had an elevated level of contact [12]. Cancer researchers interested in this hypothesis were initially intrigued by the cluster of childhood leukemia cases in Seascale, a small village 3 km from Sellafield, the principal nuclear reprocessing plant in the United Kingdom. During 1955–1983, five cases of leukemia were observed in children under the age of 10 years, when the expected number of cases was 0.5 [12]. While environmental pollution by radioactive waste and parental occupational exposure to radiation were both evaluated and considered untenable risk factors, Kinlen's population-mixing hypothesis gained traction. The local rural population of Seascale was low in density, geographically isolated, of high socioeconomic status, and likely to be susceptible to infections. The urban population that came to the area because of the nuclear plant was more likely to carry infections due to frequent contact with infectious agents in crowded cities. Although this is a small study, it stimulated a new hypothesis and has influenced the field.

The hypotheses of both Greaves and Kinlen center on the role of infection in the etiology of childhood ALL and are consistent with the disease being an abnormal response to infection. However, Greaves focuses on the barrage of infectious agents that a child is exposed to later in childhood, not on any specific agent(s), while Kinlen postulates that one or multiple specific, unidentified agents exist. These infection-related hypotheses have generated considerable scientific interest within and outside the United Kingdom, prompting many epidemiological studies conducted over the years.

13.2.1 Daycare Attendance

One of the greatest challenges to testing the infection-related hypotheses has been the difficulty of directly measuring infections in epidemiological studies. Daycare/preschool attendance, birth order, number of siblings, infections early in life, immunizations, and contact with pets and/or farm animals are some of the proxy measures that have been assessed in epidemiological studies, most of which have been case control in design given the rarity of childhood ALL. As a child's exposure to infectious agents is mostly through contact with other children, daycare attendance is an important factor to consider.

In the California Childhood Leukemia Study, incident cases of newly diagnosed childhood leukemia were rapidly ascertained from major pediatric clinical centers, and controls were randomly selected from the statewide birth records and individually matched to cases on date of birth, sex, mother's race (white, African American, or other), and ethnicity (Hispanic or not; a child was considered Hispanic if either parent was Hispanic) [10]. A personal interview with the primary caretaker of each case or control subject, usually the biological mother, was conducted to obtain information on daycare attendance among other factors of interest [10]. Child-hours at each daycare was calculated as: number of months attending a daycare × mean hours per week at this daycare × number of other children at this daycare × 4.35 (i.e., number of weeks per month) [10]. The child-hours at each daycare were added to obtain the total child-hours for each child [10]. In non-Hispanic white children, daycare attendance measured by child-hours was associated with a significantly reduced risk of ALL [10]. Compared with children who did not attend any daycare, the odds ratio (OR) for those who had >5000 child-hours during infancy was 0.42 (95% confidence interval (95% CI), 0.18–0.99) for ALL and 0.33 (95% CI, 0.11–1.01) for common ALL (i.e., ALL diagnosed in children ages 2–5 years and expressing CD10 and CD19 surface antigens, markers of neoplastic B lymphoblasts) [10]. Test for trend was also significant, supporting a dose-response relationship in which more child-hours were associated with a lower risk of ALL [10]. The magnitude of effect associated with the same number of child-hours was stronger for daycare attendance during infancy than for daycare attendance before diagnosis [10]. In addition, self-reported ear infection during infancy was associated with a significantly reduced risk of common ALL (OR = 0.32, 95% CI, 0.14–0.74) in non-Hispanic white children [10]. In Hispanic children, however, no association was observed between daycare attendance, early infections, and risk of childhood ALL or common ALL [10]. These results offer indirect yet strong support for a role of infection in protection regarding the etiology of ALL in non-Hispanic white children. The reason for the apparent ethnic difference was unclear, but one possibility could be that contact with other children in a daycare setting was not the primary source of exposure to infectious agents for the Hispanic children included in this study. Compared to non-Hispanic white children, Hispanic children had significantly more children living in the same household before they went to grade school, and fewer Hispanic children started daycare before 1 year of age [10].

This California study was the first to report a negative association between daycare attendance and risk of childhood ALL in the United States. Subsequently, a meta-analysis of 14 case-control studies from 9 countries, which included 6108 cases, suggested that daycare attendance was associated with a reduced risk of childhood ALL (OR = 0.76, 95% CI, 0.67–0.87; Fig. 13.1) [13]. Taken together, these data offer strong support for a protective role of exposure to infections in the daycare setting.

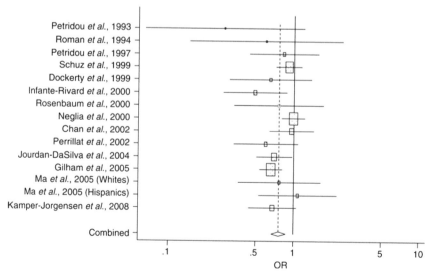

Fig. 13.1 Forest plot displaying ORs and 95% CIs of studies examining the association between daycare attendance and risk of childhood ALL. The risk estimates are plotted with boxes and the area of each box is inversely proportional to the variance of the estimated effect. The horizontal lines represent the 95% CIs of the risk estimate for each study. The solid vertical line at 1.0 represents a risk estimate of no effect. The dashed vertical line represents the combined risk estimate (OR = 0.76), and the width of the diamond is the 95% CI for this risk estimate (0.67–0.87)

13.2.2 Mode of Delivery

The early onset of childhood ALL has prompted studies on the possible etiologic role of maternal reproductive factors and birth characteristics, including the mode of delivery. Compared with vaginal delivery, cesarean section (C-section) is known to modify a newborn's first bacterial community by preventing normal exposure to the vaginal microbiome and to increase levels of stress hormone at birth [14, 15]. C-section delivery may also serve as a marker for conditions that make it difficult for a mother to deliver vaginally (e.g., infections, morphologic abnormalities). Multiple studies have observed associations between C-section and an increased risk of immune-related diseases, such as asthma [16], allergies [17], and type I diabetes [18]. In the United States, the proportion of C-section among all deliveries dramatically increased from 5.8% in 1970 [19] to 32.9% in 2009 [20], and the incidence of childhood ALL also increased continuously over the same period (although not with the same magnitude of increase) [9]. While a few earlier studies of childhood ALL assessed the role of C-section and generated inconsistent findings, recent epidemiological studies have focused on the specific type of C-section, i.e., whether the C-section was elective or emergency. This distinction may be important, since elective vs. emergency C-section reflects different scenarios of exposure. A newborn delivered by elective C-section usually does not experience rupture of the amniotic membrane until surgery, limiting microbial colonization from the birth canal [14], but many emergency C-sections are performed after physical labor has started and the membrane has broken, leading to fetal exposure to maternal vaginal flora. Furthermore, a newborn delivered by elective C-section is expected to have lower levels of stress hormones (e.g., cortisol) than a newborn delivered by emergency C-section, as the physical trauma of labor can trigger a stress response [21].

In a large population-based case-control study that linked birth records and cancer registry data from California and included over 5000 cases and almost 19,000 matched controls, no association was observed between C-section and risk of childhood ALL (age of diagnosis, 0–14 years; OR = 1.03, 95% CI, 0.96–1.10) [22]. When the analysis was restricted to cases diagnosed at 2–4 years and their controls, C-section increased the risk of ALL by 11% (OR = 1.11, 95% CI, 1.01–1.22) compared to vaginal delivery, and the magnitude of association was larger for elective C-section (OR = 1.38, 95% CI, 1.11–1.70) [22]. Emergency C-section, on the other hand, did not appear to influence the risk of childhood ALL diagnosed at 0–14 years or 2–4 years [22]. The design of this study was robust due to the large sample size, low likelihood of selection bias (no need to contact subjects for participation) and recall bias (data on mode of delivery and other covariates were obtained from preexisting record), and the adjustment of many potential confounding factors. The findings are generally consistent with those from a pooled analysis of studies from the Childhood Leukemia International Consortium [23].

While the exact mechanisms for the association between elective C-section and an increased risk of childhood ALL have not been established, the possibility of a reduced exposure to the maternal microbiome at delivery is intriguing. Since the vast majority of the increase in the proportion of C-section among all deliveries over the last few decades is due to increase in elective C-section, it is a potential modifiable risk factor. Interestingly, there is an ongoing clinical trial (ClinicalTrials.gov Identifier, NCT03298334; 2018–2025) evaluating the effect of vaginal seeding on the newborn's microbiome development, immune development, and metabolic outcomes over a 3-year follow-up. Vaginal seeding is a way to deliberately expose C-section-delivered newborns to the maternal microbiome, which involves swabbing a gauze containing the mother's vaginal flora over the face and body of the newborn shortly after cesarean delivery. Given that C-section has also been linked to other types of immune-related diseases, any positive findings from the trial may have important public health implications.

There are also ongoing studies of childhood ALL measuring the level of immunomodulatory cytokines in both maternal pregnancy sera and newborn blood specimens, as well as assessment of maternal-fetal genetic interactions in immune development, in order to elucidate the immunological mechanisms of leukemogenesis. Traditional epidemiological studies can observe an association between an exposure (e.g., daycare attendance, C-section) and a disease (e.g., childhood ALL), which is helpful but far from sufficient. Mechanistic studies aimed at clarifying the underlying biological pathways are a necessary next step to shed light on black-box associations.

13.2.3 Cytomegalovirus Infection

As discussed earlier, a major challenge to understanding the role of infection in the etiology of childhood ALL has been the difficulty in directly measuring infection exposure. Recently, investigators from the California Childhood Leukemia Study conducted a hypothesis-free, agnostic study to search for possible viruses and bacteria that may influence the risk of childhood ALL by leveraging the unique pretreatment diagnostic bone marrow specimens that they had collected from incident cases of childhood ALL and acute myeloid leukemia (AML) [24]. Accounting for about 15% of all leukemia in children, AML is considered to have a distinct etiology in which immunological factors do not play a significant role. As such, AML is sometimes treated as a control group in studies evaluating the association between infection and ALL.

A comprehensive next-generation sequencing-based virome and bacterial metagenomic analysis using pretreatment diagnostic bone marrows from incident cases of childhood ALL and AML revealed a much higher prevalence of cytomegalovirus (CMV) infection at diagnosis in ALL than in AML (OR = 18, 95% CI, 2.04–159.09) [24]. There was also active viral transcription in leukemia blasts as well as the presence of intact virions in serum [24]. Subsequently, a screening of CMV infection in newborn blood samples, which had initially been collected for the purpose of genetic screening but archived for many years, found that childhood ALL cases were significantly more likely to have in utero CMV infection than control subjects who did not have any type of cancer (OR = 3.71, 95% CI, 1.56–7.92) [24]. When the analysis was stratified by ethnicity, the OR was higher for Hispanic children (5.90, 95% CI, 1.89–25.96) than for non-Hispanic white children (2.10, 95% CI, 0.69–7.13) [24]. This study was the first to suggest a specific infectious agent in the etiology of childhood ALL. The strength of the finding was enhanced by the agnostic nature of the search for viruses and bacteria (the investigators had no a priori hypotheses), as well as the confirmation of case-control difference of CMV infection at birth. The contrast between Hispanic and non-Hispanic white children was also intriguing, given that Hispanic children have the highest incidence of ALL among all racial/ethnic groups in the United States.

The CMV finding is currently being replicated by an independent, population-based case-control study funded by the National Cancer Institute (R01CA228478, 2018–2021). If confirmed, it may motivate preventive strategies to reduce maternal transmission of CMV infection to the fetus during pregnancy. While childhood ALL is rare, congenital CMV infection is an established risk factor for sensorineural hearing loss and some other negative health outcomes such as mental retardation and microcephaly [25]. Given that CMV infection is the most common intrauterine infection in the United States and is linked to multiple negative health outcomes [25] and possibly childhood ALL, the public health impact of reducing congenital CMV infection may be substantial.

13.2.4 Immunotherapy for Childhood ALL

Children with ALL often respond well to chemotherapy. Much of the improved survival observed in childhood ALL patients over the last few decades is attributable to more effective chemotherapy regimens that usually include multiple agents. However, there are still patients who do not respond to

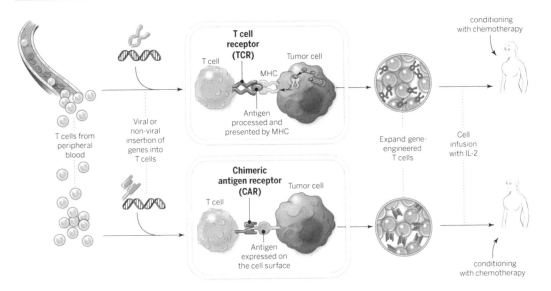

Fig. 13.2 CAR T cells and TCR T cells are engineered to produce special receptors on their surfaces. They are then expanded in the laboratory and returned to the patient. (Credit: National Cancer Institute [26])

chemotherapy or who relapse after achieving remission initially. In August 2017, the Food and Drug Administration approved a type of immunotherapy known as CAR T-cell therapy for patients up to 25 years of age with B-cell ALL that does not respond to treatment or has relapsed twice or more [26]. The treatment is customized for each patient using the patient's T cells, which are genetically modified so that they will produce a protein called a chimeric antigen receptor (CAR) [26]. The receptor has the variable domain of a heavy and light chain from an antibody which binds to the CD19 protein expressed on the tumor cells [26]. The inside of the chimeric receptor has signaling modules that lead to T-cell activation [26] (Fig. 13.2). The T cells are thus directed to the tumor via CD19 recognition and, after activation, kill the tumor. The process to produce CAR-T cells takes about 22 days and involves isolating the cells from the patient, genetically engineering and expanding them in the laboratory and then infusing the patients with these engineered immune cells [26]. With this therapy, remission rates above 80% have been observed, which is remarkable given the previously dismal clinical outcomes for such patients [26].

13.3 Glioma

13.3.1 Epidemiology of Glioma

Originating from the glial tissues in the brain, glioma accounts for approximately 81% of malignant brain tumors and has a poor prognosis [27]. Risk factors for glioma include older age, male sex, white race, radiation, genetic susceptibility, and certain dietary and lifestyle factors [27]. Interestingly, multiple studies have observed an inverse association between allergic conditions and glioma risk – cases with glioma were less likely to report a history of allergies than control subjects [27].

Given the rarity of glioma, most epidemiological studies evaluating its etiology have been case control in design, and biospecimens from cases are collected after diagnosis, sometimes after treatment has begun, which may make it challenging to interpret the level of biomarkers in posttreatment samples. For example, in a case-control study that observed an inverse relationship of allergic conditions with glioma risk, the investigators found that immunoglobulin E (IgE) levels were also lower in glioma patients than controls, but a further examination suggested that the association between IgE levels and case-control status was only limited to patients who were prescribed temozolomide, a drug that inhibits DNA replication in cancer cells, and accounted for 63% of all patients in the study [28]. It was also noted that these patients had significantly lower IgE levels than patients not prescribed temozolomide and temozolomide-taking patients whose blood draw occurred later after diagnosis had IgE levels lower than patients whose blood draw was closer to diagnosis [28]. Because of these observations, it is difficult to draw a firm conclusion about whether the cases and controls had different IgE levels prior to glioma diagnosis, that is, whether IgE levels are important from an etiological perspective. However, the finding that treatment with temozolomide may have impacted IgE levels has implications for immunotherapy.

Another study measured the levels of two serologic markers, soluble CD23 (sCD23), the low-affinity receptor for IgE, and soluble CD14 (sCD14), a macrophage product, which are part of the innate and adaptive humoral immune systems and modulate allergic responses in opposite directions, using blood samples that were drawn from 1079 glioma cases at a single point in time after diagnosis and 736 control subjects [29]. The investigators found that glioma was strongly associated with a high level of sCD14 (OR for highest vs lowest quartile = 3.94, 95% CI, 2.98–5.21) and a low level of sCD23 (OR for lowest vs highest quartile = 2.5, 95% CI, 1.89–3.23) [29]. When they assessed the impact of treatment (temozolomide, dexamethasone, and other medications) on the levels of sCD14 and sCD23, the only significant association was observed between dexamethasone treatment and sCD23 levels, where glioma cases receiving dexamethasone had lower levels of sCD23 than cases not using the same medication [29]. Nevertheless, a significant association between sCD23 and glioma risk persisted regardless of the treatment with dexamethasone [29]. After this additional scrutiny related to treatment, it was reasonable to conclude that the findings support a role of immunoregulatory proteins in the etiology of glioma.

13.3.2 Immunotherapy of Glioma

Unlike many other types of cancer that have benefited from recent progress in immunotherapy, glioma has been a difficult target due to the existence of the blood-brain barrier that prevents antibodies from getting into the brain, the frequent use of steroids as part of disease management that may suppress the immune response, and the distinctively "cold" immune microenvironment (with few immune cells) that makes it hard to activate the host immune system against tumor [30]. Multiple types of immunotherapy, including immune checkpoint inhibitors and CAR T-cell therapy, have been evaluated in glioma patients without any major progress. An area that is being actively pursued is oncolytic virus therapy, in which *a virus is used as a vaccine to stimulate host immune response to cancer*. In July 2018, the results of a Phase 1 clinical trial of a nonpathogenic, replication-competent, recombinant polio-rhinovirus chimera (PVSRIPO) oncolytic virotherapy for recurrent glioblastoma were published by the *New England Journal of Medicine* [31]. Glioblastoma is grade IV glioma and the most aggressive and common type of glioma. Historically, the survival of patients with recurrent glioblastoma is less than 12 months. In this trial, a total of 61 patients received an intratumoral infusion of PVSRIPO from May 2012 to May 2017, and the survival rate among patients who received PVSRIPO immunotherapy was higher at 24 and 36 months than the rate among historical controls [31].

The investigators chose intratumoral infusion to overcome the limitations of the blood-brain barrier, and they decided to examine the therapeutic potential of PVSRIPO, an engineered hybrid of poliovirus and rhinovirus, due to a number of intriguing findings by others in the past. PVSRIPO tropism is determined by CD155, commonly known as the poliovirus receptor [30]. PVSRIPO does not attack neurons but maintains cytotoxicity in neoplastic cells, which makes it a great candidate for the treatment of glioma [30]. PVSRIPO has been demonstrated to stimulate anticancer immunity by two mechanisms: lysing tumor cells to release a mix of tumor and viral antigens and sublethally infecting antigen-presenting cells, thereby stimulating an interferon-driven immune response in the tumor microenvironment [30]. Of course, the clinical utility of PVSRIPO is not yet clear with only a Phase 1 trial, but the initial finding is promising. More importantly, PVSRIPO is only one of many oncolytic viruses that are being actively tested in clinical trials of various phases. Other oncolytic viruses include engineered forms of herpes simplex virus type 1 and adenovirus. Collectively, these oncolytic therapies have demonstrated a capability to turn the cold immune environment to a "hot" environment with a higher level of immune cells and to elicit an immune response against tumors [32].

13.4   Concluding Remarks

For many years, cancer was considered a chronic disease that had little commenality with infectious diseases. Students interested in studying epidemiology often faced a choice of sub-specialization, and chronic disease epidemiology and infectious disease epidemiology were presented as two distinct options. However, it is now clear that these two types of diseases are intertwined and that infection plays an important role in the etiology of many types of cancer.

Treatment modalities for cancer had been limited to surgery, radiation therapy, and chemotherapy up until the 1990s. Even after the first cancer immunotherapy was approved by the Food and Drug Administration in the 1990s, immunotherapy did not enter the mainstream until the last few years. With breakthroughs in knowledge about how the immune system functions and how to harness the power of the immune system, we embrace an exciting new era for the development of paradigm-changing immunotherapies.

References

1. Nagai H, Kim YH. Cancer prevention from the perspective of global cancer burden patterns. J Thorac Dis. 2017;9(3):448–51.
2. Hanahan D, Weinberg RA. Hallmarks of cancer: the next generation. Cell. 2011;144(5):646–74.
3. Vesely MD, Kershaw MH, Schreiber RD, Smyth MJ. Natural innate and adaptive immunity to cancer. Annu Rev Immunol. 2011;29:235–71.
4. El-Serag HB. Epidemiology of viral hepatitis and hepatocellular carcinoma. Gastroenterology. 2012;142(6): 1264–73 e1.
5. Palefsky JM. Human papillomavirus infections: Epidemiology and disease associations. Available from: https://www.uptodate.com/contents/human-papillomavirus-infections-epidemiology-and-disease-associations.
6. Testerman TL, Morris J. Beyond the stomach: an updated view of helicobacter pylori pathogenesis, diagnosis, and treatment. World J Gastroenterol. 2014;20(36):12781–808.
7. Steele CB, Thomas CC, Henley SJ, Massetti GM, Galuska DA, Agurs-Collins T, et al. Vital signs: trends in incidence of cancers associated with overweight and obesity – United States, 2005–2014. MMWR Morb Mortal Wkly Rep. 2017;66(39):1052–8.
8. Alsaab HO, Sau S, Alzhrani R, Tatiparti K, Bhise K, Kashaw SK, et al. PD-1 and PD-L1 checkpoint signaling inhibition for cancer immunotherapy: mechanism, combinations, and clinical outcome. Front Pharmacol. 2017;8:561.
9. Edwards BK, Noone AM, Mariotto AB, Simard EP, Boscoe FP, Henley SJ, et al. Annual report to the nation on the status of cancer, 1975–2010, featuring prevalence of comorbidity and impact on survival among persons with lung, colorectal, breast, or prostate cancer. Cancer. 2014;120(9):1290–314.
10. Ma X, Buffler PA, Wiemels JL, Selvin S, Metayer C, Loh M, et al. Ethnic difference in daycare attendance, early infections, and risk of childhood acute lymphoblastic leukemia. Cancer Epidemiol Biomark Prev. 2005;14(8):1928–34.

11. Greaves MF, Alexander FE. An infectious etiology for common acute lymphoblastic leukemia in childhood? Leukemia. 1993;7(3):349–60.
12. Kinlen L. Evidence for an infective cause of childhood leukaemia: comparison of a Scottish new town with nuclear reprocessing sites in Britain. Lancet. 1988;2(8624):1323–7.
13. Urayama KY, Buffler PA, Gallagher ER, Ayoob JM, Ma X. A meta-analysis of the association between day-care attendance and childhood acute lymphoblastic leukaemia. Int J Epidemiol. 2010;39(3):718–32.
14. Dominguez-Bello MG, Costello EK, Contreras M, Magris M, Hidalgo G, Fierer N, et al. Delivery mode shapes the acquisition and structure of the initial microbiota across multiple body habitats in newborns. Proc Natl Acad Sci U S A. 2010;107(26):11971–5.
15. Mears K, McAuliffe F, Grimes H, Morrison JJ. Fetal cortisol in relation to labour, intrapartum events and mode of delivery. J Obstet Gynaecol. 2004;24(2):129–32.
16. Thavagnanam S, Fleming J, Bromley A, Shields MD, Cardwell CR. A meta-analysis of the association between Caesarean section and childhood asthma. Clin Exp Allergy. 2008;38(4):629–33.
17. Bager P, Wohlfahrt J, Westergaard T. Caesarean delivery and risk of atopy and allergic disease: meta-analyses. Clin Exp Allergy. 2008;38(4):634–42.
18. Cardwell CR, Stene LC, Joner G, Cinek O, Svensson J, Goldacre MJ, et al. Caesarean section is associated with an increased risk of childhood-onset type 1 diabetes mellitus: a meta-analysis of observational studies. Diabetologia. 2008;51(5):726–35.
19. Placek PJ, Taffel SM. Trends in cesarean section rates for the United States, 1970–78. Public Health Rep. 1980;95(6):540–8.
20. Martin JA, Hamilton BE, Ventura SJ, Osterman MJ, Kirmeyer S, Mathews TJ, et al. Births: final data for 2009. Natl Vital Stat Rep. 2011;60(1):1–70.
21. Hyde MJ, Mostyn A, Modi N, Kemp PR. The health implications of birth by Caesarean section. Biol Rev Camb Philos Soc. 2012;87(1):229–43.
22. Wang R, Wiemels JL, Metayer C, Morimoto L, Francis SS, Kadan-Lottick N, et al. Cesarean section and risk of childhood acute lymphoblastic leukemia in a population-based, record-linkage study in California. Am J Epidemiol. 2017;185(2):96–105.
23. Marcotte EL, Thomopoulos TP, Infante-Rivard C, Clavel J, Petridou ET, Schuz J, et al. Caesarean delivery and risk of childhood leukaemia: a pooled analysis from the Childhood Leukemia International Consortium (CLIC). Lancet Haematol. 2016;3(4):e176–85.
24. Francis SS, Wallace AD, Wendt GA, Li L, Liu F, Riley LW, et al. In utero cytomegalovirus infection and development of childhood acute lymphoblastic leukemia. Blood. 2017;129(12):1680–4.
25. Rawlinson WD, Boppana SB, Fowler KB, Kimberlin DW, Lazzarotto T, Alain S, et al. Congenital cytomegalovirus infection in pregnancy and the neonate: consensus recommendations for prevention, diagnosis, and therapy. Lancet Infect Dis. 2017;17(6):e177–e88.
26. CAR T-cell therapy approved for some children and young adults with leukemia 2017. Available from: https://www.cancer.gov/news-events/cancer-currents-blog/2017/tisagenlecleucel-fda-childhood-leukemia.
27. Ostrom QT, Bauchet L, Davis FG, Deltour I, Fisher JL, Langer CE, et al. The epidemiology of glioma in adults: a "state of the science" review. Neuro-Oncology. 2014;16(7):896–913.
28. Wiemels JL, Wilson D, Patil C, Patoka J, McCoy L, Rice T, et al. IgE, allergy, and risk of glioma: update from the San Francisco Bay Area Adult Glioma Study in the temozolomide era. Int J Cancer. 2009;125(3):680–7.
29. Zhou M, Wiemels JL, Bracci PM, Wrensch MR, McCoy LS, Rice T, et al. Circulating levels of the innate and humoral immune regulators CD14 and CD23 are associated with adult glioma. Cancer Res. 2010;70(19):7534–42.
30. Brown MC, Holl EK, Boczkowski D, Dobrikova E, Mosaheb M, Chandramohan V, et al. Cancer immunotherapy with recombinant poliovirus induces IFN-dominant activation of dendritic cells and tumor antigen-specific CTLs. Sci Transl Med. 2017;9(408). pii: eaan4220.
31. Desjardins A, Gromeier M, Herndon JE 2nd, Beaubier N, Bolognesi DP, Friedman AH, et al. Recurrent glioblastoma treated with recombinant poliovirus. N Engl J Med. 2018;379(2):150–61.
32. Galon J, Bruni D. Approaches to treat immune hot, altered and cold tumours with combination immunotherapies. Nat Rev Drug Discov. 2019;18(3):197–218.

IMMUNOEPIDEMIOLOGIC INVESTIGATIVE, THERAPEUTIC, AND PREVENTATIVE TOOLS

Modeling Approaches Toward Understanding Infectious Disease Transmission

Laura A. Skrip and Jeffrey P. Townsend

14.1 Introduction

The global burden of morbidity and mortality associated with communicable diseases is nearly three times that of cancer and 70% higher than that of cardiovascular disease [1]. Much of the infectious disease burden is caused by diseases that have a long history in human populations, such as measles, influenza, and pertussis. In recent years, additional disease burden has emerged from outbreaks of HIV, Chikungunya, Zika virus, *Ebola virus*, Middle East respiratory syndrome, coronavirus, *Nipah virus*, and Lassa fever, underscoring the continued vulnerability of human populations to novel and re-emerging threats. Mathematical models of infectious disease can be used to understand and predict epidemiological trajectories of outbreaks; they can then be applied to optimize strategies for mitigating disease transmission. These models incorporate pertinent environmental factors, such as seasonal fluctuations, that affect survival or activity of pathogens and their vectors. They can also address complexities of host behavioral change, including local and global human societal changes, health policy, clinical trial design, and resource allocation, which have been increasingly guided by modeling studies.

The epidemiology of infectious diseases and their control is complex. While models can be structured to represent the intricacies of a disease system, the quality of the information they provide depends on balancing existing data, methodological rigor, and simplifying assumptions. Here we describe factors influencing disease transmission, including both mechanisms of microbial infection and host behavior. We then discuss how model structure and parameterization are optimally used for addressing research and policy questions in the context of available information.

14.2 Biological Aspects of DiseaseTransmission

The spread and control of infectious diseases are related to biological factors that impact the magnitude, timing, and route of transmission.

L. A. Skrip
Department of Epidemiology of Microbial Disease, Yale School of Public Health, New Haven, CT, USA

J. P. Townsend (✉)
Department of Biostatistics, Yale School of Public Health, Yale University, New Haven, CT, USA
e-mail: jeffrey.townsend@yale.edu

© Springer Nature Switzerland AG 2019
P. J. Krause et al. (eds.), *Immunoepidemiology*, https://doi.org/10.1007/978-3-030-25553-4_14

14.2.1 Mode of Transmission

Transmission could result from direct contact between hosts, could require host-environment interaction, or could be mediated by a vector—often a phlebotomine insect—that transmits a pathogen between different hosts. Transmission can also vary across strata of the host population, as subgroups determined by behavioral, genetic, demographic, environmental, or other characteristics may result in differential exposure or susceptibility to specific diseases. Much of the art and science of modeling rides on critically evaluating which factors are essential to include in order to generate quantitative understanding of a focal research question.

14.2.2 Course of Infection and Infectiousness

Beyond accounting for the change in number of infected individuals over time, it can be important to also incorporate the course of infection during which microbial load, symptom severity, and contact behavior may all vary. Infection progression, or "age of infection," is associated with temporal changes in infectiousness. Microbiological studies that measure the change in pathogen load over the course of an infection are integral to parameterization of dynamic models of disease, particularly evaluating interventions as the timing of intervention during the infection period could impact predicted effectiveness.

14.3 Behavior and Disease Transmission

The behaviors of human hosts, reservoir hosts, and vectors are fundamental to risks of both infection and transmission to others. For nonhuman hosts and vectors, the geographical distribution of habitat, feeding preferences, and proximity to humans affect the rate of transmission. For human hosts, contact patterns, belief systems, attitudes about public health recommendations, and propensity to seek care impact the real-world effectiveness of infection control measures, including quarantining, school closures, handwashing, and vaccination. To some extent, behavioral effects are implicit in the measures of transmission that are used in and estimated by models. However, in many cases it can be more appropriate to treat the transmission rate as a dynamic variable that evolves in concert with behaviors associated with the epidemic. This approach has been increasingly adopted when changes in willingness to accept interventions, in public health policy, or in disease awareness are expected to impact a component (i.e., contact rate, probability of transmission given contact, or frequencies of susceptible and infectious individuals) of overall transmission [2–6].

14.3.1 Willingness to Accept Interventions

Interventions, such as vaccination, have been instrumental in reducing the prevalence and incidence of many infectious diseases, particularly those affecting children, but they are only as effective as the extent to which individuals are willing to accept them. Vaccine scares exemplify the mutual feedback between host behavior and disease dynamics: low vaccine coverage can increase the probability of disease outbreaks. As disease outbreaks occur, people can become increasingly eager to vaccinate, which in turn reduces transmission. Thus, changes in incidence are mediated by behavior-based changes in the susceptibility of population members [5].

A challenge to tackling vaccine scares and other extreme reactions is that the human mind typically overestimates the risk of highly improbable events when the thought of such events evokes fear and anxiety [7]. Human risk perception is based on potential threats to one's immediate community—historically, populations of hundreds in geographically isolated areas. However, with the shift to a more global community, our intuitive understanding of risk has adapted in ways that foster overreaction. Increased awareness of international political and health crises and a sense of connectedness to regions simply an airplane flight away have led to a "problem of scale." Teasing apart the influence of such factors from individual risk perception will be critical to determining how a model can represent elimination efforts within a given population.

14.3.2 Public Health Policy and Disease Awareness

In most cases of emerging or neglected diseases, vaccines are not available. Public health authorities must rely on other infection control methods, such as isolation of infected cases, quarantine of potentially exposed individuals, vector control, and/or social mobilization campaigns to enhance behavior change. Some authorities may enact recommendations and policies that increase social distancing, by which gatherings of individuals in affected areas are reduced through school or workplace closures. One approach to capturing how social distancing approaches reduce transmission is to model the social network explicitly, as opposed to assuming homogeneous mixing within the population. For instance, school networks could be superimposed on a dynamic model, keeping track of school-age individuals in the population and calculating their risks of infection as a function of transmission in both schools and the wider community. Even in the absence of enforced policies, individuals often spontaneously reduce their contacts in response to an outbreak by keeping children home from school, washing their hands more frequently, or avoiding public transit [8]. Such behavior change can be represented in a network model by incorporating a contact rate between network neighbors that depends on local rather than overall disease prevalence in the network [6].

Host behavioral factors are linked with epidemiological characteristics like mode of transmission. In the case of potentially airborne-transmitted and highly infectious measles, vaccination is one of the most effective interventions; therefore, population concern about vaccine safety must be addressed. In contrast, no vaccine was available in the initial phase of the 2014–2015 *Ebola* epidemic; because *Ebola virus* can easily be transmitted through close contact with the deceased, population attitudes toward funerary customs had to be addressed. Such examples also illustrate the mutual feedback that operates between host behavior and disease dynamics, wherein human behavior impacts transmission (e.g., reduced infection prevalence due to greater uptake of vaccines or participation in public health recommendations), but epidemiological trajectories can also influence behavior as perceptions of infection risk evolve. Such coupled behavior-disease systems can be represented by embedding dynamic transmission models within game theoretic or other behavioral frameworks. The resulting models can be informed by data regarding contact patterns and decision-making, as well as how the incubation period and the mode of transmission interact with host risk perception.

14.4 Infectious Disease Model Frameworks

Traditional biostatistical approaches (e.g., using regression techniques to identify predictor variables for specific epidemiological outcomes) focus on identifying associations between variables that may implicate causal relationships between them. In contrast, mathematical models of infectious disease are constructed by describing mechanistic processes that can include transmission between hosts, immunological responses to pathogens within hosts, and vector ecological dynamics, among other dynamics. Simulation of the model then demonstrates how assumptions and existing information about the disease system relate to transmission dynamics.

14.4.1 Model Structures

There are myriad model frameworks that can be employed to account for host (e.g., age, sex, immunodeficiency) and environmental (e.g., climate conditions, prevalence of disease-carrying and disease-transmitting insects) factors of disease transmission in order to answer diverse epidemiological questions (Box 14.1, Fig. 14.1). Consequently, the ideal model structure for addressing particular research questions depends on the pertinent biological aspects of disease.

Box 14.1 Recent Methodological Innovations at the Frontier of Disease Transmission Modeling

Recent methodological innovations have expanded the applicability of disease transmission modeling as a tool to inform scientists and policy-makers before they undertake field research, laboratory experimentation, or program implementation.

1. Improvements in the rigor of field study and trial design

   Epidemiological modeling techniques can be applied to simulate different trial designs and conduct power analyses prior to implementation. With the rapid development of vaccines against *Ebola virus* disease during the 2014–2015 outbreak in West Africa, field testing of the vaccines in high transmission settings was undertaken to simultaneously assess efficacy and prevent new cases among at-risk contacts. Modeling analyses determined false-positive rates and power across ranges of *Ebola* vaccine efficacy and trial start dates, comparing the stepped wedge and randomized controlled trial (RCT) designs [13]. Modeling revealed that the RCT design could achieve higher power for a given vaccine efficacy, largely due to the spatiotemporal variation in incidence and thus transmission risk.

   For interventions that have already been tested and deemed effective, modeling can be used to determine optimal population coverage levels or to evaluate targeting of subsets of the population that exhibit distinct transmission dynamics and/or disease outcomes.

2. Evaluation of endgame strategies

   Several tropical diseases are slated for local elimination or global eradication via mass administration of inexpensive drugs or via heightened awareness and the adoption of preventive behaviors. Endgame strategies to achieve and maintain elimination of disease in areas with low incidence can be evaluated using mathematical modeling. It is important to identify characteristics of remaining cases and incorporate them into the model through stratification of compartments or of individuals, in the case of an agent-based model, by risk of infection. Similarly, any individuals who are responsible for the bulk of transmission, such as due to genetic predisposition to high microbial loads, should be included within the model structure as superspreaders (Box 14.2). Modeling was used to inform onchocerciasis elimination efforts in West Africa. Administration of ivermectin was considered across transmission settings to determine what duration of treatment would be necessary to achieve local fadeout of disease [42].

(continued)

Box 14.1 (continued)

3. Guidance for health economic policy

Mathematical modeling can be used to guide decision-makers in developing policies. Cost-effectiveness analyses consider whether a particular intervention may not only have health benefits but also economic benefit. For instance, a preventative strategy may avert both adverse health outcomes as well as significant expenses associated with treatment. Traditional cost-effectiveness analysis does not incorporate ongoing transmission. Consequently, it has been assumed that when an individual is vaccinated, only that individual is protected. By combining cost-effectiveness analysis with a dynamic transmission model, the positive externality that vaccination has in terms of reducing transmission within the population can be incorporated. Such models have spurred change, such as in the case of the decision by the UK National Health Services to offer rotavirus vaccination for infants nationally [43], a policy previously deemed to be insufficiently cost-effective for the UK. As another example, results from a multi-host model of rabies transmission revealed that rabies vaccination of dogs is a cost-effective approach for preventing human disease in Tanzania, lending support for canine vaccination campaigns in the country [37].

4. Phylodynamics

Phylodynamic analysis of disease uses dated molecular sequencing of organisms to understand the implications of their evolutionary relationships on the epidemiology of disease. Specifically, such phylogenetic information provides insight into branching events or the timing of between-host transmission, such as zoonoses, and thus can inform parameters in models of disease systems [17]. Novel applications of phylodynamic approaches can estimate previously inestimable quantities such as the rates of underreporting or the numbers of subclinical infections by reconstructing transmission trees [44].

5. Big data applications

Big data refers to massive volumes of often unstructured data that require complex tools for their analysis. Evolving trends in everyday use of technology (e.g., social media, Google searches, cell phone usage) and improved computational capacity have provided novel sources of information about human interaction and behavior as well as ways to manipulate it, respectively. Open-source repositories have likewise made the data accessible for researchers of varied fields [17]. For instance, a recent modeling study investigating the global spread of *Zika virus* [45] incorporated large-scale flight itinerary data from the International Air Transport Association and a global population dataset to determine likely international dispersion pathways of the disease.

6. Probabilistic sensitivity analysis and uncertainty analysis

Uncertainty analysis (Box 14.2) and probabilistic sensitivity analysis (Box 14.2) have advanced the robustness of model fitting and the evaluation of model findings, respectively. Historically, model parameters have been calibrated to available data in an ad hoc manner [17]. Uncertainty analysis can be performed by Bayesian and semi-Bayesian approaches that evaluate a probable distribution of candidate parameter values from a prior distribution and/or their

(continued)

Box 14.1 (continued)

likelihood of producing model output that matches empirical data. Bayesian fitting methods [22] include Bayesian melding, Markov chain Monte Carlo integration, approximate Bayesian computation, particle filtering, and application of weighted Bayesian information criteria; Bayesian methods frequently supply a natural means to blend the empirical data being used for fitting (e.g., prevalence or incidence data) with other data from the literature (e.g., duration of infection, incubation period, and measures of relative infectiousness such as viral load). The posterior distributions of probable estimates that result from such methods characterize ranges of output that are appropriately influenced by but not entirely dictated by small sets of field data. Extension of Bayesian analyses to implement probabilistic sensitivity analysis is also straight-forward and provides rigorous evaluation of model assumptions by considering the change in model output when drawing from ranges of empirically supported inputs [11]. These procedures of uncertainty analysis and probabilistic sensitivity analysis allow modelers to better guide public health decision-makers on the full range of potential transmission and intervention effectiveness outcomes.

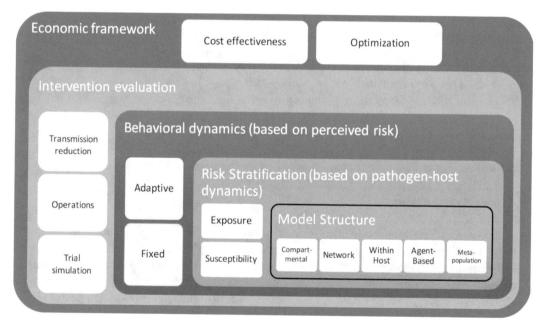

Fig. 14.1 Extension of transmission models to increase integration with field studies and public health policy relevance. The selected infectious disease model structure varies with the system being modeled and the research question, as outlined previously [9, 10]. A basic model design can be extended to include heterogeneity in biological susceptibility or exposure to infection. Exposure that varies due to behavioral dynamics can be accounted for as a fixed measure whereby a proportion of the affected population is involved in intervention with some level of adherence or as a dynamic measure that changes with time in response to increased awareness of disease. These extensions enhance the ability of the model to accurately estimate the effectiveness of interventions and thus estimate the costs of implementing strategies relative to changes in outcome measures

Box 14.2 Glossary of Terms

Superspreaders: Superspreaders are hosts that are responsible for the majority of transmission due to predisposition to high-intensity infection or behavior that results in heightened risk of exposure.

Network theory: In the context of infectious disease modeling, network models account for connections between social entities, such as individuals or groups of individuals who interact directly within the same household or community. Incorporating networks is one strategy that modelers can use to address systems where there is differential transmission risk for different groups within the network, where transmission occurs through close contact, or wherever the assumption of homogeneous mixing is inadequate.

Agent-based model: Agent-based models explicitly represent each individual in a system. For example, an outbreak of a nosocomial infection could be modeled by considering each patient and health-care worker within a hospital. The exposure history of each individual is tracked to generate probabilities of infection rather than modeling population-level rates of infection. However, the data requirements of informing parameters for each individual are often prohibitive.

Metapopulation model: A metapopulation includes many distinct subpopulations—often corresponding to spatial regions—that interact within and between themselves. Spatial meta-population models can be used to represent the geographical dissemination of diseases, potentially parameterized by mobility data. For example, disease may be eliminated in one region, but due to migration from a neighboring region, it may later resurge.

Force of infection: The force of infection (FOI) is a measure of transmission. It is the rate at which individuals (e.g., human hosts, nonhuman hosts, vectors, body cells) become infected with a pathogen. In a mathematical model, the FOI is a mathematical function that determines the rate of transition between states. It is calculated using several parameters that account for the rate of contact between infectious individuals and susceptible (i.e., uninfected and nonimmune) individuals, the probability of successful pathogen transmission given contact, and the density or frequency of susceptible and infectious individuals in the population.

Behavioral economics: The field of behavioral economics focuses on how individual decisions are affected by psychological, social, and cognitive factors. Human behavior often deviates from what simple economic models predict rational decisions should be. These deviations can impact epidemiologically pertinent factors such as vaccination decisions or risk-related behaviors.

Prospect theory: Prospect theory is a behavioral economic theory of decision-making among probabilistic alternatives when the probabilities of different outcomes are known.

Likelihood fitting procedures: Likelihood fitting procedures involve developing an equation, or likelihood function, that calculates the probability of the data given a set of model parameters. Thus, parameters—whose values are unknown—can be estimated by maximizing the likelihood of observed data. For some multiparameter models with complex likelihood surfaces, identifying the set of parameters that maximizes the likelihood can be challenging. Diverse methods, such as the Newton-Raphson optimization algorithm, Markov chain Monte Carlo (MCMC), and simulated annealing approaches, have been developed to identify peaks of the likelihood surface corresponding to parameter values that are a good fit to data.

Probabilistic sensitivity analysis: Model outputs can be determined using best-fit point estimates for model parameters, as defined by experimental or field data or by fitting procedures. In a sensitivity analysis, the model outputs are then re-evaluated by varying parameter values

(continued)

Box 14.2 (continued)

slightly above and below the point estimate. The model is considered more sensitive to parameters for which small perturbations lead to large changes in model outputs. If individual parameter values are sampled in proportion to their probability, the sensitivity analysis is probabilistic.

Joint uncertainty distribution: Data rarely provide a precise value for a model parameter; that is, its value is considered uncertain. To best represent this uncertainty, a distribution of possible parameter values can be specified based on the data that are available. Model outcomes can be calculated based on serial draws from this distribution to determine a distribution of possible outcomes. If multiple model parameters are uncertain but correlated, then a joint distribution that simultaneously represents the effect of their combined uncertainty on the model output can be used to yield a distribution of outcomes that reflects uncertainty in parameterization.

Uncertainty analysis: An uncertainty analysis produces model output that takes into account uncertain parameter estimates for which available field or experimental data are missing or sparse. By iteratively drawing from a distribution of possible parameter values and running the model each time, a distribution of probable model output (versus just a single-point estimate) is produced. A full uncertainty analysis involves drawing from distributions for all uncertain parameters with each iteration of the model. When multiple outcomes are possible, a full uncertainty analysis can provide policy-makers quantification of which outcomes are more likely than others.

Game theoretic analysis: Game theory formalizes strategic decision-making in a group. The payoff of one's decision-making process depends on what other individuals decide, the information they have, the options they are presented with, and the perceived outcomes of each decision.

Nash equilibrium: In game theory, the Nash equilibrium refers to a solution to a problem where none of the decision-makers would benefit from opting for a different choice after becoming aware of other players' choices.

One common model structure is the compartmental model (Fig. 14.2), which divides a population into compartments depending on disease or demographic states. For instance, an SIR compartmental model categorizes individuals as susceptible (S), infected (I), and recovered (R). Individuals transition between compartments at rates that reflect population-level averages and according to difference equations (for discrete time) or differential equations (for continuous time). The SIR compartments provide a dynamic framework enabling current knowledge of historical disease prevalence and/or incidence, infection duration, and immunity to inform future predictions. They can be expanded on to arbitrary complexity—for instance, to model disease progression within the compartmental framework, the infection compartments can be divided into different phases. Depending on the disease, the stratifications may include a latency period modeled by moving susceptible individuals to a transitory compartment for those who have been exposed but are not yet infectious. In this way, the standard SIR model becomes an SEIR model (Fig. 14.2). For HIV, stratifying the infectious compartment I by thresholds of CD4 levels that interplay with viral load, symptoms, and transmissibility has often been incorporated into assessments of criteria for treatment.

14.4.2 Modeling Assumptions and Approaches

A basic assumption underlying compartmental models is that the hosts within a population mix homogeneously, such that individuals interact uniformly across compartments. Nonetheless, heterogeneity within host populations can be incorporated by stratifying compartments according

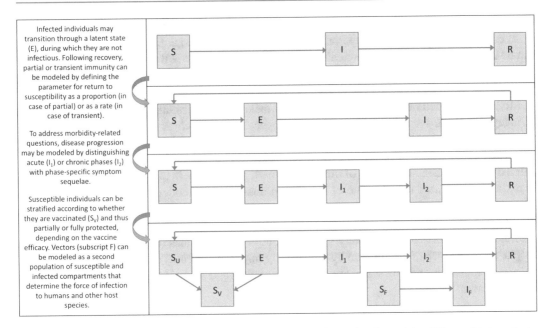

Fig. 14.2 Models are constructed with close accordance to the hypotheses that the models will be used to investigate. The structure of most disease transmission models is based on compartmentalizing individuals into categories of susceptible (S), infected (I), and—depending on the disease mechanism—recovered (R) with immunity. Additional model complexity could involve including a latency compartment (E) during which individuals are not infectious. Each arrow between compartments represents a directional rate of transition (or parameter) which is ideally informed by empirical data. Simple compartmental models are limited in their ability to capture complex disease systems; model extensions such as risk stratification and other model structures with finer units of transmission may be considered depending on the availability of sufficient data for parameterization

to, for example, age and risk factors that affect likelihoods of disease states. When a pathogen is composed of multiple antigenic strains that each elicit distinct immunological responses—such as is the case for pneumococci or human papilloma viruses—it could be important to stratify the immune state of the host according to strain-specific immunity. Stratifying by strain-specific immunity, for example, would permit accurate evaluation of the effectiveness of a vaccine that only covers a subset of the circulating strains. However, stratification should be used sparingly in deterministic compartment models, to reflect salient features of the epidemiological dynamics: as stratifications expand, the number of equations needed to describe transitions between compartments can exceed the number of host individuals in the population. If multifactorial stratification is necessary, it can become more efficient to adopt an agent-based framework (Box 14.2) in which the progression of each individual host is tracked through model states. In an agent-based model, each rate of disease transmission and progression is attributed specifically for every individual. However, agent-based models can only perform better to the extent that they can capture real information about contact mixing in the population. Availability of sufficient data with which to parameterize such individual-level specificities is a principal challenge in the development of agent-based models (Box 14.2).

For both compartmental and agent-based models, the "unit" represented could be a single human or nonhuman host or families or communities thereof, vectors that transmit pathogens between hosts, or body cells (as could be the case for within-host modeling). Other frameworks, including network models (Box 14.2), incorporate relationships between groupings of individuals, such as social connections or ecological niches of relevance to disease transmission. Scaling up from representing a single population to a group of populations, metapopulation models (Box 14.2) can be used to incorporate spatial heterogeneity in disease risk factors. Within-host models can be used to evaluate immunological responses and pharmacokinetics of treatment by simulating dynamics at the cellular or even molecular level such that population-level trends can be inferred.

Models are sometimes criticized because they make such deterministic predictions in the face of many stochastic factors that are known to impact spread, such as the location of any initial zoonotic transmission, the behavior of initial cases in an outbreak, weather conditions, or relevant failures of public health infrastructure. Such stochastic factors have a pronounced impact on population dynamics when the number of infected is small, such occurs in phases of disease emergence or extinction. Because the outcome of simulating deterministic models is always the same for a given set of parameters and initial conditions (e.g., population size and relative numbers of susceptible and infected individuals), incorporation of stochasticity into models enables probabilistic predictions that can quantify unlikely but highly important outcomes (e.g., persistence of disease despite a high chance of elimination by temporarily imposed measures). In stochastic simulations, individual transitions among states are counted explicitly and are probabilistically determined by random draws.

14.4.3　Model Outputs: Measure of Disease Transmission

A historically dominant measure of disease transmission is the basic reproductive number, R_0, defined as the average number of secondary infections caused by a single primary infection in a naïve host population. If R_0 is greater than 1, an epidemic will typically invade a population. Sustained transmission is expected in the absence of control interventions and until the population develops sufficient herd immunity; even if the population develops herd immunity from infection, recurrent epidemics are likely to occur with the waning of immunity or with incoming births that are immunologically naive. R_0 is a property of the causative agent that cannot be measured independent of the context in which contact between susceptible and infectious individuals occurs, reflecting the probability of pathogen transmission given contact as well as the duration of infectiousness.

While R_0 provides a threshold for disease emergence, it does not incorporate the length of time over which transmission occurs. For example, the R_0 values for influenza and for HIV have both been estimated at around 2 for specific settings [9], yet the epidemiological trajectories of these two diseases are dramatically different because the time period over which each infected host exposes two other hosts differs dramatically between the pathogens. Individuals with influenza remain infectious for about a week, while those with HIV can remain infectious for several months to years in the absence of treatment. Thus, to project epidemic curves and to estimate the timescales of outbreaks, the generation time (Box 14.2) of an infection is essential. Generation time, in turn, is determined by the within-host progression of infection as well as mode of transmission. R_0 can be elaborated on by quantifying the effective reproductive number, R_e, which is the average number of secondary infections caused by a single primary infection in a host population with some pre-existing immunity caused by vaccination or previous infection. Because pre-existing immunity is typically present to some degree, interventions that suppress R_e below 1 are predicted to control and ultimately eliminate the disease. This deterministic threshold is one basis for policy decisions regarding the level of interventions that should be implemented to eradicate a microbial disease. However, an intervention that brings R_e to a level just below 1 is only about 50% likely to actually do so [11] as its calculation is dependent on the accuracy of all parameters estimated.

Setting the level of intervention and calculating R_e for a set of samples from the joint uncertainty distribution (Box 14.2) of all the parameters provide the probability of disease elimination in that control scenario. Public health decision-makers—who realize that with imperfect data there is uncertainty associated with all policies—can then weigh the cost of intervention against the potential for failure based on the probabilities of specific outcomes occurring under stated scenarios of intervention [11].

Mathematical models have been developed to assess the epidemiological and health economic impact of alternative intervention approaches across a range of transmission scenarios and implementation strategies [12]. They are particularly valuable when used prior to investment in large-scale field trials or policy changes—that is, when they can be applied to evaluate likely reductions in disease burden or implementation costs. Additional innovations in modeling applications and methodologies (Box 14.1) have enabled the optimization of trial designs to maximize statistical power and feasibility [13], the evaluation of synergistic or antagonistic roles of coinfection in terms of morbidity risk [14], the incorporation of population behavior and perceptions toward vaccines and other interventions [3, 4], and the inference of previously immeasurable quantities such as the relative contributions of different host groups and subgroups to transmission [15, 16]. Compartmental, stratified compartmental, network, and agent-based models lie along a continuum of increasing resolution into individuality. Fine-grained models have an appeal because of the potential to account for inhomogeneities that cannot be easily captured with models that group individuals into classes. However, the more idiosyncratic, complex, or realistic we make a model, the less likely we will have the data to verify our assumptions are valid and the more computationally burdensome our analysis will be. Fortunately, a number of advances in infectious disease transmission modeling have broadened the utility of models by capitalizing on current knowledge and extant data to answer scientific questions and address infection control challenges.

14.4.4 Data-Driven Model Parameterization

The growing repositories of experimental, epidemiological, and clinical data, along with new and less traditional sources such as from social media, provide a wealth of information to enhance the capacity of disease transmission models to address public health questions [17, 18]. Such models are driven by a set of basic functions and parameters, including the rate of transmission, latency duration, infectious period, and waning of immunity. Values to inform parameters are derived from available surveillance data and published findings of observational studies, laboratory studies, and clinical trials, sometimes by using assumptions regarding applicability. For example, a natural history study on pneumococcal infections in children [19, 20] could be used to parameterize the attack rates for specific strains of *Streptococcus pneumoniae* across other age groups. Even small datasets that on their own do little to constrain a parameter can be informative using likelihood fitting procedures. See Box 14.2 that can draw upon that information in combination with other parameter constraints and primary epidemiological data such as prevalence and incidence rates. In Bayesian, or semi-Bayesian approaches, prior information based on small datasets can be usefully incorporated as a weak prior probability distribution for the parameter. Information from previous studies and the fit to current empirical data are increasingly being evaluated simultaneously with Bayesian or semi-Bayesian methods (see Box 14.1; [21, 22]). Incorporation of prior data that is informative about model parameters aids in the fitting of complex models with many parameters. Recent computational advances have rendered more complex models increasingly tractable; however, a healthy skepticism with regard to whether data is reliably informative must be applied to ensure predictions are well-founded. Moreover, with complexity come additional challenges adequately exploring parameter space in the performance of model fitting. A complex model without sufficient data for parameterization can yield wildly inaccurate predictions—even when it has been constructed with a highly realistic, detailed structure and an excellent perceived fit to primary epidemiological data. Therefore, structural complexity and the number of model parameters should be kept to an informative minimum [23, 24].

Infectious disease datasets are frequently limited, in which case probabilistic sensitivity analysis (Box 14.2) of parameters and full uncertainty analysis (Box 14.2) of key outcomes can be conducted to provide an overview of the robustness of model findings. Sensitivity analysis can be performed by varying the values of parameters above and below the best point estimates and re-evaluating the model output. For instance, a cost-effectiveness study of rotavirus vaccination in Canada included a sensitivity analysis to evaluate how the net benefit of vaccination was affected by changes in population-level risk of rotavirus gastroenteritis [25]. Significant seasonal variation has been observed in rotavirus disease risk, and, even when accounting for variation in season of birth, rotavirus immunization remained a highly cost-effective strategy for British Columbia, Canada [25]. When results vary significantly with perturbation to an empirically uncertain parameter (i.e., a parameter whose value has only been established by minimal field or experimental data), a distribution of probable values—rather than just a single-point estimate—can be supplied to the model to generate a credible range of model outputs. In other words, point estimates alone do not quantify the extent of uncertainty in the estimate, and arbitrarily selected degrees of perturbation can poorly represent the effects of erroneous parameter values. There can, for instance, be substantial asymmetries in the uncertainty above and below-point parameter estimates. Quantifying the extent and asymmetry of uncertainty is important for determining the robustness of estimated effectiveness of control interventions that are fundamental to policy decision-making. For example, a study investigating pre- and posttreatment efficacy of mebendazole against soil-transmitted helminth infection in Tanzania reported the mean egg reduction rate (ERR) observed with the 95% confidence interval and sample size [26]. For these data, a point estimate approach would use the mean ERR as a measure of treatment efficacy, whereas an uncertainty analysis would involve iteratively simulating the model and randomly drawing an efficacy estimate from the full distribution of empirically observed ERRs. In the latter case, the predicted impact of a treatment campaign, such as changes in population-level infection intensity, would be represented as a range of all results calculated across the distribution of efficacy. When the effects of changes to the value of a parameter on outcomes are nonlinear within the range of uncertainty—as they often are in infectious disease models—the probabilistically weighted average outcome can be surprisingly different from the outcome calculated from the best point estimates. It should further be noted that, in addition to uncertainty in parameter values due to imperfect data, some parameters have inherent variability. Susceptibility to infection or treatment efficacy may vary due to factors such as genetic constitution or acquired immunodeficiency, such that drawing from a distribution of observed efficacy values in a compartmental model will reflect inherent heterogeneity in the parameter and thus in the system being modeled.

Along with the other methodologies presented in Box 14.1, the practices of probabilistic sensitivity analysis of individual parameters (see Box 14.2) and full uncertainty analysis of outcomes (see Box 14.2) are at the forefront of disease transmission modeling. Although the procedures are technical and computationally intensive, the benefit of these novel approaches is substantial to improve the robustness of findings for policy-focused research questions (Fig. 14.3). Because these analyses provide nuance to oracular-seeming assertions and therefore enhance the credibility of results, such recent methodological innovations have facilitated the wider adoption of transmission modeling as a component of analyses historically conducted within other disciplines, fostering transdisciplinary approaches to epidemiology and the development of public health policies.

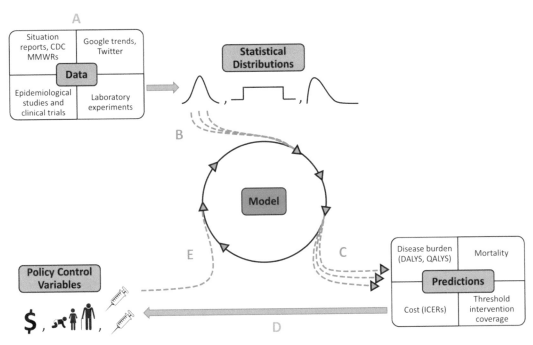

Fig. 14.3 Statistical inference to generate predictions about epidemiological trajectories, outcome measures, and likelihood of health policy effectiveness. Models can be better parameterized when (**A**) data drawn from a variety of sources, including both surveillance reports and published results of epidemiological studies, are used to inform model parameters. Rather than extracting single-point estimates, modelers can make full use of data by (**B**) constructing data-driven distributions of possible values for parameters and then sampling values from those distributions during iterative model runs. Iterations of the model are executed drawing probabilistically from distributions of data to generate (**C**) probabilistic distributions of predictions. Examples of the types of predictions that can be generated include estimates of disease burden and cost of intervention to inform policy decisions. Policy questions, such as whether to recommend a new vaccine, determine (**D**) specific variables to evaluate (e.g., cost-effectiveness). In a probabilistic framework, decision-makers are conveyed not only appropriate estimates of outcomes but also a sense of how much confidence they can have in those estimates. Settings for (**E**) variables that are under the presumed control of policy-makers can be pre-defined and can be further informed by initial model findings that lead to updated iterations of the model. Such policy variables could include cost, dosage schedule, and age of administration

14.4.5 Transdisciplinary Nature of Infectious Disease Modeling

Mathematical modeling can most effectively inform resource allocation and other health policy decisions when it is integrated with field epidemiology and basic science. In fact, the model-guided field-work paradigm [27] suggests that mathematical models can be incorporated into all phases of field research to improve our understanding of infectious disease ecology and complex biological systems. The iterative testing of hypotheses through empirical research and mathematical modeling while concurrently informing study design and model evaluation is a powerful approach for the study and control of disease (Fig. 14.3). The need for sequential data-gathering efforts and analysis and the consequent increased collaboration among experimentalists, policy-makers, and modelers are surmountable barriers to the integration of modeling evidence and public health policy. This iterative feedback approach has been increasingly advocated by researchers [12, 18] and has been demonstrated with applications in the evaluation of the rapid diagnostic test Xpert for tuberculosis [28]. An early modeling study suggested that significant reductions in TB morbidity and mortality would be associated with increases in rates of TB diagnosis due to Xpert use and the assumed corresponding increases in treatment seeking. However, clinical trials in TB-endemic areas demonstrated lower-than-expected impact of the new diagnostic since treatment coverage in such areas was already very high [29]. The new data on TB treatment practices resulted in iterative improvements in the model so that it could more accurately evaluate new diagnostic technologies across different endemic settings [28].

As host behavior is increasingly incorporated into models of infectious disease and as host behavior becomes more important to infection control in an age of patient-inclusive decision-making, the social sciences—particularly psychology—also interface with epidemiology [4]. At this interface, survey data regarding perceived risks and benefits of vaccination as well as economic data on production and administration has been integrated with epidemiological modeling and game theoretic analysis (Box 14.2) to assess the extent that vaccination recommendations will be adopted by the public. For example, this multifaceted approach yielded predictions that "Nash equilibrium" (Box 14.2) vaccination levels would be much lower than the coverage that would be socially optimal [30], projections that were consistent with the national HPV vaccination coverage actually achieved among adolescent girls several years later [31].

Rather than considering a limited number of preconceived strategies, the application of optimization algorithms to epidemiological models enables the identification of the most favorable strategies from a virtually exhaustive range of feasible options. Despite computational challenges of updating model structure to assess all strategies for a given disease system, a modeling approach for the evaluation of options is often significantly more feasible than conducting diverse field trials. To inform health policy decisions, the criteria of optimization can incorporate economic and logistical considerations, as well as mortality and morbidity outcomes. For example, a model evaluating the optimal vaccine distribution to avert influenza outbreaks in the USA determined that the distribution of 63 million vaccine doses could reduce R_e and extinguish an outbreak that had similar transmissibility and mortality patterns as historical influenza pandemics [32]. Analyses of the age-structured model optimized vaccine allocation across a range of available doses and demonstrated that vaccination of school-aged children 5–19 years would be most effective by every outcome measure considered, infections, hospitalizations, mortality, years of life lost, and economic impact, a finding that was robust to parameter uncertainty [33]. This finding challenged the efficiency of the then-current strategy behind the estimated 85 million annual vaccine doses that were being administered for seasonal influenza. The results of this modeling study spurred a shift in influenza vaccination policy in the USA [34] to focus on children and teenagers, who are responsible for the most transmission, in addition to older adults, who are at greatest risk of influenza-associated morbidity and mortality.

Data-driven real-time applications in disease forecasting and surveillance are increasingly being incorporated into modeling [35]. Such applications include web-based services to simulate the spread of disease. They depend on digital disease surveillance, which involves Internet-based data from social media, news, health department, and other sources, to provide real-time information on outbreak detection and thus increase the timeliness and relevance of studies on disease trends and intervention strategies [36]. The Texas Pandemic Flu Toolkit (http://flu.tacc.utexas.edu/), for instance, has been used to forecast trends in pandemic flu throughout Texas using data from the state health department in near real time. The web-based dashboard allows for users to input different interventions, including antiviral treatment, vaccines, and public service announcements, and observe their impact on an unfolding epidemic.

Integration of economic analyses into these real-time applications and other epidemiological models provides policy-makers with evaluations of not only intervention efficacy but also economic impact and affordability. The cost-effectiveness of distributing Texas' national stockpile of antivirals during a flu pandemic could be determined based on forecasts of final size from the Texas Pandemic Flu Toolkit. Likewise, in close collaboration with field epidemiologists who understand implementation feasibility and real-world costs, modeling has been used to investigate the cost-effectiveness of "One Health" strategies, such as vaccinating dogs to protect against human rabies infection [37] and to design innovative interventions, including the treatment of schistosomiasis to reduce HIV susceptibility in sub-Saharan Africa [38]. These examples demonstrate the plasticity of modeling to consider novel intervention strategies that inform scientists of gaps in prevention and control measures and that address the changing demands on decision-makers.

14.5   The Future of Infectious Disease Epidemiology

With the emergence of zoonotic diseases, the spread of existing diseases to new settings, and global efforts toward elimination strategies for preventable infectious diseases, dynamic modeling of infectious disease is a powerful approach to address evolving questions and inform real-time decisions in emergency situations. Recent advances in microbial disease epidemiology have involved the application of molecular techniques for source tracking [39], the investigation into implications of human-driven changes in climate and landscape on the urbanization and emergence of disease [40], and the use of big data, such as from cell phone and social media usage, for exploring contact patterns and mobility trends in growing populations [41]. Combined, these approaches hold tremendous potential to improve our forecasting of disease through data collection and analyses. The instrumental role for quantitative epidemiology in these areas of innovation underscores the continued timeliness and significance of mathematical modeling as an application that informs and facilitates the translation of scientific findings into policy implementation.

References

1. GBD 2017 DALYs and HALE Collaborators. Global, regional, and national disability-adjusted life-years (DALYs) for 359 diseases and injuries and healthy life expectancy (HALE) for 195 countries and territories, 1990–2017: a systematic analysis for the Global Burden of Disease Study 2017. Lancet. 2018;392(10159):1859–922.
2. Reluga TC. Game theory of social distancing in response to an epidemic. PLoS Comput Biol. 2010;6(5):e1000793.
3. Manfredi P, D'Onofrio A. Modeling the interplay between human behavior and the spread of infectious diseases. New York: Springer Science & Business Media; 2013. 329 p.
4. Bauch CT, Galvani AP. Epidemiology. Social factors in epidemiology. Science. 2013;342(6154):47–9.
5. Oraby T, Thampi V, Bauch CT. The influence of social norms on the dynamics of vaccinating behaviour for paediatric infectious diseases. Proc Biol Sci. 2014;281(1780):20133172.
6. Wang Z, Andrews MA, Wu Z-X, Wang L, Bauch CT. Coupled disease-behavior dynamics on complex networks: a review. Phys Life Rev. 2015;15:1–29.
7. Sunstein CR, Zeckhauser R. Overreaction to fearsome risks. Environ Resour Econ. 2011;48(3):435–49.
8. Rubin GJ, Amlôt R, Page L, Wessely S. Public perceptions, anxiety, and behaviour change in relation to the swine flu outbreak: cross sectional telephone survey. BMJ. 2009;339:b2651.
9. Anderson RM, May RM. Infectious disease of humans. Dynamics and control, vol. 1. Oxford: Oxford University Press; 1991. p. 991.
10. Keeling MJ, Rohani P. Modeling infectious diseases in humans and animals. Princeton: Princeton University Press; 2008.
11. Gilbert JA, Meyers LA, Galvani AP, Townsend JP. Probabilistic uncertainty analysis of epidemiological modeling to guide public health intervention policy. Epidemics. 2014;6:37–45.
12. Heesterbeek H, Anderson RM, Andreasen V, Bansal S, De Angelis D, Dye C, et al. Modeling infectious disease dynamics in the complex landscape of global health. Science. 2015;347(6227):aaa4339.
13. Bellan SE, Pulliam JRC, Pearson CAB, Champredon D, Fox SJ, Skrip L, et al. Statistical power and validity of Ebola vaccine trials in Sierra Leone: a simulation study of trial design and analysis. Lancet Infect Dis. 2015;15(6):703–10.

14. NdeffoMbah ML, Skrip L, Greenhalgh S, Hotez P, Galvani AP. Impact of Schistosoma mansoni on malaria transmission in Sub-Saharan Africa. PLoS Negl Trop Dis. 2014;8(10):e3234.

15. Courtenay O, Carson C, Calvo-Bado L, Garcez LM, Quinnell RJ. Heterogeneities in Leishmania infantum infection: using skin parasite burdens to identify highly infectious dogs. PLoS Negl Trop Dis. 2014;8(1):e2583.

16. Miller E, Warburg A, Novikov I, Hailu A, Volf P, Seblova V, et al. Quantifying the contribution of hosts with different parasite concentrations to the transmission of visceral leishmaniasis in Ethiopia. PLoS Negl Trop Dis. 2014;8(10):e3288.

17. Woolhouse MEJ, Rambaut A, Kellam P. Lessons from Ebola: improving infectious disease surveillance to inform outbreak management. Sci Transl Med. 2015;7(307):307rv5.

18. Knight GM, Dharan NJ, Fox GJ, Stennis N, Zwerling A, Khurana R, et al. Bridging the gap between evidence and policy for infectious diseases: how models can aid public health decision-making. Int J Infect Dis. 2016;42:17–23.

19. Sleeman KL, Griffiths D, Shackley F, Diggle L, Gupta S, Maiden MC, et al. Capsular serotype–specific attack rates and duration of carriage of Streptococcus pneumoniae in a population of children. J Infect Dis. 2006;194(5):682–8.

20. Smith T, Lehmann D, Montgomery J, Gratten M, Riley ID, Alpers MP. Acquisition and invasiveness of different serotypes of Streptococcus pneumoniae in young children. Epidemiol Infect. 1993;111(1):27–39.

21. Powers KA, Ghani AC, Miller WC, Hoffman IF, Pettifor AE, Kamanga G, et al. The role of acute and early HIV infection in the spread of HIV and implications for transmission prevention strategies in Lilongwe, Malawi: a modelling study. Lancet. 2011;378(9787):256–68.

22. Coelho FC, Codeço CT, Gomes MGM. A Bayesian framework for parameter estimation in dynamical models. PLoS One. 2011;6(5):e19616.

23. May RM. Uses and abuses of mathematics in biology. Science. 2004;303(5659):790–3.

24. Saltelli A, Ratto M, Andres T, Campolongo F, Cariboni J, Gatelli D, et al. Global sensitivity analysis: the primer. Chichester: Wiley; 2008.

25. Fisman DN, Chan CH, Lowcock E, Naus M, Lee V. Effectiveness and cost-effectiveness of pediatric rotavirus vaccination in British Columbia: a model-based evaluation. Vaccine. 2012;30(52):7601–7.

26. Albonico M, Ramsan M, Wright V, Jape K, Haji HJ, Taylor M, et al. Soil-transmitted nematode infections and mebendazole treatment in Mafia Island schoolchildren. Ann Trop Med Parasitol. 2002;96(7):717–26.

27. Restif O, Hayman DTS, Pulliam JRC, Plowright RK, George DB, Luis AD, et al. Model-guided fieldwork: practical guidelines for multidisciplinary research on wildlife ecological and epidemiological dynamics. Ecol Lett. 2012;15(10):1083–94.

28. Menzies NA, Cohen T, Murray M, Salomon JA. Effect of empirical treatment on outcomes of clinical trials of diagnostic assays for tuberculosis. Lancet Infect Dis. 2015;15(1):16–7.

29. Theron G, Zijenah L, Chanda D, Clowes P, Rachow A, Lesosky M, et al. Feasibility, accuracy, and clinical effect of point-of-care Xpert MTB/RIF testing for tuberculosis in primary-care settings in Africa: a multicentre, randomised, controlled trial. Lancet. 2014;383(9915):424–35.

30. Basu S, Chapman GB, Galvani AP. Integrating epidemiology, psychology, and economics to achieve HPV vaccination targets. Proc Natl Acad Sci U S A. 2008;105(48):19018–23.

31. CDC – Teen Vaccination Coverage – NIS – Teen – Vaccines [Internet]. [cited 2016 Jan 4]. Available from: http://www.cdc.gov/vaccines/who/teens/vaccination-coverage.html.

32. Medlock J, Galvani AP. Optimizing influenza vaccine distribution. Science. 2009;325(5948):1705–8.

33. NdeffoMbah ML, Medlock J, Meyers LA, Galvani AP, Townsend JP. Optimal targeting of seasonal influenza vaccination toward younger ages is robust to parameter uncertainty. Vaccine. 2013;31(30):3079–89.

34. Children, the Flu, and the Flu Vaccine | Seasonal Influenza (Flu) | CDC [Internet]. [cited 2016 May 18]. Available from: http://www.cdc.gov/flu/protect/children.htm.

35. Brownstein JS, Freifeld CC, Chan EH, Keller M, Sonricker AL, Mekaru SR, et al. Information technology and global surveillance of cases of 2009 H1N1 influenza. N Engl J Med. 2010;362(18):1731–5.

36. Salathé M, Freifeld CC, Mekaru SR, Tomasulo AF, Brownstein JS. Influenza A (H7N9) and the importance of digital epidemiology. N Engl J Med. 2013;369(5):401–4.

37. Fitzpatrick MC, Hampson K, Cleaveland S, Mzimbiri I, Lankester F, Lembo T, et al. Cost-effectiveness of canine vaccination to prevent human rabies in rural Tanzania. Ann Intern Med. 2014;160(2):91–100.

38. NdeffoMbah ML, Kjetland EF, Atkins KE, Poolman EM, Orenstein EW, Meyers LA, et al. Cost-effectiveness of a community-based intervention for reducing the transmission of Schistosoma haematobium and HIV in Africa. Proc Natl Acad Sci U S A. 2013;110(19):7952–7.

39. Gire SK, Goba A, Andersen KG, Sealfon RSG, Park DJ, Kanneh L, et al. Genomic surveillance elucidates Ebola virus origin and transmission during the 2014 outbreak. Science. 2014;345(6202):1369–72.

40. Neiderud C-J. How urbanization affects the epidemiology of emerging infectious diseases. Infect Ecol Epidemiol. 2015;5:27060.

41. Hay SI, George DB, Moyes CL, Brownstein JS. Big data opportunities for global infectious disease surveillance. PLoS Med. 2013;10(4):e1001413.

42. Stolk WA, Walker M, Coffeng LE, Basáñez M-G, de Vlas SJ. Required duration of mass ivermectin treatment for onchocerciasis elimination in Africa: a comparative modelling analysis. Parasit Vectors. 2015;8:552.
43. Atkins KE, Shim E, Carroll S, Quilici S, Galvani AP. The cost-effectiveness of pentavalent rotavirus vaccination in England and Wales. Vaccine. 2012;30(48):6766–76.
44. Scarpino SV, Iamarino A, Wells C, Yamin D, Ndeffo-Mbah M, Wenzel NS, et al. Epidemiological and viral genomic sequence analysis of the 2014 ebola outbreak reveals clustered transmission. Clin Infect Dis. 2015;60(7): 1079–82.
45. Bogoch II, Brady OJ, Kraemer MUG, German M, Creatore MI, Kulkarni MA, et al. Anticipating the international spread of Zika virus from Brazil. Lancet. 2016;387(10016):335–6.

Vaccines

15

Diane McMahon-Pratt

15.1 Introduction: Brief History of Vaccination

Historically, it was observed that survivors of plague and other devastating infectious diseases were relatively safe in subsequent epidemics. Thucydides [1] recorded during the Peloponnesian War (430 B.C.): "But those that were recovered had much compassion both on them that died and on them that lay sick, as having both known the misery themselves and now no more subject to the danger. For this disease never took any man the second time so as to be mortal." Historical evidence is limited but indicates that the earliest efforts to protect against disease involved the deliberate exposure/inoculation with small amounts of materials from diseased individuals; this exposure caused disease, albeit generally in a milder form [2]. For example, in the case of small pox in the early sixteenth and seventeenth centuries (possibly as early as the eighth to tenth centuries), variolation was practiced in India and China. Records from China describe methods for inoculating naïve individuals with materials contaminated with virus (pus from sores) that induced a weak form of disease. This practice of variolation was brought to England from the Ottoman Court by Lady Montague. In 1721 she, together with surgeon Thomas Maitland, convinced members of the Royal Society and College of Physicians and the Royal family that variolation conferred protection. At the same time in North America, an epidemic of small pox broke out in Boston. Through the insights concerning variolation provided by a West Indian slave, Onesimus, Cotton Mather (minister) and Dr. Zabdiel Boylston (physician) promoted inoculation/variolation in Boston; however, this was not without serious and understandable controversy. Importantly though, Mather and Boylston kept records documenting their efforts. In what may have been the first relative efficacy study, Boylston determined the comparative mortality rates among non-inoculated (14.8%) versus inoculated (2%) individuals.

However, there were obvious risks associated with variolation (inadvertent spread of disease from inoculated individuals; a remaining risk of death/serious infection). Better approaches were needed. Subsequently, the cross-protection afforded by cow pox (which caused only limited cutaneous disease) led to vaccination practiced today against small pox. Again, here it was known in the areas where cow pox circulated that dairy maids who had contracted cow pox were resistant to small pox.

D. McMahon-Pratt (✉)
Department of Epidemiology of Microbial Diseases, Yale School of Public Health, New Haven, CT, USA
e-mail: diane.mcmahon-pratt@yale.edu

© Springer Nature Switzerland AG 2019
P. J. Krause et al. (eds.), *Immunoepidemiology*, https://doi.org/10.1007/978-3-030-25553-4_15

However, it was through the work initially of Benjamin Jesty and the promotion and vaccination studies of Edward Jenner that led to adoption of cow pox vaccination against small pox.

The early work by Jenner also led to discoveries that are still important for vaccines today, especially live vaccines. Even without an understanding of germ theory, it was observed that continual passage through humans led to ineffective vaccines (attenuation). Consequently, periodic repassage through cows was performed to maintain effectiveness. Transport of cow pox also presented challenges for stability. Today vaccine stability and "cold chain" requirements still affect logistics and efficacy. Importantly, the vaccine developed through Jenner's efforts led to the WHO worldwide campaign for small pox disease eradication.

The use of a less virulent disease to protect against serious disease significantly changed thinking concerning disease prevention. However, it was the development of the germ theory (microbes cause disease) and an understanding of the pathogenesis of microbes that directed the further advancement of vaccines. The microbial basis of disease was first shown in "model systems" (silk worms; plants) in the early 1800s. Louis Pasteur was the first to propose the "germ theory" of disease for humans. The work of Robert Koch defined rigorous methods for determining the specific disease-causing organisms. Pasteur developed the first laboratory vaccine. He also proposed that vaccination could provide protection against any microbial disease and importantly that this protection was *specific* to the infecting organism. Pasteur studied microbe virulence and developed methods of *attenuation* (passage through other animal species, chemical treatment, heat). His development of a prophylactic cholera vaccine and a therapeutic rabies vaccine provided the basis for vaccine development into the twentieth century.

Ultimately, the use of killed microbes or their subcomponents or specific proteins and carbohydrate antigens (*subunit vaccines*) (as opposed to live vaccines) have been employed for the development of safe and effective vaccines. However, not all defined/killed vaccines tested have proven effective. This has led to the development of "adjuvants" and also a continuing controversy. Historically a major hypothesis of Pasteur was that only "live" vaccination could provide protection. The argument again raised today by the prominent immunologist Rolf Zinkernagel [3] is that organism persistence (in the case of live-attenuated vaccines) as well as re-exposure rather than long-term T-cell memory provides for long-lived vaccine protection. This fundamental aspect of vaccination (memory) is critical for public health and may vary depending on the vaccine and population (exposure). Nonetheless, understanding the basis for memory (as applicable to each vaccine) is important for determining the timing/requirements for revaccination.

Neither Pasteur nor his contemporaries understood the functions of the lymphocyte (B, T) or immunological memory as it is recognized today. Mechanistic understanding of vaccines began in the nineteenth century with the description in serum of disease-neutralizing antitoxins (antibodies: tetanus and diphtheria) by von Behring and Kitasato. Subsequently, studies of the bacillus Calmette-Guérin (BCG) vaccine in the early twentieth century led to the recognition of another response to vaccination: the delayed-type hypersensitivity (DTH skin test), which is known to be mediated through T cells. It can be argued that the early development of immunology was driven by discoveries and advancements in vaccines. Further reading on the historical development of vaccines is provided by Plotkin [2].

15.2   Current Vaccines

Vaccines in use today [4] are subdivided as: live (attenuated), whole cell (dead organisms), subunit (isolated protein, and/or carbohydrate molecules), and recombinant https://www.cdc.gov/vaccines/vpd/vaccines-list.html; https://www.fda.gov/biologicsbloodvaccines/vaccines/approvedproducts/ucm093833.htm) (examples found in Table 15.1). With the movement toward safer vaccination,

Table 15.1 Examples of current FDA-approved vaccines: attenuated, whole cell (killed), subunit-conjugate, subunit (purified protein and/or carbohydrate and recombinant)

Target pathogen(s) (disease)	Vaccine type	Trade name	Adjuvant	Delivery system mechanisms of action
Influenza virus (flu)	Live, cold attenuated	FluMist Quadravalent	None added; Intrinsic viral RNA and HA	Nasal delivery; 1 dose, serum and mucosal antibody and T cell responses
Rotavirus (diarrhea)	Live attenuated bovine rotavirus reassortants with human serotypes (G1, G2, G3, G4, P1 strains)	RotaTeq	None added; Intrinsic viral PAMPs	Oral delivery; 3 doses; IgA
Measles, mumps, rubella, and varicella viruses (measles, mumps, and chicken pox)	Live attenuated viruses	ProQuad	None added; intrinsic viral PAMPs	Subcutaneous injection; one dose; antibody
Vibrio cholerae serogroup O1 (cholera)	Live attenuated bacteria, V. cholerae CVD 103-HgR	VAXCHORA	None added; Intrinsic bacterial PAMPs	Oral; single dose; lyophilized; vibriocidal antibody; and possible other mechanisms
Yellow fever virus (yellow fever)	Attenuated 17D-2D4 strain of yellow fever virus	YF-VAX	None added; intrinsic viral PAMPs	Subcutaneous injection; single dose; neutralizing antibodies
Influenza virus (flu)	WHOLE: Formaldehyde inactivated "split" influenza viruses (treated with detergent)	Fluzone Quadravalent:	None added; intrinsic viral PAMPs	IM Injection; 1 dose; antibody
Rabies virus (post-exposure)	WHOLE: Flury (LEP) Rabies virus (cell culture) chemically inactivated (β-propiolactone)	Rabavert	None added; virus activates TLR7, MyD88	IM injection; 4-5 doses; neutralizing antibody
Japanese encephalitis virus (encephalitis)	WHOLE: Inactivated (formaldehyde) virus from cell culture	IXIARO	Alum (aluminum hydroxide)	IM injection; 2 doses; neutralizing antibody
Streptococcus pneumoniae (pneumococcal disease)	CONJUGATE SUBUNIT: Diphtheria CRM197 protein-carrier, chemically linked to carbohydrates of serotypes 1, 3, 4, 5, 6A, 6B, 7F, 9V, 14, 18C, 19A, 19F, and 23F	Prevnar 13	Alum (aluminum phosphate)	IM injection, 4 doses; antibody neutralization and opsonization, phagocytosis, and killing of pneumococci by leukocytes and other phagocytic cells
Haemophilus influenzae (bacteremia, pneumonia, epiglottitis, and acute bacterial meningitis)	CONJUGATE SUBUNIT: Haemophilus b capsular polysaccharide (polyribosyl-ribitol-phosphate [PRP])-tetanus toxoid conjugate	HIBERIX	None added; intrinsic bacterial PAMPs	IM injection; single dose; antibodies to polyribosyl-ribitol-phosphate (anti-PRP) ≥ 1.0 mcg/mL
Influenza virus (flu)	SUBUNIT: HA and Neuraminidase proteins isolated from egg cultured influenza viruses [3]	FLUAD	MF59C.1 adjuvant (MF59®)	IM injection; one dose; people >65 years; antibody

(continued)

Table 15.1 (continued)

Target pathogen(s) (disease)	Vaccine type	Trade name	Adjuvant	Delivery system mechanisms of action
Neisseria meningitidis (meningococcal disease)	SUBUNIT: Polysaccharides isolated from *N. meningitidis* (groups A, C, Y, W-135)	Menomune–A/C/Y/W-135	None added; potency evaluated by molecular size of polysaccharide component (WHO specifications)	Subcutaneous injection; single dose; antibody protects against invasive disease
Bacillus anthracis (anthrax)	SUBUNIT: Bacterial proteins including 83kDa protective antigen protein released during growth	BioThrax®	Alum (aluminum hydroxide)	IM injection; 5 doses; neutralizing the activities of the cytotoxic lethal toxin and edema toxin
Corynebacterium diphtheria, Clostridium tetani, Bordetella pertussis (diphtheria, tetanus and whooping cough)	SUBUNIT: Diphtheria toxoid, tetanus toxoid, and acellular pertussis antigens [detoxified pertussis toxin, filamentous hemagglutinin, pertactin, fimbriae types 2 and 3]	Daptacel	Alum (aluminum phosphate)	IM injection; five dose series; antibody- tetanus antitoxin level ≥0.1 IU/mL; diphtheria antitoxin level of >0.01 IU/mL; no established serological correlate of protection for pertussis
Human papillomavirus (cervical cancer)	SUBUNIT recombinant virus-like particles (VLP) in *Saccharomyces cerevisiae*	Gardasil 9	Alum (aluminum hydroxyphosphate sulfate)	IM injection: 3 doses; thought to be antibody to HPV types 6, 11, 16, 18, 31, 33, 45, 52, 58
Human papillomavirus (cervical cancer)	SUBUNIT recombinant L1 proteins (VLP)	Cervarix	AS04 (3-O-desacyl-4′-monophosphoryl lipid A (MPL), alum adsorbed (aluminum hydroxide)	IM injection: 3 dose; HPV types 16 and 18
Hepatitis B virus (hepatitis)	SUBUNIT purified recombinant HBsAg made in *H. polymorpha* (yeast)	HEPLISAV-B	CpG 1018	IM injection; 2 doses; antibody concentrations ≥10 mIU/mL
Varicella zoster virus (shingles)	SUBUNIT: Recombinant varicella zoster virus surface glycoprotein E (gE) antigen made in Chinese Hamster Ovary cells	SHINGRIX	AS01B (3-O-desacyl-4′-monophosphoryl lipid A (MPL), QS-21 in liposomes (cholesterol, dioleoylphosphatidylcholine)	IM injection; 2 doses; boosts immunity to herpes zoster virus

Adjuvant systems employed are indicated. Note there are multiple vaccines available for many of the infectious diseases. For a full listing visit: https://www.fda.gov/biologics-bloodvaccines/vaccines/approvedproducts/ucm093833.htm; *IM* intramuscular emphasis has been on subunit and component (isolated protein or carbohydrates) vaccines. Understanding the mechanisms of pathogenesis of microbes (points of vulnerability) as well as specific immune mechanisms of protection has directed vaccine development. However, with the subunit or component vaccine approach, immunogenicity is a challenge. To meet this need requires *adjuvants* (directing specific responses (T (Th1/Th2/Th17) and B (antibody)) and/or *delivery systems* (targeting specific tissue sites and antigen-presenting cells) that engage the innate immune system and direct the acquired immune response and provide for long-term memory.

15.3 Adjuvants

An *adjuvant* (in Latin adjuvare meaning "to help") is considered to be an agent that modifies the immune response, resulting in (1) directing toward a specific type of response (i.e., Th1, Th17, or Th2 and/or antibody; mucosal); (2) boosting/heightening the response (allowing for protection in immunocompromised or at-risk populations) or (3) providing longer-lasting protection; or (4) a requirement for less immunogen to provide protection, making a vaccine more cost-effective [5, 6].

Early vaccine adjuvants were developed empirically. Alum is the most frequently used adjuvant and has been used for vaccines for over 90 years, historically predating the establishment of the Food and Drug Administration (FDA). Alum was discovered inadvertently; Alexander Glenny found in processing diphtheria toxoid by precipitation with potash ($KAl(SO_4)_2 \cdot 12H_2O$) that the mixture induced an increased antibody response over the toxoid itself. "Alum" (named for the aluminum component) has become the primary adjuvant included in U.S. licensed vaccines. In over 60 years of monitoring, the use of alum has had an excellent safety and efficacy record. Aluminum salts are used in DTaP (diphtheria, tetanus, and pertussis combination) vaccines, the pneumococcal conjugate vaccine, and hepatitis B vaccines.

The immunological modes of action of most adjuvants are still only partly understood. Adjuvants represent a diverse range of materials from small synthetic molecules to isolated natural products and particulates of various compositions (e.g., alum). A need for new adjuvants is driven by the fact that T-cell responses (Th1, Th17, CD8 CTL) are required for optimal protection against many pathogens (especially intracellular organisms such as malaria, HIV, HCV). However, alum is best known to promote Th2 and antibody responses and would be a limited driver of the immune responses required for protection against these pathogens.

The FDA requires that the use of a new adjuvant undergo careful evaluation (safety, efficacy) and justification for use (benefit/risk to the target population) instead of alum-based adjuvant. Several vaccine formulations containing "new adjuvants" or adjuvant systems (more than one adjuvant) have been recently licensed including (1) ASO4 (contains *3-O-desacyl-4'-monophosphoryl lipid A (MPL)* and alum) in use against human papilloma virus infection (HPV; Cervarix); (2) ASO3 (*squalene-based water-in-oil emulsion containing D,L-alpha-tocopherol (vitamin E)*) in use against bird influenza (H5N1); (3) *MF59* (oil-in-water emulsion of squalene oil) in use in influenza vaccine (Fluad); and (4) *CpG 1018* in use in a hepatitis B vaccine (Heplisav-B) and ASO1B (*MPL, QS-21* (Saponin component) is used to prevent shingles (varicella-zoster virus; Shingrix)) [5].

15.3.1 Mechanisms of Adjuvant Action

Most adjuvants studied to date have several common features. They have been shown to create a local milieu at the site of injection (chemokines and cytokines), leading to cellular recruitment (PMN, monocyte, macrophages, and /or DCs, immune cells, APCs) with subsequent antigen uptake and cellular trafficking to the draining lymph node. The signaling pathways induced by adjuvants leading to these events vary significantly and can be complex.

15.3.1.1 Alum

Alum is a generic name given to *various* aluminum salts (potassium aluminum sulfate – $AlK(SO_4)_2$; aluminum oxyhydroxide (AlOOH) (erroneously called aluminum hydroxide (Alhydrogel)); and aluminum hydroxyphosphate). In part, mechanistic studies of alum adjuvants are complicated by the fact that the aluminum compounds used as adjuvants in human vaccines are *not* chemically identical and therefore differ in their absorptive capacity (based on charge of the alum, pH, and ionic strength) for antigen and equilibrium within tissues [7]. Particle size as well as shape has been found to impact the adjuvant action of alum [8], as well as other particulate adjuvants, as does the tissue site used for immunization (skin, muscle, intraperitoneal).

The original hypothesis concerning the mode of action for alum was a "depot" effect (antigen trapping and slow release at the site of injection that ensures slow, yet persistent immune stimulation); however, this has not been consistently observed. Overall, the literature examining the immunological and inflammatory mechanisms underlying alum's mode of action points *to multiple, redundant* pathways [9, 10]. No one "mechanism" alone has been found to be essential. Overall, the consensus is that alum increases antigen uptake and recognition, recruits innate cells (DCs, macrophage, monocytes, PMNs), and promotes inflammatory chemokines and cytokines. A correlation has been observed between enhanced antibody responses and the innate and inflammatory response induced by alum. Multiple inflammatory pathways have been shown to be activated (DAMP, NLRP3, TLR) by alum that can enhance APC activation, as well as antigen uptake and APC maturation. Nonetheless, neither released DNA, nor NLRP3 nor IL-1 signaling alone is essential for alum's adjuvant activity in vivo [11]. However, when alum is phagocytized by dendritic cells, activation of Src and Syk kinase activation occurs, leading to activation of NFAT, the master transcription factor regulating IL-2 expression; DC-derived IL-2 appears critical for T-cell activation and alum's action [12]. Although alum can increase levels of both Th1 and Th2 cytokines, the cytokine profile is biased toward a Th2 response. Overall, it appears that the multipronged action of alum assures its adjuvant capacity and its success as an adjuvant across populations.

15.3.1.2 TLR Ligands

The innate immune response initiates a host of inflammatory and anti-inflammatory reactions that direct the development of the acquired immune response (T and B cells). The innate immune response is engaged through pattern-recognition receptors (PRR), including the toll-like receptors (TLRs), DMAPS, RIGs, as well as polyglucans and glycolipids (stimulate NK-T, macrophages, PMNs, and DCs). Consequently, molecules known to stimulate these pathways are being used and developed as adjuvants. To date, this research has been largely focused on TLR ligands [13–16].

The first TLR ligand developed as an adjuvant was MPL (3-O-desacyl-4'-monophosphoryl lipid A), which is a TLR4 ligand and the active fragment of the LPS lipid A from *Salmonella minnesota*. Biologically derived MPL is heterogeneous and contains a mixture of molecular species (different acyl chain lengths and affinities for TLR4). MPL activates TLR4 in a TRIF-biased manner (rather than MyD88) and therefore provides a strong adjuvant effect while mitigating strong inflammatory side effects. MPL-TLR4 activation has been shown to drive Th1 T-cell responses. MPL is currently used in conjunction with alum in the ASO4 adjuvant formulation in the human papillomavirus (HPV; Cervarix) vaccine. Another related synthetic TLR 4 agonist – GLA (glucopyranosyl lipid A; hexylacylated) – that promotes Th1 and CD8 T-cell responses and IgG2c class switching has been used in conjunction with squalene (GLA-SE); GLA-SE appears to work in part through the induction of Tbet and IL-12 production and IFNαR1 signaling. GLA-SE is in clinical trials for vaccines against tuberculosis and skin melanoma.

Structure-function studies of lipid A are in process [14] to develop more effective TLR4-targeted adjuvants. Recently a new defined TLR4 agonist SLA (*second-generation lipid adjuvant*) has been synthesized which was structurally directed for the human TLR4 receptor-MD2 coreceptor; SLA induces lower inflammatory cytokine (IL-1) but higher Th1 responses (IFN-γ, TNF-α, IP-10) than GLA. Structure-function design and an understanding of signaling pathways will further enhance the specific immunomodulatory effects of TLR adjuvants in vaccines, limiting adverse side effects and optimizing immunity.

Similarly, TLR9 ligands – CpG ODNs (oligodinucleotide also called immunostimulatory sequence-ODN (ISS-ODN)) – have been incorporated into vaccines that are now in clinical trials. CpG activation has been found to drive Th1 and CD8 T-cells responses and enhance antibody levels to antigens [16]. TLR9 is highly expressed on many antigen-presenting cells (B cells and plasmacytoid DCs (pDCs)) in humans; different CpG ODN sequences preferentially activate B cells (CpG-B class; type K) or pDCs (CpG-A class; type D). CpG-C ODNs combine the effects of the other two classes, stimulating B cells, pDCs, and other immune cells such as NK cells. Selected ODNs ISS are currently in clinical trials. ODN 1018 ISS (CpG-B class) together with recombinant hepatitis B surface antigen has recently been approved by the FDA; this vaccine has shown safety profiles and high-titer seroprotective antibodies in all populations studied, including groups that are harder to immunize, such as the elderly and immunocompromised individuals. CpG adjuvants are currently in clinical trials for vaccines against malaria and hookworm infections.

TLR3 (poly I-C) ligands and TLR7/8 ligands (imiquimod; resiquimod) are known to induce innate immunity and Th1-type immune responses, increase DC maturation, and enhance IL-12 secretion. Further, TLR3 stimulation enhances cross-presentation and CD8 T-cell activation. However, toxicity caused by activation by the ligands of TLR3 and/or TLR7/8 has been noted. Nevertheless, topical treatments (HPV-induced warts, basal and squamous cell carcinomas) have been approved using imiquimod/resiquimod. Both TLR3 and TLR7/8 ligands are being used as adjuvants in clinical trials (intradermal influenza vaccine, a hepatitis B virus vaccine for patients on renal replacement therapy).

15.3.1.3 MF59

MF59 [17] is a squalene oil-in-water emulsion that is stabilized with the detergents, Tween 80 and Span 85. Squalene is an isoprenoid compound and intermediate metabolite in the synthesis of cholesterol. MF59 was originally developed as a delivery system for the NOD innate immunity ligand, muramyl-dipeptide (MDP), and antigen. However, MF59 itself (without MDP) was found to act as an adjuvant. Both squalene and Span 85 are important for MF59 activity. In contrast to water-in-oil emulsions which are long-lived and cause adverse, granulomatous responses, oil-in-water emulsions, like MF59, disperse readily and do not create long-lived depots at the site of injection.

Like alum, injected MF59 elicits multiple responses and appears to act on several cell populations (muscle, monocyte, DC, PMN). Intramuscular injection of MF59 has been shown to cause inflammatory responses (chemokines (MCP-1, IL-8, CCL3 and CCL4, CXCL10), cytokines) and stimulate antigen uptake by APCs that then migrate to the draining LN. Interestingly, MF59 appears to create an "immunostimulatory environment" as injection of MF59 twenty-four hours prior to injection of antigen still provides an adjuvant effect. MF59 action has been reported to be completely NALP3 inflammasome independent but does require ASC; MF59 also appears to require MyD88 to enhance responses but in a TLR-independent way. MF59 promotes differentiation of Mo-DCs (monocyte-derived DCs) which is a major source of antigen-loaded, activated APCs after MF59 immunization. Additionally, an MF59-adjuvanted influenza vaccine was found to induce Ig class switching, long-lived IgG antibody-producing cells, protective anti-HA antibodies, and CD8$^+$ T-cell responses in mice *deficient in CD4 T cells*. This observation has potentially important implications for human vaccines – especially for vaccines directed toward young children, the elderly, and immunocompromised populations. MF59 is used in the vaccines, Fluad (seasonal flu), Foceteria (pandemic flu), and Aflunov (pre-pandemic flu).

15.3.1.4   QS-21

Saponin adjuvants [18] are isolated from the bark from the South American tree, *Quillaja saponaria*; various saponin components, including QS-21, have been biochemically characterized. QS-21 is an amphiphilic glycoside with a lipophilic triterpene core with four structural domains (branched trisaccharide, a quillaic acid triterpene, bridging linear oligosaccharide, pseudodimeric acyl chain) [19].

Studies indicate that QS-21 elicits CD4$^+$ and CD8$^+$ cells and antibody responses. After intramuscular injection, liposomal QS-21 rapidly accumulates in resident CD169$^+$ macrophages (subcapsular sinus) of the draining lymph node; these cells apparently control the adjuvant effect. In CD169$^+$ macrophages, QS-21 induces caspase-1 activation and HMGB1 (high-mobility group protein B1) release, DAMP activation, and the production of IL-1β, resulting in the recruitment of innate immune cells and activation of dendritic cells and antigen uptake, and leading to antigen-specific cellular and humoral responses. Interestingly, the trapping of QS-21 within subcapsular sinus macrophages mimics the trapping and responses of these cells to bacteria and other pathogens. Therefore, these cells may represent potential additional adjuvant targets in vaccine development.

QS-21 has several problems as an adjuvant, including scarcity, chemical instability, and dose-limiting toxicity (hemolysis). Moreover, its immunological mode of action is not completely understood. Chemical synthesis studies are currently investigating structure–activity relationships of QS-21. These studies have resulted in the development of more stable adjuvants and pointed to structures responsible for the activity of the QS-21 adjuvant (carbohydrate, triterpene, C-16 hydroxyl). The type of CD4 T-cell response elicited (Th1, Th2) varies depending on the presence of the fucopyranosyl residue. Further, modification of the acyl group can significantly reduce toxicity without mitigating adjuvant efficacy. These synthetic studies should provide for better and more readily available saponin-based adjuvants.

QS-21 has been used as part of the AS01 adjuvant to prevent shingles (varicella-zoster virus; Shingrix) and in conjunction with several vaccines in clinical trials (HIV, tuberculosis) in the adjuvant formulation AS02, an oil-in-water nanoemulsion that also contains MPL, a TLR4 ligand.

15.3.2 Adjuvants: Future

There are a number of additional adjuvants in preclinical and early clinical trials – such as chitosan, alpha-galatosylceramide (a NK-T cell agonist), and heat-labile enterotoxin, which potentially may result in new vaccine adjuvants for future use. It is clear that the use of synthetic defined molecules as adjuvants should allow large-scale production, higher safety profiles, and reduced costs in comparison to naturally derived materials.

15.4   Vaccine Delivery Systems

Current vaccine delivery systems primarily consist of particulate materials, termed nanoparticles [20]. The size (between 1 and 100 nanometers) of the particles optimally allows for APC uptake and trafficking to the lymph node. These systems also allow for incorporation of adjuvants. Although not well understood, nanoparticle size, shape, and charge can determine the APC cellular uptake mechanism and hence the level of MHC class I and/or class II presentation and activation. Overall, progress made in the use of nanoparticle delivery systems (immune-engineering) has prompted the design of novel materials that interact with the immune system and direct its response. Nanoparticles are divided into two classes: biologic (VLPs, liposomes) and polymeric (synthetic).

15.4.1 Biologic Nanoparticles

15.4.1.1 Virus-Like Particles

Virus-like-particles (VLPs) [21, 22] are subviral particles generated through the self-assembly of viral structural proteins. VLPs resemble the morphology and size (20–200 nm) of the originating virus, but lack viral genetic material and are therefore unable to replicate or cause infection. Given their viral origin, many of the biological/immunological actions of the VLPs are conserved: (1) recognition by antigen-presenting cells; (2) trafficking from the site of injection to the lymph nodes; and (3) VLP repetitive structural features that allow for presentation of repetitive antigens (in recombinant virions). This facilitates B-cell activation (cross-linking BCRs), resulting in a stronger humoral immune response. Furthermore, a class of VLPs called *virosomes* can be assembled in vitro using engineered biomolecules such as liposomes and purified viral proteins and additional adjuvants (MPL).

VLP technology has provided the basis of approved multivalent vaccines as, for example, the HPV vaccine Gardasil 9 (Merck), which provides protection against nine different HPV strains/serotypes. VLPs are also employed for the formulation of vaccines in clinical trial (norovirus, Chikungunya Fever). *Heterologous* VLP-based vaccine platforms (fusion protein VLP or a chemical conjugation to a VLP) have been developed and are currently in clinical trials. For instance, the HBV core protein has been employed as a VLP carrier (using T- and B-cell epitopes from the *Plasmodium falciparium* circumsporozoite protein) for the first vaccine against the malaria parasite (RTS,S (Mosquirix, GSK)).

VLPs can be deliberately loaded with or linked to adjuvants to enhance their immunogenicity; this has been done in the case of the HPV Cervarix vaccine, which is a VLP vaccine that utilizes the AS04 adjuvant (alum, MPL). Other adjuvants (CpG, imiquimod, GLA-SE) have been utilized in clinical trials of VLP-based vaccines.

15.4.1.2 Liposomes

Liposomes [23, 24] are lipid vesicles that can encapsulate proteins/antigens through either membrane-anchoring (surface) or entrapment within the vesicle. Liposomes act as antigen-delivery vehicles, facilitating antigen stability and uptake. Surface-exposed antigens are available and may directly stimulate B-cells for antibody production. Antigens (surface-exposed and/or encapsulated) require intracellular liposome disruption upon delivery to APCs to induce T cell as well as B-cell responses.

Liposomes, in general, have been shown to have little to no adjuvant effect when used alone. However, liposomes incorporating bioactive lipids can activate signaling pathways to promote phagolysosomal fusion and phagosome maturation and enhance antigen presentation and immune activation. Liposomes employed in vaccine clinical trials have been used together with various adjuvants, for targets such as HIV (MPL), malaria (MPL and QS-21 (AS01); GLA-QS-21 (GLA-LSQ)), and breast cancer (3D-MPL, QS-21, CpG). CAF01 is a liposome-adjuvant formulation that is composed of dimethyldioleoylammonium (DDA) stabilized with trehalose 6,6-dibehenate (TDB). TDB activates macrophages and dendritic cells (DCs) via Syk signaling pathway. CAF01 has been employed in clinical vaccine trials for tuberculosis, HIV, and *Chlamydia trachomatis*. An advantage of liposomal-adjuvant combinations has been the lower toxicities observed for the adjuvants, providing for reduced adverse reactions. Notably, liposome formulations were shown to reduce the toxic effects of QS-21 (hemolytic activity) and MPL (endotoxic activity).

Immune-stimulating complexes (*ISCOMs; MATRIX-M*) [25] are liposomes consisting of cholesterol, phospholipids, and the adjuvant *QS-21*. ISCOMs form *perforated* bilayer vesicles with icosahedral, ellipsoid, or round structures. Although the mechanisms underlying the effectiveness of ISCOMs are not completely understood, ISCOMs induce local inflammation, with recruitment of neutrophils, mast cells, macrophages, dendritic cells, and lymphocytes, which release inflammatory mediators (IL-1, IL-6, IL-12, IFN-γ, reactive oxygen intermediates). ISCOMs achieve efficient antigen delivery into DCs, resulting in the induction of antigen-specific T-cell responses (Th1/Th2) and antibody responses. ISCOMs can also be used in combination with other immune-stimulating molecules (TLR ligands or cholera toxin A). ISCOMs have been used in clinical trials of malaria, influenza, and Ebola vaccines.

Virosomes (combinations of VLP and liposomes) [26] are employed in vaccine formulations as antigen delivery and antigen-adjuvant vaccine systems. An influenza virosome is also used as the *delivery system for a hepatitis A* virus vaccine (HAV; Epaxal Berna); the HAV is adsorbed onto the influenza virosome. An HA influenza virosome platform is now being tested as a heterologous vaccine platform for vaccines against HIV and hepatitis C. The mechanisms involved in the immunological enhanced responses by the HA virosomes to heterologous antigens are not clear and may involve properties of the HA protein (activation of innate immunity, receptor binding (CD44, RHAMM, ICAM-1) to APCs). Additionally, the fusogenic properties of the HA may help elicit cytotoxic T-cell responses to the incorporated antigen. The contribution of population exposure (priming) due to previous exposure to the flu virus is unclear.

15.4.2 Polymeric Nanoparticles

15.4.2.1 Synthetic Nanoparticles

The development of polymeric nanoparticles (pNP) [20, 27] for vaccines began in the late 1960s, shortly after the development of pNPs for drug delivery. Vaccine nanoparticles are made of materials selected for their biological safety and slowly degrade in water and tissue. These polymers (e.g., D,L-lactide-co-glycolide (PLGA), poly(lactic acid) (PLA), poly(glutamic acid) (PGA)) can be designed to incorporate antigen as well as adjuvant/immunomodulatory agent and are thought to create a "depot effect" – allowing for a slow, continuous release of cargo (antigen and adjuvant) for a period of time. Polymeric nanoparticles (pNPs) may also induce innate immune responses; various pNP formulations have been shown to activate complement, DAMP and PRR pathways resulting in the local recruitment of inflammatory cells (PMNs and macrophages). Polymeric nanoparticles are engulfed by APCs (resident DCs), trafficked and/or entrapped within draining lymph nodes, priming the immune response. Given these properties, pNPs have been found to enhance the immune response to antigen. Further, pNPs can be chemically modified, offering flexibility to target specific immune responses (Th1, Th2, antibody) as well as enhance immunogenicity.

Recently a *novel PLGA-based nanoparticle formulation* using cationic polymers as excipients to stabilize the inactivated polio vaccine (IPV) antigens [28] was designed to *release two bursts of IPV 1 month* apart, mimicking a typical vaccination schedule. In an animal model, the single vaccination was found to elicit high titers of neutralizing antibody, comparable to that found for the traditional IPV vaccine. This type of *controlled release technology* could potentially serve as a platform for delivery of different types of vaccines and potentially improve global public health.

15.4.2.2 Dissolvable Microneedles

Dissolvable microneedles (dMNs) [29], similar to pNPs, are made from polymeric materials (e.g., poly(vinylalcohol) (PVA), poly(vinylpyrrolidone) (PVP), sodium hyaluronate). dMNs provide transdermal delivery systems (TDDS) for intradermal vaccination. The polymeric needles are arranged in assemblies which are mounted on a base substrate that is attached to a patch backing to facilitate handling. The dMNs penetrate the skin and over time deliver antigen and adjuvant to dermal dendritic cells (Langerhans, pDCs, MoDCs) and other skin immune cells (dermal macrophages, T cells, keratinocytes). The dMNs also cause local cell death and inflammation, which further amplify the local host immune response. Various adjuvants have been incorporated into dMNs including CpG, Quil-A (QS-21), and monophosphoryl lipid A (MPLA). dMNs have been utilized in a clinical trial of a flu vaccine and appear to be as effective as FDA-approved vaccines delivered through intramuscular injection.

The advantages of dMN are ease of delivery, cost-effectiveness, stability, and safety (no needle disposal). The dMNs have been found to be less painful than needle delivery and reduce the expertise needed for administration. These advantages are important for vaccine uptake by populations and delivery, especially in developing countries. Vaccines using microneedle formulations for a variety of infectious diseases (hepatitis B, varicella, poliomyelitis) are currently in human clinical trials.

15.5 Immunologic and Epidemiologic Challenges for Vaccines: Targets for Innovation

Not all infectious diseases have proven amenable to vaccine development. For many pathogens, there is uncertainty about what is the functional protective response and appropriate target antigens. Further, new (Ebola, chikungunya, Zika, and West Nile) and re-emerging (dengue, mumps, measles) infectious diseases as well as those with poorly effective vaccines (tuberculosis) require the development of new or next-generation vaccines. Additionally, some vaccines require several doses to be fully effective (e.g., measles-mumps-rubella (MMR), hepatitis A and B, varicella, and *Haemophilus influenzae* type B). Therefore, there remain challenges ahead for vaccine development.

15.5.1 Genetic Variability of Target Pathogens

Current vaccines are against infectious disease targets that have mutation rates for key pathogenic molecules and antigens that are relatively slow in comparison to those of organisms for which we do not have a vaccine. Genetic variability presents formidable challenges and requires new approaches for diseases caused by organisms, such as HIV or *Plasmodium* (malaria).

15.5.1.1 Malaria

In 2016, the WHO estimated that 216 million cases of malaria occurred worldwide and an estimated 445,000 malaria deaths. Increased prevention and control measures have led to a reduction in malaria mortality rates; however, a vaccine is needed for disease control. The RTS,S vaccine (Mosquirix™) for malaria, which has progressed the furthest uses the adjuvant AS01 and the hepatitis B (HBsAg) viral envelope protein as a "carrier" and targets relatively conserved epitopes on the *P. falciparum* circumsporozoite protein (CSP). The Mosquirix™ vaccine provides significant but limited protection (ranges 26–50% in infants and young children). The fact that CSP is predominantly expressed in pre-erythrocytic and not erythrocytic stages biologically limits vaccine effectiveness. Alternate vaccine candidate molecules as well as whole parasite vaccines (irradiated sporozoites, whole blood stage organisms) are in clinical trials.

Although a conjugate 23-valent polysaccharide pneumococcal vaccine was formulated to overcome a worldwide genetic diversity of 90 serotypes, malaria parasites are considerably more complex, with numerous life cycle stages and surface proteins with extensive diversity. Epidemiological data indicate that *Plasmodium* antigenic variants are related to the geographic area. Hence a concerted epidemiological, biological, genetic, and immunological approach (protective immune responses and immune evasion mechanisms) is required for effective vaccine development [30, 31].

15.5.1.2 HIV

The world Health Organization estimates that approximately 37 million individuals are living with AIDS. However, 30 years after the discovery of the virus, no effective vaccine is available [32]. Neutralizing antibodies and ADCC mechanisms as well as NK cell and T-cell immunity (CD4 and CD8) are known to contribute to control of infection. However, the quasi-species nature (clades) and high mutation rate of HIV have made it an elusive and challenging vaccine target.

Although several clinical vaccine trials have been undertaken, only one to date has provided even limited protection. A clinical trial in Thailand of the RV144 [33] vaccine involved over 16,000 individuals 18–65 years of age. The vaccine was a combination of 2 previously tested vaccines (ALVAC-HIV (Sanofi Pasteur) and AIDSVAX B/E (Genetech)), requiring 6 injections. In the modified intention-to-treat analysis (excluding enrollees who contracted AIDS before their first vaccination), the vaccine efficacy was highest at 12 months (60%) and after 3 years was 31.2%. However, there was no difference between the viral load or CD4 T-cell levels in the two cohorts; further, there was no clear correlate of protection. The results, although hopeful, have been controversial and remain to be confirmed in at-risk populations; currently, a trial in South Africa is planned using a modified protocol. Further development is required to achieve the higher levels of protection required for HIV elimination.

Current HIV vaccine approaches include a focus on the transmitted/founder viruses, as bottlenecks at the mucosal and skin surfaces biologically limit transmission; only certain HIV variants are successful and these are being targeted for vaccination. Another strategy is to attempt to increase the depth of variant coverage. This has been shown in other systems to overcome issues with failure to elicit immune responses to closely related antigens/epitopes and could enhance the ability of the T-cell response to respond to escape mutations.

Clinical trials have demonstrated that T-cell response alone does not provide the protection; hence, multiple arms of the host immune response will need to be engaged. A profile of the "protective" response and development of immunological markers are needed. It is clear that HIV remains a challenge and an understanding of the in vivo biology (viral and human) is critical for vaccine development.

15.5.1.3 Hepatitis C Virus

High genetic/antigenic variability has posed a barrier to vaccine development against hepatitis C virus (HCV). HCV causes most of the acute and chronic liver diseases (cirrhosis and hepatocellular carcinoma) occurring worldwide. HCV has seven distinct genotypes and more than 100 subtypes; HCV mutates at a rate of nearly one nucleotide per replication cycle. Although newly developed antiviral therapies have cure rates of 90%, these are prohibitively expensive and consequently not generally available in the developing world, where the disease burden is the most severe. Both antibody and T cell (CD4 and CD8)-mediated responses are considered important for protection; however, the lack of specific immunologic markers of protection and lack of good preclinical models hamper vaccine development. Further understanding of pathogenesis is needed; the virus is known to promote immune exhaustion and negative regulatory immunity. Overcoming these features through vaccination of infected individuals may require specific activation mechanisms and adjuvant/delivery systems. Prophylactic and therapeutic vaccines against HCV are currently in clinical trial [34].

15.5.2 Improving Current Vaccines

Most current vaccines appear to provide protection for a period of approximately 9 years. There are notable exceptions. The diphtheria vaccine appears to provide protection for 4–5 years; the tetanus and diphtheria vaccines are not as effective in the elderly. It is possible that adjuvant or delivery systems that potentiate these vaccines could overcome these deficiencies. Additionally, both the influenza and tuberculosis vaccines do not currently provide optimal protection.

15.5.2.1 Influenza Virus (A and B)

Influenza-associated respiratory illness remains a major global burden (http://www.who.int/immunization/topics/influenza/en/). The influenza virus is the most variable pathogen against which we have an effective vaccine. Influenza virus undergoes significant antigenic change (shift, drift, mutation) within one season, particularly in the vaccine-targeted HA antigen. Consequently, each year/flu season requires a "new" vaccine whose formulation is based on the viruses in circulation.

Production time for the flu vaccine remains a concern, especially during pandemics, as it is not amenable to rapid responses. The process of WHO selection of the influenza virus variants for the annual vaccine and egg-based production takes 6 months. Alternate approaches, such as cell culture-based influenza propagation or recombinant antigen vaccines, can be faster to scale up. Recently Flublok, a recombinant HA vaccine which is produced in Sf9 insect cells, has been approved by the FDA and is as effective as egg-based vaccines. Several other cell culture-based vaccines are undergoing evaluation. It is likely that the egg-based system may be replaced in the coming years.

Flu vaccines [35, 36], targeted to provide protection over multiple seasons, are under development. These are focused on cross-reactive antibody epitopes as well as CD8 T-cell and local (lung) memory responses. For example, the recombinant M-001 flu vaccine contains *conserved* antigenic peptides from the NP and M1 proteins (conserved among many different influenza viruses) as well as the more variable HA protein. The objective is to induce cross-reactive immunity (antibody and T cell) to these conserved epitopes; the M-001 vaccine [37] is currently in phase III clinical trials. A flu vaccine that is cross-protective against multiple influenza strains and effective in vulnerable populations (elderly, children, immune impairment) would be a major public health contribution.

15.5.2.2 Tuberculosis Vaccine

In 2016 the WHO indicated that globally, 10.4 million people became infected with tuberculosis (TB), with 1.7 million dying from the disease; about one-quarter of the world's population has latent TB. It is estimated that the current bacillus Calmette-Guérin (BCG) vaccine prevents 120,000 childhood TB deaths each year. However, the current vaccine has variable efficacy and does not prevent infection in adult populations. This is complicated by the frequent co-HIV-tuberculosis infections. Furthermore, multidrug-resistant TB (MDR-TB) is increasing. A tuberculosis vaccine that could enhance protection duration or provide protection in adulthood would have a significant impact on global TB rates. Although the results from recent vaccine trials of the Ag85 antigen have been disappointing, current progress on understanding the immune response to *Mycobacteria* infection, the development of biomarkers for various stages of disease (latent versus active), and new studies delineating new antigenic targets are promising. However, biomarkers of vaccine-mediated protection, further vaccine candidate antigens, and new animal models will be important to advance new vaccines. Concerted global efforts

(TuBerculosis Vaccine Initiative (TBVI) and Aeras, WHO) are in progress; prophylactic and thera-peutic vaccines against TB are currently in phase II/III clinical trials [38, 39].

15.6   Population Genetic Variability and Vaccine Responses

Genetic information could potentially be used to predict vaccine effectiveness and used to develop more effective vaccination strategies, possibly in conjunction with immunological systems approaches (discussed above). Twin studies of varicella-zoster [40] as well as other specific vaccines (diphtheria, tetanus, measles, mumps, rubella, hepatitis B, *H. influenzae* type B) have indicated that vaccine responses appear to be largely genetically determined (38–90%). As vaccine failure (as defined by little/no antibody response after immunization) can occur for 5–15% of a population, an understand-ing of the underlying mechanisms is important to assure vaccine coverage/efficacy. Genetic studies (GWAS, SNP approach) of vaccine responses/nonresponses are challenging, requiring well-considered study design and sufficient size for analysis, and results may vary depending on the population (geo-graphic area). A further challenge to assessing the specific contributions of genes is the robustness of the immune system (functional redundancy of genes and proteins). However, it has been established that polymorphisms in immune-response genes (e.g., MHC Class I and II, TLRs, NLRs) [41–43] contribute to responses to vaccination. Although no investigation to date has examined vaccine response genetics across large numbers of multiple, distinct populations, the available studies do per-suasively point to immunogenetic factors in vaccine responses.

Polymorphisms in HLA class II molecules have been observed to modulate the human immune response to infection and vaccination. Interestingly, analyses indicate that *certain HLA genotypes commonly* lead to decreased antibody responses to vaccination, while others are associated with increased responses. For example, DRB1∗07, DQB1∗02:01, and DQB1∗03:03 were associated with a significant decrease of antibody responses to measles, mumps, and rubella (MMR-II), hepatitis B, and influenza vaccines. On the other hand, DRB1∗13 and DRB1∗13:01 were associated with a sig-nificant increase of antibody responses to these same vaccines. These results suggest that targeting certain populations could be beneficial. In certain instances, an additional immunization boost was found to provide antibody levels (titers) within the "protective" range for those inadequately respond-ing to the usual vaccination protocols.

Various TLR genes [41] have been found to be associated with vaccine responses. Particular TLR4 polymorphisms have been correlated with responses (cytokine and/or antibody responses) to measles and meningococcal and pertussis vaccination. Although mechanisms involved are not fully under-stood, SNPs have been found to be associated with specific responses (e.g., cytokine but not anti-body). For example, in response to the measles vaccine, TLR4 SNP (rs4986790) in the TLR4 gene was associated with higher IL-4 production, while rs5030710 was found to be associated with the level of measles virus-specific antibodies. However, replicated studies and further research is required to establish the contribution of specific TLR4 polymorphisms to vaccine-mediated protection. Given the use of MPL (and related synthetic TLR4 ligands) in new-generation vaccines, it will be important to understand the consequence of various TLR4 polymorphisms on vaccine responses.

Cytokine and cytokine-receptor genes have not been extensively studied to date in terms of response to vaccination. Although functional redundancies exist, cytokine and cytokine receptor genes (e.g., IL10RB, IL-6, IL-18, IL-12A, IFNG, IL-1R, IL2RG, IL4R, IL12RB, IFNAR2, TNFRSF1A) have been implicated in vaccine responses (influenza, MMR, hepatitis B). However, these have not yet been replicated in multiple studies and more research is required to establish the contribution to protection.

Importantly, the immune responses to current vaccines based on whole organisms (killed, attenuated) would be expected to mimic those of infection within the population; genetic variability can result in differential susceptibility to infection and consequent host response. For example, TLR receptor polymorphisms have been related to susceptibility/host response to infection to a wide variety of organisms (e.g., gram-positive and gram-negative bacteria, HIV, *Mycobacterium*, *Plasmodium*, *Hepatitis C virus*). Notably, TLR4 polymorphisms/SNPs have also been related to susceptibility to measles, meningococcal disease, and pertussis and as indicated above to vaccination for these diseases. Additionally, MHC polymorphisms have been related to disease susceptibility and vaccine responses. For example, *HLA-DPB1* alleles (as mentioned above) influence the hepatitis B vaccine response as well as HBV persistence (disease susceptibility). Additionally, genetic variation in receptors or pathways utilized by pathogens for survival has been related to susceptibility and vaccine response. As an example, studies in the USA and Mozambique have linked polymorphisms in a measles virus receptor (CD46) [44], which have been related to measles virus caused febrile seizure, to failure of the measles vaccine antibody response. Consequently, understanding genetics of disease susceptibility can inform vaccinology and provide targets for public health intervention. It is important to note here that the same individuals at risk for disease severity are also poor responders to vaccination. Whether adjuvants or other delivery systems approaches could modify these outcomes remains to be determined. Although genetic approaches have been successfully employed in the susceptibility and treatment of cancer, studies of genetic associations with vaccine outcomes are limited; however, genetic approaches in conjunction with systems approach should prove a powerful tool in vaccine development, assuring better efficacy.

15.7 Vaccines: The Future

Most current vaccines have been developed empirically and are generally based upon antibody responses, assuming neutralization as the key effector mechanism for protection. However, it is clear that this is an oversimplification of the processes involved in protection, even in the case of vaccines (e.g., influenza, hepatitis B) where antibody obviously can play a major role. The immune system is complex and interactive (innate, acquired immunity; T cells, B cells) and co-operation and cross-regulation determine overall response; response can also be tissue-specific. The mechanisms underlying our most effective vaccines are only now beginning to be appreciated.

15.7.1 Systems Biology

Recently a number of tools [45] (proteomics, metabolomics, genomics, transcriptomics, single-cell analyses, BCR and TCR repertoire analyses, microbiome sequencing) and high-throughput technologies have been developed that allow the ability to perform multiparameter analyses on very small amounts of precious sera or tissue samples; these have begun to be applied to understanding of an integrative immune response and successful vaccination (vaccinomics) [46, 47] and also adverse reactions to vaccines (adversomics) [48].

Additional computational tools and improved databases are being developed; these should allow for standardization and more global accessibility to raw data. Studies (employing some of these tools) are beginning to generate novel correlates of vaccination outcome and insights into mechanisms of vaccine action. To date these approaches have been largely applied to the influenza vaccine and the highly successful yellow fever vaccine. In the case of yellow fever, gene signatures were uncovered that allowed an accurate prediction of antibody and CD8 T-cells responses. Interestingly flu vaccine studies have found human variability in responding to immunization; notably, factors found affecting flu disease pathogenesis (sex, age, host immune genetics (innate and acquired immune responses)) [49] as well as baseline immune status (prevaccination antibody titers) have been shown to affect vaccine efficacy [50].

The ability to combine five influenza data sets (disease and vaccine responses) also allowed the detection of a "meta-gene signature" of 11 genes that was associated with both higher vaccine efficacy (antibody neutralization titers) and reduced disease pathogenesis [51]. This signature was not evident in each individual study but was in the collective data set; further, this gene signature was able to predict outcomes for 11 independent influenza studies.

Multiple/distinct immunologic gene signatures have been found to lead to successful vaccination, depending in part on the microbiological target (bacterial, viral). Systems vaccinology is promising and still in a developmental phase. An understanding of the immunological mechanisms underlying correlations extracted from high-throughput data analyses is important for vaccine development. This will require hypothesis-driven studies to determine mechanistic and causal relationships and to generate a meaningful understanding of the protective immune response. Such studies should help guide successful vaccine development for at-risk populations (infants, immunocompromised, elderly).

15.7.2 Adjuvants and Delivery Systems

As indicated above, adjuvant mechanisms of action are beginning to be understood; delivery systems formulated to target specific immune effectors and target APCs are being developed. However, further research and understanding is needed to help develop a new generation of adjuvants and delivery systems that minimize adverse reactions while optimizing for the specific immunologic responses needed for protection.

15.7.3 Environmental Factors Impacting Vaccine Effectiveness

We are beginning to understand that environmental factors such as nutrition, BMI, and coinfection (pathogenic and/or symbiotic microbiome organisms) may affect responses to vaccination [52–54]. For example, individuals with high BMI have been found to have poor responses to both hepatitis B and influenza vaccines. However, the immunologic mechanisms are not fully understood but obviously could provide for interventions to improve vaccine efficacy.

In the case of helminth and malaria infection (which together impact nearly 30% of the world's population), the immunoregulation and cytokine milieu created by these infections have been found to impact the course of other infectious diseases and vaccine responses [53]. Notably, helminth infections exacerbate tuberculosis and diminish responses to the BCG vaccine. Studies have revealed that helminth infection results in epigenetic changes (DNA methylation) in the human genome that perturb the immune response (low IL-12, IFN-γ, IFNγ R1/2, IL-12Rβ responses) [55]. In the case of schistosomiasis, these changes can persist for at least 6 months after therapeutic cure. It is of interest to note that these effects in the case of schistosomiasis have been extended to prenatal (in utero) exposure, emphasizing the importance of control and prevention of parasitic infections among pregnant women [56]. Latent or chronic viral infection has also been shown to impact vaccine responses and efficacy. Studies to date have mainly been concerned with EBV (Epstein Barr virus) and CMV (cytomegalovirus) infections [45]. The mechanisms underlying these effects are not understood; however, the local immune environment created by latent/chronic infection and, possibly, cross-reactivity between the pathogens may contribute.

Overall further understanding of the effects of host-pathogen interactions, chronic infection, and duration of epigenetic changes induced will be important for improving vaccine efficacy.

15.7.4 Nonspecific Unintended Vaccine Effects

Studies [57, 58] have shown vaccines can provide unexpected effects that either reduce or exacerbate disease caused by *nontargeted pathogens*. These effects have been termed "generalized herd effects." Although epidemiological findings showing nonspecific effects of vaccines have been questioned, as these appear to contradict the definition of a vaccine (specificity), investigations are beginning to bring the biological underpinnings of these observations into focus. These studies reveal the further complexities of the host immune response and dynamics of pathogens within populations. For example, measles vaccination prevents disease and, as a consequence, the deleterious immunosuppressive effects of infection; measles virus infection depletes T and B cells, notably memory populations, resulting in impaired host resistance for up to 2–3 years post infection for *multiple* pathogens. Epidemiological data indicate that measles vaccination protects polymicrobial herd immunity [59]. Similarly, observational studies [60] suggest that BCG vaccination (tuberculosis) enhances the survival of infants in Africa; this effect is not related to protection against tuberculosis and appears to be highest for low-birth-weight infants. Recent studies suggest that BCG vaccination may induce epigenetic reprograming of monocytes; one study demonstrated that this effect protected against experimental infection with an attenuated yellow fever virus vaccine strain in humans. However, these studies require further validation [61].

It is now evident that vaccines (live or attenuated) can alter the ecological niche and dynamics of phylogenetically distinct microbes, altering the human microbiome. Therefore, vaccines may unintentionally affect transmission of non-vaccine-targeted pathogens. However, these effects can be complex as demonstrated by the live attenuated influenza vaccine (LAIV) [62]. LAIV has been shown (as flu, but to a *lower level*) to increase carriage of staphylococcal and pneumococcal bacteria. However, LAIV vaccination actually prevents influenza infection and consequent flu-associated increases in bacterial transmission, prevalence, and disease; it does so at the expense of a limited increased bacterial transmission earlier in the year, when risk of severe bacterial complications is low.

15.7.5 Tissue Site-Specific Immunity and Memory

Immunological memory is the cornerstone of vaccine development. The biological basis for generation and maintenance of long-lived populations (T and B cells) remains to be fully understood [3, 63, 64]. Cytokines, physiological milieu, and re-exposure or microbe persistence may contribute to "immunological memory," and these could vary across populations and pathogens. There is functional and molecular diversity in the memory B-cell repertoire. Further, in addition to central memory T cells (T_{CM}) residing in lymphoid tissues (LN, spleen), there are populations of resident memory T cells (T_{RM}) specific for different organs (e.g., skin, lung, kidney). These tissue-dwelling cells are considered to be the "first responders" of host defense upon infection. Although T effector memory cells (T_{EM}) circulate between the blood and tissues sites, T_{RM} cells comprise the majority of memory T cells in the nonlymphoid tissues. The roles and contributions and interactions of these various populations are currently being investigated and will be important for vaccine development.

15.7.6 Vaccine Hesitancy

In 2019, the World Health Organization (https://www.who.int/emergencies/ten-threats-to-global-health-in-2019) named "vaccine hesitancy" (defined as the reluctance or refusal to vaccinate despite the availability of vaccines) as one of its top ten global health threats along with diseases such as pandemic flu, Ebola, dengue, and HIV. WHO notes that the reasons why people choose not to vaccinate are complex and vary depending on the community. The Vaccines Advisory Group to WHO identified lack of confidence, complacency, and inconvenience in accessing vaccines as key reasons underlying hesitancy (https://www.who.int/immunization/sage/meetings/2014/october/1_Report_WORKINGGROUP_vaccine_hesitancy_final.pdf). Confidence involves in part trust in the effectiveness and safety of vaccines. The WHO Advisory Group also noted that the precise level at which hesitancy becomes a problem ("disrupting immunization programs and/or contributing to vaccine preventable disease outbreaks") in general "cannot be precisely determined with current measurement and diagnostic tools." Although vaccination (with currently available vaccines) is a major effective preventative measure against infectious diseases, public health communication and community engagement as well as development of safer, more effective vaccines are important to assure vaccine uptake and coverage [65].

References

1. Thucydides (translation Thomas Hobbs). History of the Peloponnesian war. Chicago: University of Chicago Press; 1989. p. 608.
2. Plotkin SA, editor. History of vaccine development. New York: Springer; 2011. p. 338.***
3. Zinkernagel RM. What if protective immunity is antigen-driven and not due to so-called "memory" B and T cells? Immunol Rev. 2018;283:238–46.
4. Plotkin S, Orenstein W, Offit P, Edward KM, editors. Plotkin's vaccines. 7th ed. Philadelphia: Elsevier; 2018. p. 1720. https://doi.org/10.1016/C2013-0-18914-3.*****
5. Bonam SR, Partidos CD, Halmuthur SKM, Muller S. An overview of novel adjuvants designed for improving vaccine efficacy. Trends Pharmacol Sci. 2017;38:771–93.
6. van Aalst SI, Ludwig S, van Kooten PJS, van der Zee R, van Eden W, Broere F. Dynamics of APC recruitment at the site of injection following injection of vaccine adjuvants. Vaccine. 2017;35:1622–9.****
7. Cain DW, Sanders SE, Cunningham MM, Kelsoe G. Disparate adjuvant properties among three formulations of "alum". Vaccine. 2013;31:653–60.
8. Sun B, Ji Z, Liao YP, Wang M, Wang X, Dong J, et al. Engineering an effective immune adjuvant by designed control of shape and crystallinity of aluminum oxyhydroxide nanoparticles. ACS Nano. 2013;7:10834–49.
9. Ghimire TR. The mechanisms of action of vaccines containing aluminum adjuvants: an in vitro vs in vivo paradigm. Springerplus. 2015;4:181.
10. Wen Y, Shi Y. Alum: an old dog with new tricks. Emerg Microbes Infect. 2016;5:e25.**
11. Noges LE, White J, Cambier JC, Kappler JW, Marrack P. Contamination of DNase preparations confounds analysis of the role of DNA in alum-adjuvanted vaccines. J Immunol. 2016;197:1221–30.
12. Khameneh HJ, Ho AW, Spreafico R, Derks H, Quek HQ, Mortellaro A. The Syk-NFAT-IL-2 pathway in dendritic cells is required for optimal sterile immunity elicited by alum adjuvants. J Immunol. 2017;198:196–204.
13. O'Hagan DT, Friedland LR, Hanon E, Didierlaurent AM. Towards an evidence based approach for the development of adjuvanted vaccines. Curr Opin Immunol. 2017;47:93–102.
14. Carter D, Fox CB, Day TA, Guderian JA, Liang H, Rolf T, et al. A structure-function approach to optimizing TLR4 ligands for human vaccines. Clin Transl Immunol. 2016;5:e108.
15. Ignacio BJ, Albin TJ, Esser-Kahn AP, Verdoes M. Toll-like receptor agonist conjugation: a chemical perspective. Bioconjug Chem. 2018;29:587–603.
16. Campbell JD. Development of the CpG adjuvant 1018: a case study. Methods Mol Biol. 2017;1494:15–27.
17. O'Hagan DT, Ott GS, De Gregorio E, Seubert A. The mechanism of action of MF59 – an innately attractive adjuvant formulation. Vaccine. 2012;30:4341–8.**
18. Marciani DJ. Elucidating the mechanisms of action of saponin-derived adjuvants. Trends Pharmacol Sci. 2018;39:573–85.**

19. Fernandez-Tejada A, Tan DS, Gin DY. Development of improved vaccine adjuvants based on the saponin natural product QS-21 through chemical synthesis. Acc Chem Res. 2016;49:1741–56.**

20. Silva AL, Peres C, Conniot J, Matos AI, Moura L, Carreira B, et al. Nanoparticle impact on innate immune cell pattern-recognition receptors and inflammasomes activation. Semin Immunol. 2017;34:3–24.**

21. Mohsen MO, Gomes AC, Vogel M, Bachmann MF. Interaction of viral capsid-derived virus-like particles (VLPs) with the innate immune system. Vaccine. 2018;6:37–50.****

22. Fuenmayor J, Godia F, Cervera L. Production of virus-like particles for vaccines. New Biotechnol. 2017;39:174–80.

23. Schwendener RA. Liposomes as vaccine delivery systems: a review of the recent advances. Ther Adv Vaccines. 2014;2:159–82.

24. De Serrano LO, Burkhart DJ. Liposomal vaccine formulations as prophylactic agents: design considerations for modern vaccines. J Nanobiotechnol. 2017;15:83.****

25. Sun HX, Xie Y, Ye YP. ISCOMs and ISCOMATRIX. Vaccine. 2009;27:4388–401.**

26. Moser C, Amacker M, Kammer AR, Rasi S, Westerfeld N, Zurbriggen R. Influenza virosomes as a combined vaccine carrier and adjuvant system for prophylactic and therapeutic immunizations. Expert Rev Vaccines. 2007;6:711–21.

27. Silva AL, Soema PC, Slutter B, Ossendorp F, Jiskoot W. PLGA particulate delivery systems for subunit vaccines: linking particle properties to immunogenicity. Hum Vaccin Immunother. 2016;12:1056–69.

28. Tzeng SY, McHugh KJ, Behrens AM, Rose S, Sugarman JL, Ferber S, et al. Stabilized single-injection inactivated polio vaccine elicits a strong neutralizing immune response. Proc Natl Acad Sci U S A. 2018;115:E5269–78.**

29. Leone M, Monkare J, Bouwstra JA, Kersten G. Dissolving microneedle patches for dermal vaccination. Pharm Res. 2017;34:2223–40.**

30. Draper S, Sack BK, King CR, Nielsen CM, Rayner JC, Higgins MK, et al. Malaria vaccines: recent advances and new horizons. Cell Host Microbe. 2018;24:43–56.****

31. Ouattara A, Barry AE, Dutta S, Remarque EJ, Beeson JG, Plowe CV. Designing malaria vaccines to circumvent antigen variability. Vaccine. 2015;33:7506–12.****

32. Rios A. Fundamental challenges to the development of a preventive HIV vaccine. Curr Opin Virol. 2018;29:26–32.**

33. Kim JH, Excler JL, Michael NL. Lessons from the RV144 Thai phase III HIV-1 vaccine trial and the search for correlates of protection. Annu Rev Med. 2015;66:423–37.

34. Guo X, Zhong JY, Li JW. Hepatitis C virus infection and vaccine development. J Clin Exp Hepatol. 2018;8:195–204.

35. Soema PC, Kompier R, Amorij JP, Kersten GF. Current and next generation influenza vaccines: formulation and production strategies. Eur J Pharm Biopharm. 2015;94:251–63.****

36. Zhou F, Trieu MC, Davies R, Cox RJ. Improving influenza vaccines: challenges to effective implementation. Curr Opin Immunol. 2018;53:88–95.****

37. Atsmon J, Caraco Y, Ziv-Sefer S, Shaikevich D, Abramov E, Volokhov I, et al. Priming by a novel universal influenza vaccine (Multimeric-001)-a gateway for improving immune response in the elderly population. Vaccine. 2014;32:5816–23.

38. Voss G, Casimiro D, Neyrolles O, Williams A, Kaufmann SHE, McShane H, et al. Progress and challenges in TB vaccine development. F1000Res. 2018;7:199.****

39. Moliva JI, Turner J, Torrelles JB. Immune responses to bacillus Calmette-Guerin vaccination: why do they fail to protect against Mycobacterium tuberculosis? Front Immunol. 2017;8:407.****

40. Wang C, Liu Y, Cavanagh MM, Le Saux S, Qi Q, Roskin KM, et al. B-cell repertoire responses to varicella-zoster vaccination in human identical twins. Proc Natl Acad Sci U S A. 2015;112:500–5.

41. Pellegrino P, Falvella FS, Cheli S, Perrotta C, Clementi E, Radice S. The role of Toll-like receptor 4 polymorphisms in vaccine immune response. Pharmacogenomics J. 2016;16:96–101.

42. Poland GA, Ovsyannikova IG, Jacobson RM, Smith DI. Heterogeneity in vaccine immune response: the role of immunogenetics and the emerging field of vaccinomics. Clin Pharmacol Ther. 2007;82:653–64.****

43. Posteraro B, Pastorino R, Di Giannantonio P, Ianuale C, Amore R, Ricciardi W, Boccia S. The link between genetic variation and variability in vaccine responses: systematic review and meta-analyses. Vaccine. 2014;32:1661–9.****

44. Haralambieva IH, Ovsyannikova IG, Kennedy RB, Larrabee BR, Zimmermann MT, Grill DE, et al. Genome-wide associations of CD46 and IFI44L genetic variants with neutralizing antibody response to measles vaccine. Hum Genet. 2017;136:421–35.

45. Tsang JS. Utilizing population variation, vaccination, and systems biology to study human immunology. Trends Immunol. 2015;36:479–93.****

46. Hagan T, Pulendran B. Will systems biology deliver it's promise and contribute to the development of new or improved vaccines? From data to understanding through systems biology. Cold Spring Harbor perspectives in biology. Cold Spring Harb Perspect Biol. 2017. https://doi.org/10.1101/cshperspect.a028894.

47. Bragazzi NL, Gianfredi V, Villarini M, Rosselli R, Nasr A, Hussein A, et al. Vaccines meet big data: state-of-the-art and future prospects. From the classical 3Is ("isolate-inactivate-inject") Vaccinology 1.0 to Vaccinology 3.0, vaccinomics, and beyond: a historical overview. Front Public Health. 2018;6:62.

48. Whitaker JA, Ovsyannikova IG, Poland PA. Adversomics: a new paradigm for vaccine safety and design. Expert Rev Vaccines. 2015;14:935–47.

49. Gounder AP, Boon ACN. Influenza pathogenesis: the effect of host factors on severity of disease. J Immunol. 2019;202:341–50.∗∗

50. Tsang JS, Schwartzberg PL, Kotliarov Y, Biancotto A, Xie Z, Germain RN, et al. Global analyses of human immune variation reveal baseline predictors of postvaccination responses. Cell. 2014;157:499–513.

51. Andres-Terre M, McGuire H, Pouliot Y, Bongen E, Sweeney TE, Tato CM, et al. Systems analysis of immunity to influenza vaccination across multiple years and in diverse populations reveals shared molecular signatures. Immunity. 2015;43:1199–211.

52. Bhattacharjee A, Hand TW. Role of nutrition, infection, and the microbiota in the efficacy of oral vaccines. Clin Sci. 2018;132:1169–77.

53. Li XX, Zhou XN. Co-infection of tuberculosis and parasitic diseases in humans: a systematic review. Parasit Vectors. 2013;6:79.∗∗∗∗

54. Smith AD, Panickar KS, Urban JF Jr, Dawson HD. Impact of micronutrients on the immune response of animals. Annu Rev Anim Biosci. 2018;6:227–54.

55. DiNardo AR, Nishiguchi T, Mace EM, Rajapakshe K, Mtetwa G, Kay A, et al. Schistosomiasis induces persistent DNA methylation and tuberculosis-specific immune changes. J Immunol. 2018;201:124–33.

56. Malhotra I, Mungai P, Wamachi A, Kioko J, Ouma JH, Kazura JW, King CL. Helminth- and Bacillus Calmette-Guerin-induced immunity in children sensitized in utero to filariasis and schistosomiasis. J Immunol. 1999;162:6843–8.

57. Benn CS, Netea MG, Selin LK, Aaby P. A small jab – a big effect: nonspecific immunomodulation by vaccines. Trends Immunol. 2013;34:431–9.∗∗∗∗

58. Jensen KJ, Benn CS, van Crevel R. Unravelling the nature of non-specific effects of vaccines-A challenge for innate immunologists. Semin Immunol. 2016;28:377–83.

59. Mina MJ, Metcalf CJ, de Swart RL, Osterhaus AD, Grenfell BT. Long-term measles-induced immunomodulation increases overall childhood infectious disease mortality. Science. 2015;348:694–9.

60. Nankabirwa V, Tumwine JK, Mugaba PM, Tylleskar T, Sommerfelt H, PROMISE- EBF Study Group. Child survival and BCG vaccination: a community based prospective cohort study in Uganda. BMC Public Health. 2015;15:175.

61. Arts RJW, Moorlag SJCFM, Novakovic B, Li Y, Wang SY, Oosting M, et al. BCG vaccination protects against experimental viral infection in humans through the induction of cytokines associated with trained immunity. Cell Host Microbe. 2018;23:89–100.

62. Mina MJ. Generalized herd effects and vaccine evaluation: impact of live influenza vaccine on off-target bacterial colonisation. J Infect. 2017;74(Suppl 1):S101–7.

63. Good-Jacobson K. Strength in diversity: phenotypic, functional, and molecular heterogeneity within the memory B cell repertoire. Immunol Rev. 2018;284:67–78.

64. Takamura S. Niches for the long-term maintenance of tissue-resident memory T cells. Front Immunol. 2018;9:1214.∗∗∗∗

65. Hickler B, Guirguis S, Obregon R. Special issue on vaccine hesitancy. Vaccine. 2015;33:4155–217.

Readings Key

∗∗∗∗∗Plotkin's vaccines – ultimate reference on vaccines and vaccination
∗∗∗∗Required readings
∗∗Recommended readings
Other references of interest

Immunotherapy for Infectious Diseases, Cancer, and Autoimmunity

16

Peter J. Krause, Paula B. Kavathas, and Nancy H. Ruddle

16.1 Introduction

Medicine is poised to take advantage of directed immunotherapy now that the basic mechanisms of immunology are being elucidated. The goal of immunotherapy is to harness the immune system to combat disease. Specific reagents, including antibodies, can be directed against infectious organisms, against tumors, against particular tissue-damaging cells, or against cytokines in autoimmunity or allergy. In other settings, it is important to overcome inhibition of the immune response in situations where a robust response is needed, as in cancer. The ultimate goal is the use of directed immunotherapy with minimal side effects. The field of immunotherapeutics has employed the lessons of bench to bedside, applying key concepts from the laboratory and epidemiological studies to drug design and treatments.

16.2 Immunotherapy for Infectious Diseases

16.2.1 Introduction

The earliest recorded use of immune therapy was in China in the eleventh century when physicians used crusts from smallpox lesions to protect others against the disease, a process called variolation [1]. In the late eighteenth century, Edouard Jenner developed a smallpox vaccine using material from cowpox lesions and demonstrated its efficacy. In 1901 Emil von Behring and Shibasaburo Kitasato

P. J. Krause
Department of Epidemiology of Microbial Diseases, Yale School of Public Health and Departments of Medicine and Pediatrics, Yale School of Medicine, New Haven, CT, USA
e-mail: peter.krause@yale.edu

P. B. Kavathas
Departments of Laboratory Medicine and Immunobiology, Yale School of Medicine, New Haven, CT, USA
e-mail: paula.kavathas@yale.edu

N. H. Ruddle (✉)
Department of Epidemiology of Microbial Diseases, Yale School of Public Health, New Haven, CT, USA
e-mail: nancy.ruddle@yale.edu

© Springer Nature Switzerland AG 2019
P. J. Krause et al. (eds.), *Immunoepidemiology*, https://doi.org/10.1007/978-3-030-25553-4_16

discovered that transfer of immune sera in animals provided immunity against diphtheria and tetanus in humans. Behring won the first Nobel prize in Physiology or Medicine for this work. Subsequently, sera from animals (horses, sheep, and chickens) and humans vaccinated against specific pathogens were used to treat more than 15 different infections. Hyperimmune serum therapy consists of polyclonal antibody but has many disadvantages: for example, only a small proportion of the antibody is directed against the target pathogen. The advent of antibiotics in the 1940s decreased interest in the use of serum therapy; nonetheless, hyperimmune human sera are still used today for prevention and/ or treatment of several infections including cytomegalovirus (CMV), hepatitis A and B, rabies, tetanus, and varicella [1–4].

Although several hyperimmune polyclonal antibody preparations have been very effective, monoclonal antibodies (mAbs) are generally superior for several reasons. These include fewer side effects, minimal lot variation, and ease of use. Both hyperimmune polyclonal antibodies and mAbs are especially useful for treatment of antibiotic-resistant pathogens or other pathogens for which antibiotic therapy is not effective, including viral infections. Unlike antibiotics, polyclonal and mAb therapy target a specific pathogen and do not alter normal microflora or lead to the development of antibiotic-resistant organisms. Important disadvantages of polyclonal and mAb therapy over antibiotics include the need to make a specific pathogen diagnosis before use, the need to treat early in the course of infection, increased cost, and the need for systemic administration. Microbial antigenic variation can render mAbs ineffective, although this problem can be overcome either through the use of Mab therapy that targets conserved regions of the microbe or the use of multiple mAbs against multiple pathogen epitopes [1–4].

16.2.2 Production of Monoclonal Antibodies

In 1975, Kohler and Milstein developed a technique for making mAbs (Fig. 16.1) [5]. In brief, mice are immunized several times with the target antigen, which can be protein from a pathogen or tumor cell or another protein, such as a cytokine, until a sufficient titer of antibody is generated as assessed by an evaluation of the sera. The mice are euthanized, the spleen is removed, and a single-cell suspension is prepared that includes antibody-producing B cells. The spleen cells are then added in special media containing polyethylene glycol to an immortal cell line of a mouse plasma cell tumor (myeloma). Some of the two cell types fuse and are placed in special media where only myeloma-lymphocyte hybrids and replicating (hybridoma) cells survive. The media containing the cells is diluted and placed into 96-well plates so that each well contains a single clone of cells producing a single antibody type. The cells are then screened for production of antibodies against the original immunizing antigen. Each hybridoma cell produces an antibody against a particular epitope of the antigen. Antibody is harvested and purified. The various mAbs are tested for efficacy against the immunizing antigen, and the most promising Mab clones are selected for use.

Newer methods have been developed to produce mAbs that allow for mass production of highly specific and fully human antibody. Second-generation mAbs are chimeric so that the constant region of the mouse immunoglobulin is replaced by a human constant region or they contain murine CDR loop sequences and the rest is human. These antibodies more closely resemble those of humans (humanized mAbs) and minimize antiglobulin responses to nonhuman proteins in mAb molecules (Fig. 16.2) [6]. Third-generation mAbs are fully human antibodies. Several methods have been developed to produce these mAbs including (i) phage display, (ii) PCR or direct RNA sequencing of single plasma cells or B-cell blasts, and (iii) immunization of transgenic mice with

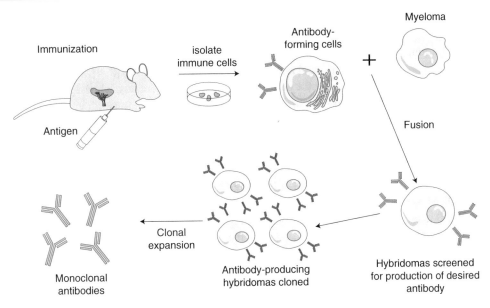

Fig. 16.1 Monoclonal antibody preparation. Mice are immunized several times with the target antigen and euthanized and antibody-producing spleen cells (splenocytes) are harvested. They are placed in polyethylene glycol along with immortal mouse B-lymphocyte tumor (myeloma) cells. The two types of cells fuse to form myeloma-lymphocyte hybridoma cells. The hybridoma cells are selected in medium and screened for production of antibody to the immunizing antigen. Individual hybridoma cells are cloned and expanded. Those mAb clones with highest affinity for the target antigen are selected for use. (©Krause 2020)

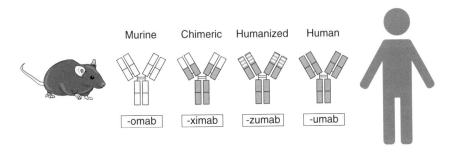

Fig. 16.2 Types of genetically modified monoclonal antibodies starting from a mouse mAb. The chimeric antibody has human constant domains and a murine variable domain. The humanized antibody retains the CDR loops from the murine sequence. The human antibody is identical to human sequences. The antibody name endings indicate the degree to which the Mab is humanized or is fully human. (©Kavathas 2020)

human Ig genes substituted for the mouse Ig genes. (iv) immortalization of human B cells using one of several methods including Epstein-Barr virus (EBV); IL-2, IL-21, and irradiated 3T3-msCD40L feeder cells; or a retrovirus containing BCL-6 and BCL-XL [7, 8]. These methods yield fully human mAbs and avoid the cost and time required for humanization of murine mAbs.

In this chapter, we will concentrate on the use of mAbs in immunotherapy, but it must be pointed out that their utility goes far beyond that function. Monoclonal Abs also have been of great use in diagnostics as the basis of measuring the presence of particular pathogens and in elucidating the nature of immune cell subsets (e.g., T-cell subsets) and pathogen components.

16.2.3 Examples of Antibody Treatment of Infectious Diseases

Monoclonal antibodies have been licensed for use for the following infectious diseases: anthrax, *Clostridium difficile* (toxin B), HIV, and respiratory syncytial virus (RSV) [3, 4]. The first of these to be developed was antibody treatment for protection against RSV infections, which has been available since 1998 [7, 8]. RSV is the most important respiratory tract pathogen in children less than 5 years of age worldwide and is *the* major cause of hospitalization for bronchiolitis and pneumonia among infants less than 2 years of age [9]. It causes life-threatening illness in immunocompromised patients, predisposes to asthma and chronic lung disease in older children and adults, and can cause repeated respiratory infections into adulthood. The use of intravenous polyclonal RSV immunoglobulin obtained from healthy people with high-titer RSV antibody was licensed for prophylaxis against RSV in 1996 [10]. Monthly administration of this product during the RSV season (November to May in the United Sates) decreased hospitalizations for RSV infection by more than 50% in premature infants and infants with chronic lung disease. Several problems associated with this treatment included no benefit or even worsened outcome in children with congenital heart disease (one of the high-risk groups for severe RSV disease), interference with immune response to live attenuated vaccines for other infections, and risk of infectious diseases transmitted through this plasma-derived product. In 1998, a humanized anti-RSV mAb (palivizumab) was licensed for use. Several placebo-controlled trials showed that this mAb had greater efficacy with fewer side effects and greater ease of use (lower volume of infusion) than the high-titer intravenous polyclonal antibody product [10]. Palivizumab also was shown to be effective in treating RSV infection in infants with congenital heart disease.

There is enormous potential for mAb therapy of infectious disease and promising mAb preparations are being developed for HIV, hepatitis C, influenzae, rabies, *Cryptococcus neoformans*, and West Nile virus, as well as for toxins produced by *E. coli*, *C. difficile*, and *B. anthracis* [1–4].

16.3 Immunotherapy for Cancer

Immune cells normally eliminate cancer cells in a process called cancer immunosurveillance. This was originally proposed by F. MacFarlane Burnet and Lewis Thomas in the 1950s [11]. However, definitive evidence to support this theory was not obtained until genetically altered mice were developed that specifically lost T cells and NK cells [12]. The incidence of tumor initiation and metastasis in chemically induced tumors was much higher in those animals than in genetically matched immunocompetent mice. This indicated that the tumor cells could be recognized as nonself. Cells acquire multiple genetic alterations as they attain malignancy and exhibit dysregulated proliferation. Malignantly transformed cells often express new antigens called neoantigens that result from mutations that can be recognized by T cells. While neoantigens are the prime target of tumor-specific T cells, tumor-associated antigens can arise from abnormal expression of self-antigens or expression of those that are normally found in immunologically privileged sites (no tolerance). These can potentially be detected by CD8 cytotoxic T cells (CTLs) which kill the tumor cells. Natural killer (NK) cells are another important cytotoxic cell and are activated when the tumor cells have reduced or eliminated HLA expression ("missing self") and express stress-induced ligands or other ligands recognized by NK cell receptors.

Those tumor cells that grow are able to evade immune attack. There are multiple means for this escape. One mechanism is through tumor immunoediting, whereby additional mutations result in the loss of the original target antigens for CTLs [13]. The state of the tumor microenvironment is an important factor [14]. A suppressive microenvironment in the vicinity of the tumor can occur with the presence of CD4 T regulatory cells and/or myeloid suppressor cells. Expression of ligands, either on the tumor or on cells in the microenvironment, that bind inhibitory receptors on T cells or NK cells deliver "stop" signals. Secretion of inhibitory cytokines such as TGF-β, as well as metabolic changes that starve the immune cells of nutrients, can create an inhospitable environment for immune cells. Another mechanism is the acquisition of an "exhausted" state by immune cells in the tumor microenvironment resulting in functional impairment. Other changes in the microenvironment can lead to the exclusion of the CTLs or NK cells from reaching the tumor cells. Infiltrating immune cells can sometimes be observed near the tumor but are unable to penetrate into the tumor. Therefore, different therapeutic approaches are required to address the different mechanisms of tumor escape.

An important advantage of cancer immunotherapy is its ability to harness the specificity of antibodies and T and B cells to target tumor cells, in contrast to chemotherapy which generally targets all dividing cells. Antibodies or immune cells can travel throughout the body, potentially targeting even small numbers of cancer cells. This is particularly important for those cancers where the tumor cells have left the original site, usually through lymphatic or blood vessels, to metastasize or spread to other tissues. About 90% of patients who die of cancer have metastases. In addition, because the T and B cells of the adaptive immune system can develop into memory cells, there is the potential for lasting immunity. This section will focus on some of the approaches to cancer immunotherapy and what might account for variability in differences in the success of different treatments between people. This is a growing field, so many more advances are expected in the future.

The main immunotherapeutic approaches for cancer patients are (1) monoclonal antibodies that bind to the tumor cells and target them for destruction or modulate the tumor microenvironment; (2) infusion of immune cells that have been expanded and/or genetically engineered outside the body (Chap. 15); (3) treatment with immune checkpoint inhibitors (ICIs), which are antibodies that prevent inhibitory receptors from being activated on immune cells; (4) injection of substances directly into the tumor to enhance the immune response and (5) administration of tumor vaccines to stimulate tumor immunity.

One of the first monoclonal antibodies approved for therapy in 1997 was Rituximab, a mAb directed against the cell surface protein CD20 found on mature B lymphocytes. It has been used for targeting and destroying B-cell tumors. Once the antibody binds to the surface of tumor cells, natural killer cells with an Fc receptor for the IgG antibody kill the tumor cells in a process called antibody-dependent cell-mediated cytotoxicity (ADCC). Variability in response to rituximab has been linked to polymorphisms in the IgG Fc receptor [15]. Individuals who have an Fc receptor with stronger (higher affinity) binding to IgG show a better response to rituximab treatment. Normal mature B cells are also affected, but not long-lived antibody-secreting plasma cells, because CD20 is downregulated on those cells. Rituximab does not always induce a cure however, as tumor variants develop over time that lose expression of the CD20 protein and become resistant to the therapy. Interestingly, this antibody has also been found to be effective in the treatment of multiple sclerosis, an autoimmune disease described below. Additional antibodies targeting tumor cells were subsequently developed, such as an antibody binding to the surface epidermal growth factor 2 (ERBB2, formerly HER2), which is elevated in a subset of breast cancer cells due to genetic amplification of the ERBB2/HER2 gene.

A radically new approach for antibody therapy was developed in the late 1990s: the use of immune checkpoint inhibitors (ICIs). Rather than employing antibodies for tumor destruction, these antibodies are used to *modulate* the immune response so as to exert an antitumor effect. When tumor cells die, antigen-presenting cells such as dendritic cells can potentially pick up antigen and cross-prime T cells. Because T cells express inhibitory receptors after activation such as CTLA-4 (Chap. 5), Dr. James Allison and his research team reasoned that blocking this receptor with an anti-CTLA4 antibody could promote a stronger T-cell response against the tumor. This was the case in a mouse cancer model that they reported in 1996 [16]. In 2011 the FDA approved a humanized monoclonal anti-CTLA-4 antibody, ipilimumab, for cancer therapy based on the positive results in the animal models and human clinical trials. An antibody against the PD-1 receptor (nivolumab, pembrolizumab) was approved in 2014 for the treatment of melanoma and in 2015 for lung cancer, based on improvement in patient survival. PD-1 is an inhibitory receptor on activated T and NK cells. Its ligand, PDL-1, is induced on cells in the presence of IFN-γ (see Chap. 5). Anti-PDL-1 mAb was subsequently approved (e.g., Atezolizumab) [17]. Blocking this receptor-ligand interaction releases the "brakes" on CD8 cytotoxic cells (Fig. 16.3). A small subset of patients with advanced melanoma or lung cancer have had increased long-term survival (years) when anti-CTLA-4 is given in combination with anti-PD-1 compared with anti-PD-1 alone. Antibodies blocking other inhibitory receptor-ligand pairs are currently being tested in clinical trials, as are different combinations of antibodies. Subsets of patients manifest neurological, respiratory, musculoskeletal, cardiac, ocular [18], and/or autoimmune side effects [19]. Regardless, ICI therapy holds great promise for cancers that previously had very low survival rates such as melanoma or late-stage lung cancer. Such therapies have dramatically improved the long-term survival of patients from less than a year to more than 5 years; however, many patients do not respond. Rizvi et al. found a correlation between antigen load and response to pembrolizumab in non-small cell lung cancer (NSCLC). They reported that smokers had significantly more mutations in NSCLC tumors than nonsmokers [20]. Thus, the antigen load of a tumor could be one variable affecting response to ICIs.

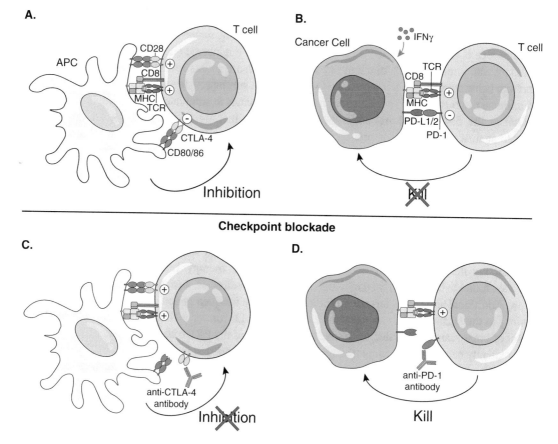

Fig. 16.3 Inhibitory receptors CTLA-4 and PD-1. (**a**) CTLA4 normally functions as an inhibitory receptor on activated T cells binding to the costimulatory proteins CD80/86 or B7.1/B7.2 on APCs. It competes for binding with the costimulatory protein CD28. (**b**) PD-1 also functions as an inhibitory receptor on T cells whose ligand, PD-L1 or PD-L2, is expressed on cells of the body in the presence of IFN-γ. (**c**) In checkpoint blockade immunotherapy, anti-CTLA-4, or (**d**) anti-PD-1, or anti-PD-L1 mAbs are used to block receptor-ligand interaction. This removes the "brakes" or inhibitory signals transmitted by these two receptors. (©Kavathas 2020)

Cancers can acquire resistance to immune-based therapies through multiple mechanisms. One mechanism is the loss or reduction of HLA class I from the cell surface. In order to kill a target cell, a CD8 cytotoxic T cell needs a signal from its receptor after binding to a specific peptide bound to HLA class I. In the absence HLA class I, cytotoxic T cells are not effective against tumors. Some lung cancer tumors in patients with acquired resistance after checkpoint blockade therapy were found to have lost β2-microglobulin, required for expression of HLA class I [21]. Thus, they lacked HLA class I expression on their tumor cells, which explains the development of resistance.

One variable that affects therapeutic efficacy of immune checkpoint inhibitors against cancer appears to be the composition of the gut microbiome (Chap. 2). The gut microbiome is composed of trillions of bacteria along with fungi, archaea, protozoa, and viruses. Individuals are exposed to the microbiome during the birthing process and subsequent environmental exposure. It can be modulated by diet and antibiotics. Antibiotics can cause temporary or persistent changes in the composition of the microbiome. Patients with lung, kidney, and bladder cancer who take antibiotics before starting PD-1 immunotherapy relapse sooner and do not live as long as those who do not [22]. Another group reported that ICI responders had a more diverse microbiome and the presence of certain bacterial strains. Transfer of bacteria into mice from patients who responded or not led to similar results in the animals [23]. Efforts to modulate the composition of the gut microbiome before ICI therapy are being explored.

The use of neoantigen cancer vaccines is another potential therapeutic approach. With advances in genetic sequencing and RNA expression analysis, as well as the development of in silico programs to predict binding of peptides to HLA proteins, potential peptide neoantigens can be determined. Creating vaccines by immunizing against tumor-specific mutant peptides is being explored to either generate or expand existing neoantigen-reactive T cells [24]. In the case of tumors containing a high-risk human papilloma virus (HPV) strain, individuals that can present peptides derived from the oncogenic HPV proteins E6 and E7 can potentially mount a T-cell response against the cancer cells after vaccination against the oncoproteins. Cell therapy is emerging as a promising therapeutic modality spearheaded by the clinical success of chimeric antigen receptor (CAR)-modified T cells for B cell malignancies approved by the FDA in 2017. The hybrid receptors were derived from an antibody single-chain variable fragment with intracellular signaling domains derived from endogenous TCRs and costimulatory proteins. Next generation modifications include enhancing in vivo persistence and overcoming T cell dysfunction. Immunotherapy for cancer has made tremendous advances as reflected both in publications but also in the growth of biotechnology companies working on these types of therapies. There is clearly much to learn, and the future is bright.

16.4 Immunotherapy for Autoimmunity

16.4.1 Introduction

The goal of immunotherapy in autoimmune diseases is to inhibit the destructive role of lymphocytes directed toward self-antigens while maintaining the integrity of the immune system in its critical function of defense against pathogens, with a minimum of side effects. Many of the original therapies that are still in use have nonspecific anti-inflammatory activity. These include nonsteroidal anti-inflammatory drugs (NSAIDS), such as aspirin and indomethacin; glucocorticoids such as prednisone, dexamethasone, and Leflunomide; and disease-modifying anti-rheumatic drugs (DMARDS), such as methotrexate. All have side effects, although many remain in use alone (in some cases to reduce pain) or in combination with other therapies. None act directly on the particular effector molecules or cells

Table 16.1 Immunotherapeutics for autoimmune diseases

Trade name ®	Common name	Molecular form	Target/mechanism	Diseases
BETASERON	IFN-beta-1β	IFN-beta-1β	Anti-inflammatory	MS
AVONEX	IFN-beta-1α	IFN-beta-1α	Anti-inflammatory	MS
CIMZIA	Certolizumab	Anti-TNF-α mAb (pegol)	TNF-α	CD, RA, PSA, AS, PS
SIMPONI	Golimumab	Anti-TNF-α mAb	TNF-α	RA
ENBREL	Etanercept	TNFRII-Fc	TNF-α, LT-α	RA, PS, AS
KINRERET	Anakinra	IL-1R antagonist	IL-1	RA
ACTEMRA	Tocilizumab	Anti-IL-6RmAb	IL-6	RA
TALTZ	Ixekizumab	Anti-IL-17 mAb	IL-17	PS
STELARA	Ustekinumab	Anti-IL12/23 mAb	IL-12/23	PS
PRV-031	Teplizumab	Anti-CD3	T cells	T1D
ORENCIA	Abatacept	CTLA4-Fc	T cells	RA
GILENYA	Fingolimod	FTY-720	Lymphocyte egress from SLOs	MS
RITUXAN	Rituximab	Anti-CD20 mAb	B cells	RA, MS
COPAXONE	Glatiramer acetate	Myelin basic protein peptides	Decoy?	MS
TECFIDERA	Dimethyl-fumarate		Blocking cytokines and chemokines?	MS

Abbreviations: *CD* Crohn's disease, *RA* rheumatoid arthritis, *MS* multiple sclerosis, *PS* psoriasis, *AS* ankylosing spondylitis, *PSA* psoriatic arthritis, *T1D* type 1 diabetes

Information provided by manufacturer's websites. Many of these reagents are use in other diseases as well.

of the immune system. In this section, we will concentrate on the recent development of drugs whose target is selective inhibition of particular cell types or cytokines that appear to be key to the pathogenesis of autoimmunity. A partial list of the commercially available therapies that fall into this category are summarized in Table 16.1.

16.4.2 Cytokine Therapies

The interferons were the first cytokine therapies to be used in autoimmunity. Several forms of type 1 interferon are available (Table 16.1). All appear to act as general anti-inflammatory agents.

16.4.3 Anti-cytokine Therapies

16.4.3.1 TNF Inhibitors

The original pharma interest in TNF was based on the possibility that the cytokine could be used in combating tumors. However, when administered systemically, profound adverse events were noted that resembled sepsis, due to the fact that TNF is a major cytokine released after gram-negative infection. TNF had some efficacy when delivered locally to easily accessible tumors. The further observation that high levels of TNF were present in the circulation in bacterial-induced sepsis in humans and animal models gave rise to the idea that TNF inhibitors, rather than agonists, might be useful in treating overwhelming bacterial infections. Furthermore, treatment with anti-TNF antibody resulted in enhanced survival of LPS-treated mice, but only if the TNF inhibitor was given *before* exposure to the inciting agent [25]. Clinical trials in humans failed, as it was not possible to predict who would benefit from anti-TNF therapy. This was so because in order to be effective, the anti-TNF had to be administered before bacterial exposure. Concurrently, Maini and Feldmann realized that high levels of TNF were present in the synovial fluid of rheumatoid arthritic joints in humans and also found that treatment with anti-TNF was effective in mouse models of rheumatoid arthritis (RA). Thus, the first clinical trials of a TNF inhibitor used a chimeric (partially humanized mouse mAb) anti-TNF antibody to treat RA patients. The treatment group exhibited an improved joint score and reduced joint erosion [26]. This initial success has given rise to a revolution in treatment with TNF inhibitors for a variety of autoimmune diseases.

16.4.3.2 Other Cytokine Inhibitors

Many cytokines besides TNF have been implicated in autoimmune diseases. In some cases, such as IL-1, they may be downstream targets of TNF. In others, they are effector molecules with very distinct pathways of activation and biologic activities, including IL-17. As indicated in Table 16.1, monoclonal antibodies are available against almost all of the inflammatory cytokines and are used in particular autoimmune diseases.

16.4.3.3 Factors Influencing Treatment Failure

Despite the tremendous increase in the availability of immunotherapeutic agents to treat autoimmune disease (Table 16.1), treatment failure is not uncommon. This may be due to an initial unresponsiveness to the agent, a later tolerance to that agent, or adverse events such as activation of latent infections. Tuberculosis reactivation is a particular problem with these immunosuppressive agents. Here we will concentrate on studies that have investigated the reasons for failure of TNF inhibitors, but similar problems exist for all of the cytokine inhibitors.

It has been reported that 10–40% of the Crohn's disease (CD) patients do not respond to anti-TNF therapy and that 24–46% show a loss of response in the course of treatment. What is the underlying cause of the failures, particularly nonresponsiveness? An analysis of the PANTS (personalized anti-TNF therapy in CD) study evaluated this question in 1610 patients treated with TNF inhibitors, infliximab or adalimumab [27]. The main conclusion of the study was that primary (evaluated at 14 weeks) or secondary (evaluated at 56 weeks) treatment failure was correlated with a low concentration of the inhibitor and high titers of antibody directed against it, even though the agents had been engineered to be predominately of human origin. It is also possible that the study subjects were producing antibodies against their own TNF, although this was not investigated specifically in this study. The more interesting question that needs to be addressed is why these individuals might be producing antibody to the TNF inhibitors. It is interesting that there is a higher likelihood of the production of such antibodies in smokers or obese individuals. It must be kept in mind that the TNF gene complex (TNF-α, LT-α, LT-β) is highly polymorphic [28]. Thus, it is likely that responsiveness to therapy is influenced by polymorphisms in individual cytokines and their receptors.

Even if the reasons for treatment failure are not completely understood, it is possible to treat with inhibitors of other cytokines, as was the case with a study of RA patients who failed anti-TNF treatment but were successfully treated with an inhibitor of the IL-6 receptor (tocilizumab) plus methotrexate [29]. In another study of RA patients who were intolerant or unresponsive to TNF inhibitors, 604 patients received rituximab and 507 received a second TNF inhibitor. Those treated with rituximab were significantly improved compared to those treated with a second TNF inhibitor [30]. This was particularly true for those individuals who had initially been unresponsive to TNF inhibitors. This suggests that either they had very high anti-TNF inhibitor antibodies [27], that the mechanism of their disease varied, or that additional genetic or epigenetic factors influenced their lack of responsiveness.

16.4.4 Cell-Directed Immunotherapies

16.4.4.1 T Cells

T cells play a major role in many autoimmune diseases. One approach could be to induce tolerance in T cells to particular autoantigens. Teplizumab, a humanized, non-Fc-binding mouse monoclonal antibody against CD3 (a molecule expressed on T cells), has shown some promise in trials designed to preserve pancreatic beta-cell function in patients with new-onset type 1 diabetes. Transcriptomic analysis of peripheral blood samples from patients in the AbATE (Autoimmunity-Blocking Antibody for Tolerance) trial was carried out in a longitudinal study that involved analysis of beta-cell function over time by evaluating C-peptide levels in the blood (a marker of endogenous insulin production) [31]. Those patients who showed the greatest preservation of islet function (i.e., responders) had an accumulation of a population of CD8 T cells that expressed exhaustion markers and thus reduced function, suggesting that changing the phenotype of CD8 CTLs could be a promising approach. It remains to be determined why some individuals responded positively to the therapy and others did not.

T cells require 3 signals for activation, TCR (binding peptide MHC), CD28 (binding CD80 or CD86), and a cytokine-cytokine receptor. The inhibitory receptor, CTLA-4, can bind to CD80 or CD86 on the antigen-presenting cells and thus prevent activation of the T cell. ORENCIA (abatacept) is a fusion protein between the extracellular domain of CTLA-4 that binds to CD80 or CD86 and the Fc region of IgG1. Abatacept interferes with signal 2, preventing activation of T cells. This drug is used in RA.

16.4.4.2 Lymphocyte Trafficking

Activated T cells express surface molecules that direct them out of lymph nodes and to sites of their cognate antigen. One such surface molecule is alpha-4 integrin that combined with the beta-4 chain as a heterodimer becomes VLA-4. VCAM-1, the ligand for VLA-4, is expressed on activated endothelium at sites of inflammation. TYSABRI (natalizumab) is a monoclonal antibody that recognizes alpha-4 integrin, and thus interferes with the ability of cells that express it to access sites of VCAM-1 expression, thus blocking their entry into inflamed sites. It has proven effective in MS but in a small number of cases has been associated with progressive multifocal leukoencephalopathy (PML) that is caused by activation of latent JC virus, particularly in patients who have been on other forms of immunosuppression and/or who have titers of anti-JC virus.

Lymphocyte traffic through the body is guided by chemokines and in part by the lipid chemoattractant, sphingosine-1-phosphate (S1P), present in blood and lymph. S1P1, a receptor for S1P, is expressed on activated T cells in lymph nodes. Thus, their egress from that organ is encouraged by their ligand, S1P, in the lymph [32]. FTY-720, also known as fingolomid, is an agonist of the receptor, causing its internalization. The cells of patients treated with fingolomid are no longer responsive to the S1P gradient and accumulate in lymphoid organs rather than in the circulation, resulting in a functional lymphopenia. This agent was first used in transplantation but is now used in autoimmune diseases, especially MS. The rationale is that the activated T cells will be "stuck" in the lymph nodes and incapable of accessing the autoimmune site.

16.4.4.3 B Cells

In recent years, an interest in the role of B cells in the pathogenesis of autoimmune diseases has arisen, even in those traditionally thought to be of an inflammatory T-cell nature. As noted above, RITUXAN (rituximab) is a chimeric murine/human monoclonal antibody directed against CD20, a molecule expressed on B cells. It was originally used in non-Hodgkin's lymphoma. It has shown some efficacy in RA and in MS. Its mode of action in autoimmune diseases is unclear but is probably not due to the destruction of the antibody-forming capacity of plasma cells, which no longer express CD20. One possibility is that it is directed against the cytokine-producing capacity of B cells or their antigen-presenting activity. RITUXAN has also been associated with development of progressive multifocal leukoencephalopathy (PML) as noted above.

RITUXAN treatment has been used in a clinical trial to treat newly diagnosed type 1diabetes patients. Whole genome RNA-seq and flow cytometric analyses of whole blood were carried out to evaluate progression (responders) and lack of progression (nonresponders) using serum C-peptide levels. A population of T cells was transiently increased in the peripheral blood of those patients with lower C-peptide levels. The cells in this population were hypoproliferative to islet cell antigens [33]. A recently reported 7-year follow-up of these patients showed that the responders had an increase in PD-1[+] central memory and anergic CD8[+] T cells [34]. These data indicate that a useful approach for monitoring different populations of patients could involve noninvasive analysis of peripheral blood. They also suggest that an approach that utilizes combination therapies could be beneficial.

16.4.5 Additional Therapies

COPAXONE (glatiramer acetate) is a synthetic protein that is somewhat similar to myelin basic protein, a component of myelin. Since myelin is a target of the immune response in MS, the substance was hypothesized to act as a decoy for immune attack. This drug appears to block myelin-damaging T-cells through a mechanism that is not completely understood.

TECFIDERA (dimethyl fumarate) is an orally available drug that has recently been approved for relapsing MS. Although its mechanism of action is unclear, it appears to act by blocking cytokine action. A recent report [35] suggests that the drug inhibits a micro-RNA that is necessary for activation of CCR6, a chemokine receptor required for T cell homing to the brain.

16.5 Conclusions

The explosion in pharmaceuticals available to treat autoimmune diseases has come about in part from numerous studies in animal models and in human diseases aimed at understanding mechanisms, and then applying inhibitors of immune cells and cytokines to human diseases. As noted above, some of these advances have been serendipitous with mechanistic insights still to be determined. What is clear is that treatment failures, unresponsiveness, and nonspecific immunosuppression resulting in activation of latent diseases, such as tuberculosis or JC virus, and activation of autoimmune disease in checkpoint inhibition remain as serious issues. Immunoepidemiologic studies, as noted in the case of TNF inhibitors, have provided important information. Much needs to be learned.

References

1. Doherty M, Robertson MJ. Some early trends in immunology. Trends Immunol. 2004;25(12):623–31.
2. Marasco WA, Sui J. The growth and potential of human antiviral monoclonal antibody therapeutics. Nat Biotechnol. 2007;25(12):1421–34.
3. Pelfrene E, Mura M, Cavaleiro Sanches A, Cavaleri M. Monoclonal antibodies as anti-infective products: a promising future? Clin Microbiol Infect. 2019;25(1):60–4.
4. Saylor C, Dadachova E, Casadevall A. Monoclonal antibody-based therapies for microbial diseases. Vaccine. 2009;27(Suppl 6):G38–46.
5. Kohler G, Milstein C. Continuous cultures of fused cells secreting antibody of predefined specificity. Nature. 1975;256(5517):495–7.
6. Riechmann L, Clark M, Waldmann H, Winter G. Reshaping human antibodies for therapy. Nature. 1988;332(6162):323–7.
7. Huang J, Doria-Rose NA, Longo NS, Laub L, Lin CL, Turk E, et al. Isolation of human monoclonal antibodies from peripheral blood B cells. Nat Protoc. 2013;8(10):1907–15.
8. Kwakkenbos MJ, van Helden PM, Beaumont T, Spits H. Stable long-term cultures of self-renewing B cells and their applications. Immunol Rev. 2016;270(1):65–77.

9. Welliver RC. Review of epidemiology and clinical risk factors for severe respiratory syncytial virus (RSV) infection. J Pediatr. 2003;143(5 Suppl):S112–7.

10. Born AAoPCoIDaCoFaN. Prevention of respiratory syncytial virus infection: indications for use of palivizumab and update on the use of RSV-IVIG. Pediatrics. 1998;102:1211–6.

11. Burnet M. Cancer; a biological approach. I. The processes of control. Br Med J. 1957;1(5022):779–86.

12. Street SE, Cretney E, Smyth MJ. Perforin and interferon-gamma activities independently control tumor initiation, growth, and metastasis. Blood. 2001;97(1):192–7.

13. Schreiber RD, Old LJ, Smyth MJ. Cancer immunoediting: integrating immunity's roles in cancer suppression and promotion. Science. 2011;331(6024):1565–70.

14. Binnewies M, Roberts EW, Kersten K, Chan V, Fearon DF, Merad M, et al. Understanding the tumor immune microenvironment (TIME) for effective therapy. Nat Med. 2018;24(5):541–50.

15. Weng WK, Levy R. Two immunoglobulin G fragment C receptor polymorphisms independently predict response to rituximab in patients with follicular lymphoma. J Clin Oncol. 2003;21(21):3940–7.

16. Leach DR, Krummel MF, Allison JP. Enhancement of antitumor immunity by CTLA-4 blockade. Science. 1996;271(5256):1734–6.

17. Weiss SA, Wolchok JD, Sznol M. Immunotherapy of melanoma: facts and hopes. Clin Cancer Res. 2019; https://doi.org/10.1158/1078-0432.CCR-18-1550.

18. Zimmer L, Goldinger SM, Hofmann L, Loquai C, Ugurel S, Thomas I, et al. Neurological, respiratory, musculo-skeletal, cardiac and ocular side-effects of anti-PD-1 therapy. Eur J Cancer. 2016;60:210–25.

19. Stamatouli AM, Quandt Z, Perdigoto AL, Clark PL, Kluger H, Weiss SA, et al. Collateral damage: insulin-dependent diabetes induced with checkpoint inhibitors. Diabetes. 2018;67(8):1471–80.

20. Rizvi NA, Hellmann MD, Snyder A, Kvistborg P, Makarov V, Havel JJ, et al. Cancer immunology. Mutational landscape determines sensitivity to PD-1 blockade in non-small cell lung cancer. Science. 2015;348(6230):124–8.

21. Gettinger S, Choi J, Hastings K, Truini A, Datar I, Sowell R, et al. Impaired HLA class I antigen processing and presentation as a mechanism of acquired resistance to immune checkpoint inhibitors in lung cancer. Cancer Discov. 2017;7(12):1420–35.

22. Routy B, Le Chatelier E, Derosa L, Duong CPM, Alou MT, Daillere R, et al. Gut microbiome influences efficacy of PD-1-based immunotherapy against epithelial tumors. Science. 2018;359(6371):91–7.

23. Helmink BA, Khan MAW, Hermann A, Gopalakrishnan V, Wargo JA. The microbiome, cancer, and cancer therapy. Nat Med. 2019;25(3):377–88.

24. Palucka K, Banchereau J, Mellman I. Designing vaccines based on biology of human dendritic cell subsets. Immunity. 2010;33(4):464–78.

25. Sheehan KC, Ruddle NH, Schreiber RD. Generation and characterization of hamster monoclonal antibodies that neutralize murine tumor necrosis factors. J Immunol. 1989;142(11):3884–93.

26. Elliott MJ, Maini RN, Feldmann M, Long-Fox A, Charles P, Katsikis P, et al. Treatment of rheumatoid arthritis with chimeric monoclonal antibodies to tumor necrosis factor alpha. Arthritis Rheum. 1993;36(12):1681–90.

27. Kennedy NA, Heap GA, Green HD, Hamilton B, Bewshea C, Walker GJ, et al. Predictors of anti-TNF treatment failure in anti-TNF-naive patients with active luminal Crohn's disease: a prospective, multicentre, cohort study. Lancet Gastroenterol Hepatol. 2019;4(5):341–53.

28. Hajeer AH, Hutchinson IV. TNF-alpha gene polymorphism: clinical and biological implications. Microsc Res Tech. 2000;50(3):216–28.

29. Emery P, Keystone E, Tony HP, Cantagrel A, van Vollenhoven R, Sanchez A, et al. IL-6 receptor inhibition with tocilizumab improves treatment outcomes in patients with rheumatoid arthritis refractory to anti-tumour necrosis factor biologicals: results from a 24-week multicentre randomised placebo-controlled trial. Ann Rheum Dis. 2008;67(11):1516–23.

30. Emery P, Gottenberg JE, Rubbert-Roth A, Sarzi-Puttini P, Choquette D, Taboada VM, et al. Rituximab versus an alternative TNF inhibitor in patients with rheumatoid arthritis who failed to respond to a single previous TNF inhibitor: SWITCH-RA, a global, observational, comparative effectiveness study. Ann Rheum Dis. 2015;74(6):979–84.

31. Long SA, Thorpe J, DeBerg HA, Gersuk V, Eddy J, Harris KM, et al. Partial exhaustion of CD8 T cells and clinical response to teplizumab in new-onset type 1 diabetes. Sci Immunol. 2016;1(5):eaai7793.

32. Matloubian M, Lo CG, Cinamon G, Lesneski MJ, Xu Y, Brinkmann V, et al. Lymphocyte egress from thymus and peripheral lymphoid organs is dependent on S1P receptor 1. Nature. 2004;427(6972):355–60.

33. Linsley PS, Greenbaum CJ, Rosasco M, Presnell S, Herold KC, Dufort MJ. Elevated T cell levels in peripheral blood predict poor clinical response following rituximab treatment in new-onset type 1 diabetes. Genes Immun. 2019;20(4):293–307.

34. Perdigoto AL, Preston-Hurlburt P, Clark P, Long SA, Linsley PS, Harris KM, et al. Treatment of type 1 diabetes with teplizumab: clinical and immunological follow-up after 7 years from diagnosis. Diabetologia. 2019;62(4):655–64.

35. Ntranos A, Ntranos V, Bonnefil V, Liu J, Kim-Schulze S, He Y, et al. Fumarates target the metabolic-epigenetic interplay of brain-homing T cells in multiple sclerosis. Brain. 2019;142(3):647–61.

Appendix

Jane O'Bryan, Kara Fikrig, Peter J. Krause and Kate Nyhan

Introduction

Immunoepidemiology is a relatively new field with the first published studies appearing in the late 1950s. Although there are a few excellent review papers on the topic, a broad review with a comprehensive bibliography that could aid researchers and scholars in identifying important papers on the topic does not yet exist. Accordingly, we carried out a scoping review using optimal literature search strategies developed by a professional medical librarian. Scoping reviews address broad, complex, and exploratory research questions, while systematic reviews are designed to answer more precisely defined and narrower questions. Our objectives were to determine the number of articles with the words "immunoepidemiology" or "immune-epidemiology" in the title or abstract that have been published each year over the past six decades and to identify articles written since 1980 that are most relevant to the field using predefined screening and list these in a bibliography. Here we present the methodology and results of a scoping review of the extant immunoepidemiology literature from 1959 to 2019. We describe the search strategy, article selection process, and findings of the review in detail.

Methods

A scoping review of the immunoepidemiology literature was conducted using the online databases Ovid MEDLINE, Embase, PubMed, Scopus, and Web of Science in November 2015. The database searches were conducted using the following search strategy:

J. O'Bryan · K. Fikrig
Department of Epidemiology of Microbial Diseases, Yale School of Public Health, New Haven, CT, USA
e-mail: jane.obryan@yale.edu; kmfikrig@gmail.com

P. J. Krause
Department of Epidemiology of Microbial Diseases, Yale School of Public Health and Departments of Medicine and Pediatrics, Yale School of Medicine, New Haven, CT, USA
e-mail: peter.krause@yale.edu

K. Nyhan
Harvey Cushing/John Hay Whitney Medical Library, Yale University, New Haven, CT, USA
e-mail: kate.nyhan@yale.edu

© Springer Nature Switzerland AG 2019
P. J. Krause et al. (eds.), *Immunoepidemiology*, https://doi.org/10.1007/978-3-030-25553-4

Table A.1 Inclusion and exclusion criteria of the Scoping reviews of 2015 and 2019

Inclusion criteria	Exclusion criteria
Human studies	Non-human/animal studies
Articles published in the English language	Articles written in a language other than English
Review papers, book chapters, journal articles	Conference/committee reports
Reference to immunology and to populations and/or epidemiology in abstract	Missing either reference to immunology or epidemiology in abstract
Abstract went beyond describing prevalence/incidence of disease for epidemiology component	Abstract did not go beyond describing prevalence/incidence of disease
Abstract went beyond describing general diagnostics or vaccine efficacy	Abstract did not go beyond describing general diagnostics or vaccine efficacy
Paper was published after 1980	Paper was published before 1980 and/or contained outdated information
Complete record	Incomplete record (i.e. figure or table, not an article)

"immunoepidemiological" OR "immunoepidemiology" OR (immunoepidemiology[All Fields] OR immunoepidemiological[All Fields])

Articles that were included were human studies, review papers, book chapters, and journal articles that referenced immunology and populations and/or epidemiology in the abstract. Articles that did not reference both immunology and epidemiology in the abstract, articles that did not go beyond describing disease incidence/prevalence, and articles that did not go beyond describing general diagnostics and/or vaccine efficacy were excluded. Additionally, articles that were published before 1980 and contained outdated information, incomplete records (i.e., figure or table alone), and committee reports and meetings were excluded. The inclusion and exclusion criteria are summarized in Table A.1.

The review was updated with a search in Scopus (chosen for its wide coverage) on March 21, 2019, with the query TITLE-ABS-KEY (immuno-epidemiolog* OR immunoepidemiolog*). A total of 282 references were retrieved and screened in Covidence. A linear regression model was created in SAS v.9.4 to test whether the number of publications on the topic of immunoepidemiology has increased significantly over time.

Results

Determining the Number of Immunoepidemiology Papers Over Time

The number of articles with "immunoepidemiology" in the title or abstract published since 1959 is relatively small but has increased markedly over time. Figure A.1 (Fig. 1.3 in the text) shows the number of documents published each year from 1959 to present that were retrieved using the following Scopus query: TITLE-ABS-KEY (immuno-epidemiolog* OR immunoepidemiolog*). This query identified articles in which the hyphenated or unhyphenated term "immunoepidemiology" appeared in either the title or abstract, or as one of the article's key words. Figure A.1 clearly shows an upward trend in the number of articles published on the topic of immunoepidemiology over time. A linear regression model confirmed that the trend is statistically significant ($p < 0.0001$).

Of note, many articles which are relevant to the topic of immunoepidemiology do not include the term itself in the title or abstract, which presents some challenges for literature searching. The types of documents retrieved by the Scopus query are shown in Fig. A.2. The majority of documents were articles (224/279 documents; 80%), and 14% of documents were of a single disease or condition-specific reviews (38/279). Conference papers, book chapters, articles in press, short surveys, editorials, and letters accounted for the remaining 6% of documents. These results indicate that most published works on the topic of immunoepidemiology exist in the form of peer-reviewed articles and reviews.

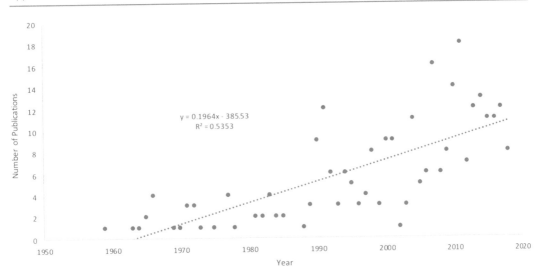

Fig. A.1 (Fig. 1.3) The number of documents published each year with the word "immunoepidemiology" in the title or abstract since 1959, which were retrieved by a Scopus search. A linear regression model was created in SAS v.9.4 and confirmed that the number of publications on this topic has increased significantly over time ($p < 0.0001$). The number of publications in the year 2019 represents the months of January to April only, and is expected to increase during the remainder of the year. Publications that investigated the field of immunoepidemiology but did not specifically use the term in the title or abstract are not included in the counts. (©Krause 2020)

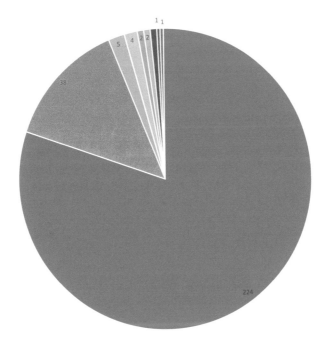

■ Article ■ Review ■ Note ▫ Conference Paper ▪ Book Chapter ▫ Article in Press ■ Short Survey ■ Editorial ■ Letter

Fig. A.2 Immunoepidemiology publications by type (1959–2019). The document types of records retrieved by the Scopus query that captured publications with the word "immunoepidemiology" in the title or abstract, or listed as a keyword. (©Krause 2020)

Identifying the Most Relevant Immunoepidemiology Papers Using Predefined Criteria

2015 Scoping Review

The Ovid MEDLINE search identified a total of 148 articles, Embase identified 161, PubMed identified 228, Scopus identified 229, and Web of Science identified 328 for a total of 1094 articles. The database results were merged in EndNote X7, and duplicate articles were removed. The relevance of the remaining 178 articles was then assessed using prespecified inclusion and exclusion criteria (Table A.1), based on the article titles and available abstracts. The abstract screening process involved two researchers (J.O. and K.F.) who evaluated each individual record and came to consensus about inclusion or exclusion.

After screening the 178 abstracts that remained after de-duplication, 39 records were excluded because they did not meet inclusion criteria, leaving 139 records for full-text PDF download. EndNote X7's PDF search function located 51 full-text PDFs. An additional 59 full-text PDF articles were located using Yale University Library's databases and Google Scholar. PDFs of 29 articles were not available for download, nor were they accessible through Yale University's interlibrary loan. Many of these articles were conference papers and as such, published full-text papers did not exist for review. These articles were excluded from further review.

A total of 110 full-text PDFs were available for abstraction at the end of the screening process. Articles were sorted based on disease category (viral, parasitic, fungal, autoimmune, chronic) and disease outcome. Data fields relating to immunology (i.e., innate vs. adaptive immune system, antibodies, T-cell involvement, cytokines, and other immune functions) and epidemiology (i.e., population and disease significance) were abstracted. Each article was given a rating based on its relevance to the field of immunoepidemiology (1 = Not Applicable; 2 = Moderately Applicable; 3 = Highly Relevant). To receive a rating of "highly relevant," the paper must have addressed both the immunologic response and mechanisms of the disease outcome investigated and the epidemiologic dynamics and implications for the population(s) studied. A PRISMA flow-chart diagram representing the study selection process of this 2015 review and a table of the inclusion and exclusion criteria are shown in Fig. A.3 and Table A.1.

Spring 2019 Update of the Scoping Review

A total of 279 publications with immunoepidemiology in the title or abstract that were published since 1959 (about 5 articles per year over 60 years) were identified during the Spring 2019 Scopus update review. Of these publications, 23 met the selection criteria. A combined list of references (133 total) from the 2015 review (110 articles) and 2019 update (23 articles) is included at the end of this Appendix.

Conclusions

The number of publications with "Immunoepidemiology" in the title or abstract since 1959 is relatively small with less than 300 publications identified. In comparison, the number of publications with either epidemiology or immunology in the title or abstract (and indexed under the medical subject heading (MeSH) tag "human") over the same time period each exceed 150,000 publications. Nonetheless, the number of publications on immunoepidemiology (term used in title or abstract) is increasing over time (Fig. A.1), indicating increasing interest in and recognition of the interdisciplinary field of immunoepidemiology.

The search strategy of the 2015 scoping review included all fields of the bibliographic records instead of being limited to titles, abstract, and subject headings (as is conventional). This strategy captured

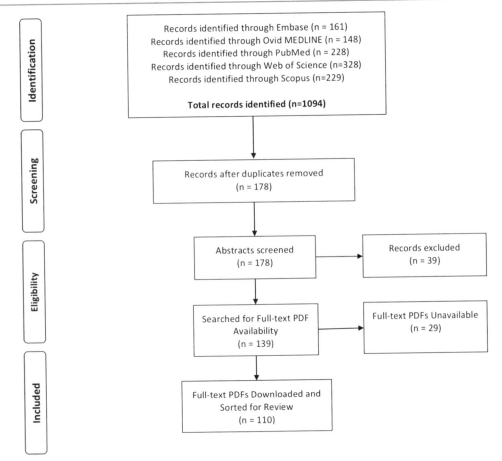

Fig. A.3 PRISMA flow-chart diagram of study selection. (based on protocol of Moher D, Liberati A, Tetzlaff J, Altman DG, The PRISMA Group (2009). Preferred Reporting Items for Systematic Reviews and Meta-Analyses: The PRISMA Statement. PLoS Med 6(7): e1000097. doi:10.1371/journal.pmed1000097). (©Krause 2020)

papers with authors affiliated with, for example, the Infections and Immunoepidemiology Branch of the Division of Cancer Epidemiology and Genetics (National Cancer Institute of the National Institutes of Health (NIH)) or the Genomic Immunoepidemiology Laboratory of HUMIGEN LLC. This search strategy, in combination with the rigorous selection process, identified relevant papers where the word "immunoepidemiology" was absent from the abstract.

There are several strategies that could be utilized in future searches of the immunoepidemiology literature. These are outlined in Table A.2. In combining searches, one would use the parentheses for nesting, or enter queries on separate lines, to preserve the logic. The decision of which queries to include in a search will depend on the information needed and the time available for screening potentially relevant references. It is advisable to combine with the Boolean operator OR the "all fields" search and the "subject heading" search, at least.

A relatively small number of immunoepidemiology articles were identified in the 2019 update of the 2015 scoping review, but the number has progressively increased over the past half century. A total of 133 articles ultimately met all of the inclusion criteria. These results indicate that immunoepidemiology is truly an emerging field. The authors hope that the content of this Appendix will be a welcome addition and that the information and guidance provided will be both useful and instructive to researchers working in the field of immunoepidemiology.

Table A.2 Strategies for searching the immunoepidemiology literature

Fields	Notes	PubMed syntax	Ovid MEDLINE syntax
Textword or keyword	Note the truncation. This conventional query, which doesn't include author addresses, will not retrieve all the papers screened as relevant by JO and KF	Immunoepidemiolog*[tw] OR immuno-epidemiolog*[tw]	(Immunoepidemiolog* or immuno-epidemiolog*).mp.
All fields	"All fields" includes author addresses and, in Embase, candidate terms. Some 22 articles identified as relevant by KF and JO had been included in the screening process because of their author affiliations, not because of anything in their titles/abstracts	Immunoepidemiolog*[all fields] OR immuno-epidemiolog*[all fields]	(Immunoepidemiolog* or immuno-epidemiolog*).af.
Author addresses	Papers featuring authors from immunology departments collaborating with authors from epidemiology departments may be relevant. Out of six papers in the original screening set that happen to be retrieved by this query, one was included	Immunolog*[ad] AND epidemiolog*[ad]	(immunolog* and epidemiolog*).ia,in.
Subject headings	In some bibliographic databases, indexers apply subject headings from hierarchical controlled vocabularies. No papers retrieved by this query were included in the original screening set, but it is a small set to screen (under 150 citations in MEDLINE), and I believe it may repay investigation	Epidemiology[mh] AND "allergy and immunology"[mh]	exp epidemiology/ and exp "allergy and immunology"/
Adjacency	In some databases, you can search for a term near another term. This query retrieves less than 1000 MEDLINE citations, but further testing would be necessary to establish the best adjacency statement and truncation	Not available	(immunolog* adj2 epidemiolog*).af.
Subheadings	In some bibliographic databases, indexers apply subheadings to further contextualize subject headings. This query is relatively sensitive; two-thirds of the papers screened in by KF and JO have this characteristic. However, it is not specific; more than 80,000 other MEDLINE citations do. In practice, its utility is limited	Epidemiology[fs] AND immunology[fs]	(epidemiology and immunology).fs.

Bibliography

1. Abe M, Ozawa T, Minagawa F, Yoshino Y. Immunoepidemiological studies on subclinical infection in leprosy: II. Geographical distribution of seropositive responders with special reference to their possible source of infection. Jpn J Lepr. 1990;59(3–4):162–8.
2. Abraham AG, D'Souza G, Jing Y, Gange SJ, Sterling TR, Silverberg MJ, et al. Invasive cervical cancer risk among HIV-infected women: a North American multicohort collaboration prospective study. J Acquir Immune Defic Syndr. 2013;62(4):405–13.
3. Acosta E. Antibodies to the metacestode of Taenia solium in the saliva from patients with neurocysticercosis. J Clin Lab Anal. 1990;4(2):90–4.
4. Addai-Mensah O, Seidel M, Amidu N, Maskus DJ, Kapelski S, Breuer G, et al. Acquired immune responses to three malaria vaccine candidates and their relationship to invasion inhibition in two populations naturally exposed to malaria. Malar J. 2016;15(1):65.
5. Adegnika AA, Breitling LP, Agnandji ST, Chai SK, Schutte D, Oyakhirome S, et al. Effectiveness of quinine monotherapy for the treatment of Plasmodium falciparum infection in pregnant women in Lambarene, Gabon. Am J Trop Med Hyg. 2005;73(2):263–6.
6. Aidoo M, McElroy PD, Kolczak MS, Terlouw DJ, Ter Kuile FO, Nahlen B, et al. Tumor necrosis factor-alpha promoter variant 2 (TNF2) is associated with pre-term delivery, infant mortality, and malaria morbidity in western Kenya: Asembo bay cohort project IX. Genet Epidemiol. 2001;21(3):201–11.
7. Aka PV, Kuniholm MH, Pfeiffer RM, Wang AS, Tang W, Chen S, et al. Association of the IFNL4-DeltaG allele with impaired spontaneous clearance of Hepatitis C virus. J Infect Dis. 2014;209(3):350–4.
8. Anderson LA, Li Y, Graubard BI, Whitby D, Mbisa G, Tan S, et al. Human herpesvirus 8 seroprevalence among children and adolescents in the United States. Pediatr Infect Dis J. 2008;27(7):661–4.
9. Arama C, Maiga B, Dolo A, Kouriba B, Traore B, Crompton PD, et al. Ethnic differences in susceptibility to malaria: what have we learned from immuno-epidemiological studies in West Africa? Acta Trop. 2015;146((Miller) Laboratory of Malaria and Vector Research, National Institute of Allergy and Infectious Diseases, National Institutes of Health, Rockville, MD 20852, United States):152–6.
10. Arndts K, Specht S, Debrah AY, Tamarozzi F, Klarmann Schulz U, Mand S, et al. Immunoepidemiological profiling of onchocerciasis patients reveals associations with microfilaria loads and ivermectin intake on both individual and community levels. PLoS Negl Trop Dis. 2014;8(2):e2679.
11. Aucan C, Traore Y, Fumoux F, Rihet P. Familial correlation of immunoglobulin G subclass responses to Plasmodium falciparum antigens in Burkina Faso. Infect Immun. 2001;69(2):996–1001.
12. Barbedo MB, Ricci R, Jimenez MC, Cunha MG, Yazdani SS, Chitnis CE, et al. Comparative recognition by human IgG antibodies of recombinant proteins representing three asexual erythrocytic stage vaccine candidates of Plasmodium vivax. Mem Inst Oswaldo Cruz. 2007;102(3):335–9.
13. Baum E, Jain A, Prachumsri JS, Sirichaisinthop J, Yan G, Felgner P. Seroprevalence to malaria parasites in tak province, Thailand reveals more frequent exposure to plasmodium sp. than estimated by epidemiological surveys. Am J Trop Med Hyg. 2013;89(5 Suppl. 1):204–5.
14. Bhatia K, Goedert JJ, Modali R, Preiss L, Ayers LW. Merkel cell carcinoma subgroups by Merkel cell polyomavirus DNA relative abundance and oncogene expression. Int J Cancer. 2010;126(9):2240–6.
15. Bloch P, Simonsen PE. Immunoepidemiology of Dracunculus medinensis infections I. Antibody responses in relation to infection status. Am J Trop Med Hyg. 1998;59(6):978–84.

16. Bloch P, Simonsen PE. Immunoepidemiology of Dracunculus medinensis infections II. Variation in antibody responses in relation to transmission season and patency. Am J Trop Med Hyg. 1998;59(6):985–90.

17. Bourke CD, Maizels RM, Mutapi F. Acquired immune heterogeneity and its sources in human helminth infection. Parasitology. 2011;138(2):139–59.

18. Bradley JE, Jackson JA. Immunity, immunoregulation and the ecology of trichuriasis and ascariasis. Parasite Immunol. 2004;26(11–12):429–41.

19. Bueno LL, Lobo FP, Morais CG, Mourao LC, de Avila RAM, Soares IS, et al. Identification of a highly antigenic linear B cell epitope within Plasmodium vivax apical membrane antigen 1 (AMA-1). PLoS One. 2011;6(6):e21289.

20. Bundy DAP, Medley GF. Immuno-epidemiology of human geohelminthiasis: ecological and immunological determinants of worm burden. Parasitology. 1992;104(Suppl):S105–S19.

21. Campbell AR. Immunoepidemiology of schistosomiasis in ancient Nubia. Am J Phys Anthropol. 2009;101:290–98.

22. Castellsague X, Naud P, Chow SN, Wheeler CM, Germar MJ, Lehtinen M, et al. Risk of newly detected infections and cervical abnormalities in women seropositive for naturally acquired human papillomavirus type 16/18 antibodies: analysis of the control arm of PATRICIA. J Infect Dis. 2014;210(4):517–34.

23. Chaturvedi AK, Caporaso NE, Katki HA, Wong HL, Chatterjee N, Pine SR, et al. C-reactive protein and risk of lung cancer. J Clin Oncol. 2010;28(16):2719–26.

24. Chaturvedi AK, Gaydos CA, Agreda P, Holden JP, Chatterjee N, Goedert JJ, et al. Chlamydia pneumoniae infection and risk for lung cancer. Cancer Epidemiol Biomark Prev. 2010;19(6):1498–505.

25. Chaturvedi AK, Madeleine MM, Biggar RJ, Engels EA. Risk of human papillomavirus-associated cancers among persons with AIDS. J Natl Cancer Inst. 2009;101(16):1120–30.

26. Chavez JM, Vicetti Miguel RD, Cherpes TL. Chlamydia trachomatis infection control programs: lessons learned and implications for vaccine development. Infect Dis Obstet Gynecol. 2011;2011:754060.

27. Cohen CR, Koochesfahani KM, Meier AS, Shen C, Karunakaran K, Ondondo B, et al. Immunoepidemiologic profile of Chlamydia trachomatis infection: importance of heat-shock protein 60 and interferon-gamma. J Infect Dis. 2005;192(4):591–9.

28. Cooper PJ. Intestinal worms and human allergy. Parasite Immunol. 2004;26(11–12):455–67.

29. Davis CF, Dorak MT. An extensive analysis of the hereditary hemochromatosis gene HFE and neighboring histone genes: associations with childhood leukemia. Ann Hematol. 2010;89(4):375–84.

30. Day KP. The endemic normal in lymphatic filariasis: a static concept. Parasitol Today. 1991;7(12):341–3.

31. de Sousa TN, Kano FS, de Brito CF, Carvalho LH. The Duffy binding protein as a key target for a Plasmodium vivax vaccine: lessons from the Brazilian Amazon. Mem Inst Oswaldo Cruz. 2014;109(5):608–17.

32. Do TN, Ucisik-Akkaya E, Davis CF, Morrison BA, Dorak MT. An intronic polymorphism of IRF4 gene influences gene transcription in vitro and shows a risk association with childhood acute lymphoblastic leukemia in males. Biochim Biophys Acta. 2010;1802(2):292–300.

33. Dodoo D. Antibody levels to Msp1-Block 2 Hybrid, GLURP R2 and As202.11 and the risk of malaria in under 5 year old children of Burkina Faso and Ghana: an Afro-Immuno Assay project. Trop Med Int Health. 2012;17(Suppl. 1):44.

34. Dodoo D, Aikins A, Kusi KA, Lamptey H, Remarque E, Milligan P, et al. Cohort study of the association of antibody levels to AMA1, MSP1 19, MSP3 and GLURP with protection from clinical malaria in Ghanaian children. Malar J. 2008;7:142.

35. Duncan CJA, Hill AVS, Ellis RD. Can growth inhibition assays (GIA) predict blood-stage malaria vaccine efficacy? Hum Vaccin Immunother. 2012;8(6):706–14.

36. Dunne DW, Riley EM. Immunity, morbidity and immunoepidemiology in parasite infections. Parasite Immunol. 2004;26(11–12):425–8.

37. Egan AF, Morris J, Barnish G, Allen S, Greenwood BM, Kaslow DC, et al. Clinical immunity to Plasmodium falciparum malaria is associated with serum antibodies to the 19-kDa C-terminal fragment of the merozoite surface antigen, PfMSP-1. J Infect Dis. 1996;173(3):765–9.

38. Elfaki TEM, Arndts K, Wiszniewsky A, Ritter M, Goreish IA, Atti El Mekki MEYA, et al. Multivariable regression analysis in Schistosoma mansoni-infected individuals in the Sudan reveals unique immunoepidemiological profiles in uninfected, egg+ and non-egg+ infected individuals. PLoS Negl Trop Dis. 2016;10(5):e0004629.

39. Emmanuel B, Kawira E, Ogwang MD, Wabinga H, Magatti J, Nkrumah F, et al. African Burkitt lymphoma: age-specific risk and correlations with malaria biomarkers. Am J Trop Med Hyg. 2011;84(3):397–401.

40. Engels EA. Epidemiology of thymoma and associated malignancies. J Thorac Oncol. 2010;5(10 Suppl 4):S260–5.

41. Engels EA, Biggar RJ, Hall HI, Cross H, Crutchfield A, Finch JL, et al. Cancer risk in people infected with human immunodeficiency virus in the United States. Int J Cancer. 2008;123(1):187–94.

42. Engels EA, Pfeiffer RM, Landgren O, Moore RD. Immunologic and virologic predictors of AIDS-related non-hodgkin lymphoma in the highly active antiretroviral therapy era. J Acquir Immune Defic Syndr. 2010;54(1):78–84.

43. Fowkes FJ, Richards JS, Simpson JA, Beeson JG. The relationship between anti-merozoite antibodies and incidence of Plasmodium falciparum malaria: a systematic review and meta-analysis. PLoS Med. 2010;7(1):e1000218.

44. Gabrie JA, Rueda MM, Rodriguez CA, Canales M, Sanchez AL. Immune profile of Honduran schoolchildren with intestinal parasites: the skewed response against geohelminths. J Parasitol Res. 2016;2016:e1769585.

45. Geiger SM. Immuno-epidemiology of Schistosoma mansoni infections in endemic populations co-infected with soil-transmitted helminths: present knowledge, challenges, and the need for further studies. Acta Trop. 2008;108(2–3):118–23.

46. Gilchrist JJ, MacLennan CA. Invasive nontyphoidal Salmonella disease in Africa. EcoSal Plus. 2019;8(2):1–23.

47. Goedert JJ, Bower M. Impact of highly effective antiretroviral therapy on the risk for Hodgkin lymphoma among people with human immunodeficiency virus infection. Curr Opin Oncol. 2012;24(5):531–6.

48. Goedert JJ, Swenson LC, Napolitano LA, Haddad M, Anastos K, Minkoff H, et al. Risk of breast cancer with CXCR4-using HIV defined by V3 loop sequencing. J Acquir Immune Defic Syndr. 2015;68(1):30–5.

49. Gottstein B, Felleisen R. Protective immune mechanisms against the metacestode of Echinococcus multilocularis. Parasitol Today. 1995;11(9):320–6.

50. Graham AL, Cattadori IM, Lloyd-Smith JO, Ferrari MJ, Bjornstad ON. Transmission consequences of coinfection: cytokines writ large? Trends Parasitol. 2007;23(6):284–91.

51. Greenhouse B, Ho B, Hubbard A, Njama-Meya D, Narum DL, Lanar DE, et al. Antibodies to Plasmodium falciparum antigens predict a higher risk of malaria but protection from symptoms once parasitemic. J Infect Dis. 2011;204(1):19–26.

52. Griffiss JM. Epidemic meningococcal disease: synthesis of a hypothetical immunoepidemiologic model. Rev Infect Dis. 1982;4(1):159–72.

53. Griffiss JM, Broud DD, Silver CA, Artenstein MS. Immunoepidemiology of meningococcal disease in military recruits. I. A model for serogroup independency of epidemic potential as determined by serotyping. J Infect Dis. 1977;136(2):176–86.

54. Heaton T, Rowe J, Turner S, Aalberse RC, De Klerk N, Suriyaarachchi D, et al. An immunoepidemiological approach to asthma: identification of in-vitro T-cell response patterns associated with different wheezing phenotypes in children. Lancet. 2005;365(9454):142–9.

55. Hellriegel B. Immunoepidemiology—bridging the gap between immunology and epidemiology. Trends Parasitol. 2001;17(2):102–6.

56. Helmby H. Schistosomiasis and malaria: another piece of the crossreactivity puzzle. Trends Parasitol. 2007;23(3):88–90.

57. Hildesheim A, Wang CP. Genetic predisposition factors and nasopharyngeal carcinoma risk: a review of epidemiological association studies, 2000–2011: Rosetta Stone for NPC: genetics, viral infection, and other environmental factors. Semin Cancer Biol. 2012;22(2):107–16.

58. Hollams EM, Deverell M, Serralha M, Suriyaarachchi D, Parsons F, Zhang G, et al. Elucidation of asthma phenotypes in atopic teenagers through parallel immunophenotypic and clinical profiling. J Allergy Clin Immunol. 2009;124(3):463.

59. Hviid L. The immuno-epidemiology of pregnancy-associated Plasmodium falciparum malaria: a variant surface antigen-specific perspective. Parasite Immunol. 2004;26(11–12):477–86.

60. Hviid L. The role of Plasmodium falciparum variant surface antigens in protective immunity and vaccine development. Hum Vaccin. 2010;6(1):84–9.

61. Jaenisch T. A description of the evolution of clinical features in 1916 dengue-infected patients across four Southeast Asian and three Latin American countries: are particular syndromes identifiable? Trop Med Int Health. 2011;16(Suppl. 1):75.

62. Jaoko WG, Michael E, Meyrowitsch DW, Estambale BBA, Malecela MN, Simonsen PE. Immunoepidemiology of Wuchereria bancrofti infection: parasite transmission intensity, filaria-specific antibodies, and host immunity in two East African communities. Infect Immun. 2007;75(12):5651–62.

63. Karunaweera ND, Dewasurendra R, Fernando D, Sereejaitham P, Suriyaphol P. Genetic markers and risk of malaria infections: genetic-epidemiology study in a low malaria endemic area of Sri Lanka. Am J Trop Med Hyg. 2010;83(5 Suppl. 1):219–20.

64. Koshiol J, Kreimer AR. Lessons from Australia: human papillomavirus is not a major risk factor for esophageal squamous cell carcinoma. Cancer Epidemiol Biomark Prev. 2010;19(8):1889–92.

65. Kreuels B, Verra F. Haemoglobinopathies: natural selection at work against Plasmodium falciparum malaria. In: Malaria: etiology, pathogenesis and treatments. New York: Nova Biomedical; 2012. p. 339–62.

66. Lawn SD, Bangani N, Vogt M, Bekker L-G, Badri M, Ntobongwana M, et al. Utility of interferon-gamma ELISPOT assay responses in highly tuberculosis-exposed patients with advanced HIV infection in South Africa. BMC Infect Dis. 2007;7:99.

67. Li D, Zhu Y, Wang M. Immuno-epidemiological investigation of recurrent spontaneous abortion. Zhonghua Yi Xue Za Zhi. 1998;78(2):94–7.

68. Lundblom K, Murungi L, Nyaga V, Olsson D, Rono J, Osier F, et al. Plasmodium falciparum infection patterns since birth and risk of severe malaria: a nested case-control study in children on the coast of Kenya. PLoS One. 2013;8(2):e56032.

69. MacDonald TT, Spencer J, Murch SH, Choy MY, Venugopal S, Bundy DAP, et al. Immunoepidemiology of intestinal helminthic infections 3. Mucosal macrophages and cytokine production in the colon of children with Trichuris trichiura dysentery. Trans R Soc Trop Med Hyg. 1994;88(3):265–8.

70. Mandal NN, Achary KG, Kar SK, Bal MS. Immuno-epidemiology of bancroftian filariasis: a 14-year follow-up study in Odisha, India. Southeast Asian J Trop Med Public Health. 2014;45(3):547–55.

71. Marks MA, Rabkin CS, Engels EA, Busch E, Kopp W, Rager H, et al. Markers of microbial translocation and risk of AIDS-related lymphoma. AIDS. 2013;27(3):469–74.

72. Michael E, Simonsen PE, Malecela M, Jaoko WG, Pedersen EM, Mukoko D, et al. Transmission intensity and the immunoepidemiology of bancroftian filariasis in East Africa. Parasite Immunol. 2001;23(7):373–88.

73. Moncunill G, Mayor A, Bardaji A, Puyol L, Nhabomba A, Barrios D, et al. Cytokine profiling in immigrants with clinical malaria after extended periods of interrupted exposure to Plasmodium falciparum. PLoS One. 2013;8(8):e73360.

74. Morrison BA, Ucisik-Akkaya E, Flores H, Alaez C, Gorodezky C, Dorak MT. Multiple sclerosis risk markers in HLA-DRA, HLA-C, and IFNG genes are associated with sex-specific childhood leukemia risk. Autoimmunity. 2010;43(8):690–7.

75. Mpairwe H, Amoah AS. Parasites and allergy: observations from Africa. Parasite Immunol. 2018;41(6):e12589.

76. Murungi LM, Kamuyu G, Lowe B, Bejon P, Theisen M, Kinyanjui SM, et al. A threshold concentration of anti-merozoite antibodies is required for protection from clinical episodes of malaria. Vaccine. 2013;31(37):3936–42.

77. Mutapi F. Heterogeneities in anti-schistosome humoral responses following chemotherapy. Trends Parasitol. 2001;17(11):518–24.

78. Mutapi F, Bourke C, Harcus Y, Midzi N, Mduluza T, Turner CM, et al. Differential recognition patterns of Schistosoma haematobium adult worm antigens by the human antibodies IgA, IgE, IgG1 and IgG4. Parasite Immunol. 2011;33(3):181–92.

79. Mutapi F, Mduluza T, Gomez-Escobar N, Gregory WF, Fernandez C, Midzi N, et al. Immuno-epidemiology of human Schistosoma haematobium infection: preferential IgG3 antibody responsiveness to a recombinant antigen dependent on age and parasite burden. BMC Infect Dis. 2006;6:96.

80. Mutapi F, Mduluza T, Roddam AW. Cluster analysis of schistosome-specific antibody responses partitions the population into distinct epidemiological groups. Immunol Lett. 2005;96(2):231–40.

81. Mutapi F, Ndhlovu PD, Hagan P, Woolhouse ME. Anti-schistosome antibody responses in children coinfected with malaria. Parasite Immunol. 2000;22(4):207–9.

82. Mutapi F, Ndhlovu PD, Hagan P, Woolhouse MEJ. A comparison of humoral responses to Schistosoma haematobium in areas with low and high levels of infection. Parasite Immunol. 1997;19(6):255–63.

83. Nahrevanian H, Gholizadeh J, Farahmand M, Assmar M, Sharifi K, Ayatollahi Mousavi SA, et al. Nitric oxide induction as a novel immunoepidemiological target in malaria-infected patients from endemic areas of the Islamic Republic of Iran. Scand J Clin Lab Invest. 2006;66(3):201–9.

84. Nakachi K, Hayashi T, Imai K, Kusunoki Y. Perspectives on cancer immuno-epidemiology. Cancer Sci. 2004;95(12):921–9.

85. Needham CS, Lillywhite JE. Immunoepidemiology of intestinal helminthic infections 2. Immunological correlates with patterns of Trichuris infection. Trans R Soc Trop Med Hyg. 1994;88(3):262–4.

86. Nurjadi D, Kain M, Marcinek P, Gaile M, Heeg K, Zanger P. Ratio of T-helper type 1 (Th1) to Th17 cytokines in whole blood is associated with human beta-defensin 3 expression in skin and persistent Staphylococcus aureus nasal carriage. J Infect Dis. 2016;214(11):1744–51.

87. Odegaard JI, Hsieh MH. Immune responses to Schistosoma haematobium infection. Parasite Immunol. 2014;36(9):428–38.

88. Oeuvray C, Roussilhon C, Theisen M, Muller-Graf C, Tall A, Rogier C, et al. Long-term clinical protection from falciparum malaria is strongly associated with IgG3 antibodies to merozoite surface protein 3. PLoS Med. 2007;4(11):e320.

89. Offeddu V, Olotu A, Osier F, Marsh K, Matuschewski K, Thathy V. High sporozoite antibody titers in conjunction with microscopically detectable blood infection display signatures of protection from clinical malaria. Front Immunol. 2017;8:488.

90. Oliveira RG, Easton A, Kepha S, Njenga SM, Mwandawiro CS, Lamberton PH, et al. Immuno-epidemiology of soil-transmitted helminth infections after repeated school-based deworming: a community-wide cross-sectional study in Western Kenya. Am J Trop Med Hyg. 2015;93(4 Supplement):138.

91. Oradovskaya IV, Fadeeva ID, Ulyanova NV, Chernetsova LF, Nikonova MF, Litvina MM. Six-year observation of immune state of persons affected by the Chernobyl accident. Radiat Prot Dosim. 1995;62(1–2):63–7.

92. Periasamy M, Datta M, Kannapiran M, Ramanathan VD, Venkatesan P. Neonatal bacillus Calmette-Guerin vaccination and environmental mycobacteria in sensitizing antimycobacterial activity of macrophages. Am J Med Sci. 2014;348(1):57–64.

93. Petridou ET, Chavelas C, Dikalioti SK, Dessypris N, Terzidis A, Nikoulis DI, et al. Breast cancer risk in relation to most prevalent IgE specific antibodies: a case control study in Greece. Anticancer Res. 2007;27(3 B):1709–13.

94. Pit DSS, Polderman AM, Baeta S, Schulz-Key H, Soboslay PT. Parasite-specific antibody and cellular immune responses in humans infected with Necator americanus and Oesophagostomum bifurcum. Parasitol Res. 2001;87(9):722–9.

95. Pritchard DI, Quinnell RJ, Slater AFG, McKean PG, Dale DD, Raiko A, et al. Epidemiology and immunology of Necator americanus infection in a community in Papua New Guinea: humoral responses to excretory-secretory and cuticular collagen antigens. Parasitology. 1990;100(2):317–26.

96. Quinnell RJ, Bethony J, Pritchard DI. The immunoepidemiology of human hookworm infection. Parasite Immunol. 2004;26(11–12):443–54.

97. Quinnell RJ, Woolhouse MEJ, Walsh EA, Pritchard DI. Immunoepidemiology of human necatoriasis: correlations between antibody responses and parasite burdens. Parasite Immunol. 1995;17(6):313–8.

98. Rehman MQ, Beal D, Liang Y, Noronha A, Winter H, Farraye FA, et al. B cells secrete eotaxin-1 in human inflammatory bowel disease. Inflamm Bowel Dis. 2013;19(5):922–33.

99. Remoue F, Cisse B, Ba F, Sokhna C, Herve JP, Boulanger D, et al. Evaluation of the antibody response to anopheles salivary antigens as a potential marker of risk of malaria. Trans R Soc Trop Med Hyg. 2006;100(4):363–70.

100. Robinson RD, Lindo JF, Neva FA, Gam AA, Vogel P, Terry SI, et al. Immunoepidemiologic studies of Strongyloides stercoralis and human T lymphotropic virus type I infections in Jamaica. J Infect Dis. 1994;169(3):692–6.

101. Ryan BM, Pine SR, Chaturvedi AK, Caporaso N, Harris CC. A combined prognostic serum interleukin-8 and interleukin-6 classifier for stage 1 lung cancer in the prostate, lung, colorectal, and ovarian cancer screening trial. J Thorac Oncol. 2014;9(10):1494–503.

102. Sagna AB, Biram Sarr J, Gaayeb L, Senghor S, Poinsignon A, Faye N, et al. Use of the immuno-epidemiological biomarker of human exposure to anopheles bites in the monitoring of malaria transmission in (pre) elimination areas. Am J Trop Med Hyg. 2017;97(5 Supplement 1):96–7.

103. Samudio M, Montenegro-James S, De Cabral M, Martinez J, Rojas De Arias A, Woroniecky O, et al. Differential expression of systemic cytokine profiles in Chagas' disease is associated with endemicity of Trypanosoma cruzi infections. Acta Trop. 1998;69(2):89–97.

104. Shiels MS, Chaturvedi AK, Katki HA, Gochuico BR, Caporaso NE, Engels EA. Circulating markers of interstitial lung disease and subsequent risk of lung cancer. Cancer Epidemiol Biomark Prev. 2011;20(10):2262–72.

105. Shiels MS, Engels EA, Shi J, Landi MT, Albanes D, Chatterjee N, et al. Genetic variation in innate immunity and inflammation pathways associated with lung cancer risk. Cancer. 2012;118(22):5630–6.

106. Shiels MS, Pfeiffer RM, Hildesheim A, Engels EA, Kemp TJ, Park JH, et al. Circulating inflammation markers and prospective risk for lung cancer. J Natl Cancer Inst. 2013;105(24):1871–80.

107. Simonsen PE, Meyrowitsch DW, Jaoko WG, Malecela MN, Michael E. Immunoepidemiology of Wuchereria bancrofti infection in two East African communities: antibodies to the microfilarial sheath and their role in regulating host microfilaraemia. Acta Trop. 2008;106(3):200–6.

108. Skowronski DM, Chambers C, De Serres G, Sabaiduc S, Winter AL, Dickinson JA, et al. Age-related differences in influenza B infection by lineage in a community-based sentinel system, 2010–2011 to 2015–2016, Canada. J Infect Dis. 2017;216(6):697–702.

109. Skowronski DM, Hottes TS, McElhaney JE, Janjua NZ, Sabaiduc S, Chan T, et al. Immuno-epidemiologic correlates of pandemic H1N1 surveillance observations: higher antibody and lower cell-mediated immune responses with advanced age. J Infect Dis. 2011;203(2):158–67.

110. Soboslay PT, Geiger SM, Weiss N, Banla M, Luder CG, Dreweck CM, et al. The diverse expression of immunity in humans at distinct states of Onchocerca volvulus infection. Immunology. 1997;90(4):592–9.

111. Stirnadel HA, Al-Yaman F, Genton B, Alpers MP, Smith TA. Assessment of different sources of variation in the antibody responses to specific malaria antigens in children in Papua New Guinea. Int J Epidemiol. 2000;29(3):579–86.

112. Stirnadel HA, Beck HP, Alpers MP, Smith TA. Genetic analysis of IgG subclass responses against RESA and MSP2 of Plasmodium falciparum in adults in Papua New Guinea. Epidemiol Infect. 2000;124(1):153–62.

113. Taylor-Robinson AW. A model of development of acquired immunity to malaria in humans living under endemic conditions. Med Hypotheses. 2002;58(2):148–56.

114. Tertipis N, Hammar U, Nasman A, Vlastos A, Nordfors C, Grun N, et al. A model for predicting clinical outcome in patients with human papillomavirus-positive tonsillar and base of tongue cancer. Eur J Cancer. 2015;51(12):1580–7.

115. Thomson GT, Chiu B, De Rubeis D, Falk J, Inman RD. Immunoepidemiology of post-Salmonella reactive arthritis in a cohort of women. Clin Immunol Immunopathol. 1992;64(3):227–32.

116. Tindall B, Cooper DA, Burcham J, Gold J, Penny R. Clinical and immunologic sequelae of AIDS retrovirus infection. Aust NZ J Med. 1986;16(6):749–56.

117. Tindall B, Cooper DA, Donovan B, Barnes T, Philpot CR, Gold J, et al. The Sydney AIDS Project: development of acquired immunodeficiency syndrome in a group of HIV seropositive homosexual men. Aust NZ J Med. 1988;18(1):8–15.

118. Tsang RSW, Bruce MG, Lem M, Barreto L, Ulanova M. A review of invasive Haemophilus influenzae disease in the Indigenous populations of North America. Epidemiol Infect. 2014;142(7):1344–54.

119. Ucisik-Akkaya E, Davis CF, Gorodezky C, Alaez C, Dorak MT. HLA complex-linked heat shock protein genes and childhood acute lymphoblastic leukemia susceptibility. Cell Stress Chaperones. 2010;15(5):475–85.

120. Ucisik-Akkaya E, Dorak MT. A study of natural killer cell lectin-like receptor K1 gene (KLRK1/NKG2D) region polymorphisms in a European population sample. Tissue Antigens. 2009;73(2):177–83.

121. Vestergaard LS, Lusingu JP, Nielsen MA, Mmbando BP, Dodoo D, Akanmori BD, et al. Differences in human antibody reactivity to Plasmodium falciparum variant surface antigens are dependent on age and malaria transmission intensity in Northeastern Tanzania. Infect Immun. 2008;76(6):2706–14.

122. Wang AS, Pfeiffer RM, Morgan TR, O'Brien TR. Hepatitis C genotype 1 virus with low viral load and rapid virologic response to peginterferon/ribavirin obviates a protease inhibitor. Hepatology. 2014;59(6):2423–4.

123. Wickramarachchi T, Illeperuma RJ, Perera L, Bandara S, Holm I, Longacre S, et al. Comparison of naturally acquired antibody responses against the C-terminal processing products of Plasmodium vivax merozoite surface protein-1 under low transmission and unstable malaria conditions in Sri Lanka. Int J Parasitol. 2007;37(2):199–208.

124. Wilson S, Vennervald BJ, Dunne DW. Chronic hepatosplenomegaly in African school children: a common but neglected morbidity associated with schistosomiasis and malaria. PLoS Negl Trop Dis. 2011;5(8):e1149.

125. Wipasa J, Okell L, Sakkhachornphop S, Suphavilai C, Chawansuntati K, Liewsaree W, et al. Short-lived IFN-gamma effector responses, but long-lived IL-10 memory responses, to malaria in an area of low malaria endemicity. PLoS Pathog. 2011;7(2):e1001281.

126. Wojcik GL, Thio CL, Kao WH, Latanich R, Goedert JJ, Mehta SH, et al. Admixture analysis of spontaneous hepatitis C virus clearance in individuals of African descent. Genes Immun. 2014;15(4):241–6.

127. Woolhouse MEJ. Immunoepidemiology of intestinal helminths: pattern and process. Parasitol Today. 1992;8(4):111.

128. Woolhouse MEJ. A theoretical framework for the immunoepidemiology of helminth infection. Parasite Immunol. 1992;14(6):563–78.

129. Woolhouse MEJ. A theoretical framework for the immunoepidemiology of blocking antibodies to helminth infection. Parasite Immunol. 1994;16(8):415–24.

130. Woolhouse MEJ. Immunoepidemiology of human schistosomes: taking the theory into the field. Parasitol Today. 1994;10(5):196–202.

131. Yobo CM, Sadia-Kacou AM, Adja AM, Eilanga-Ndile E, Sagna AB, Guindo-Coulibaly N, et al. Influence of rubber and palm cultivations on human exposure to Aedes aegypti evaluated by using an immuno epidemiological biomarker. Am J Trop Med Hyg. 2017;97(5 Supplement 1):192–3.

132. Yobo CM, Sadia-Kacou CAM, Adja MA, Elanga-Ndille E, Sagna AB, Guindo-Coulibaly N, et al. Evaluation of human exposure to Aedes bites in rubber and palm cultivations using an immunoepidemiological biomarker. Biomed Res Int. 2018;2018:3572696.

133. Yu G, Fadrosh D, Ma B, Ravel J, Goedert JJ. Anal microbiota profiles in HIV-positive and HIV-negative MSM. AIDS. 2014;28(5):753–60.

Index

© Springer Nature Switzerland AG 2019
P. J. Krause et al. (eds.), *Immunoepidemiology*, https://doi.org/10.1007/978-3-030-25553-4

Printed in the United States
By Bookmasters